SACRED
DANCE
MEDITATIONS

SACRED DANCE MEDITATIONS

365 Globally Inspired Movement Practices Enhancing Awakening, Clarity, and Connection

CARLA STALLING WALTER, PHD

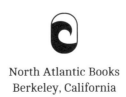

North Atlantic Books
Berkeley, California

Published by
North Atlantic Books
Berkeley, California

Cover photo © Zolotarevs/Shutterstock.com
Cover art © gettyimages.com/jakkaje808
Cover design by Rob Johnson
Book design by Happenstance Type-O-Rama

Printed in the United States of America

Sacred Dance Meditations: 365 Globally Inspired Movement Practices Enhancing Awakening, Clarity, and Connection is sponsored and published by the Society for the Study of Native Arts and Sciences (dba North Atlantic Books), an educational non-profit based in Berkeley, California, that collaborates with partners to develop cross-cultural perspectives, nurture holistic views of art, science, the humanities, and healing, and seed personal and global transformation by publishing work on the relationship of body, spirit, and nature.

North Atlantic Books' publications are available through most bookstores. For further information, visit our website at www.northatlanticbooks.com or call 800-733-3000.

Library of Congress Cataloging-in-Publication Data

Names: Walter, Carla Stalling, 1961– author.
Title: Sacred dance meditations : 365 globally inspired movement practices enhancing awakening, clarity, and connection / Carla Stalling Walter.
Description: Berkeley, California : North Atlantic Books, [2020] | Includes bibliographical references and index. | Summary: "365 dances from around the globe that are sacred conduits for hope, love, connection, community, and spirituality"—Provided by publisher.
Identifiers: LCCN 2020031794 (print) | LCCN 2020031795 (ebook) | ISBN 9781623174811 (paperback) | ISBN 9781623174828 (ebook)
Subjects: LCSH: Religious dance. | Movement, Psychology of—Religious aspects. | Spirituality.
Classification: LCC GV1783.5 .W35 2020 (print) | LCC GV1783.5 (ebook) | DDC 793.3/1—dc23
LC record available at https://lccn.loc.gov/2020031794
LC ebook record available at https://lccn.loc.gov/2020031795

1 2 3 4 5 6 7 8 9 VERSA 25 24 23 22 21 20

For My Parents, Alma and Donald

CONTENTS

FOREWORD

WE KNOW THAT SACRED dance has told the story of the human Spirit since before recorded time. In this book, the author has responded to a hunger I have had for many years but was not even fully aware of. Just reading the Introduction and the Table of Contents caused a quickening of my heart with a feeling that I was coming home to re-experience something that my body, mind, and Soul had always known and was longing to be reacquainted with. It was somewhat like driving into a town that you grew up in as a young person and had the opportunity to revisit as an elder—memories flood back, and you begin to breathe deeply into the history of who you are, all the while connecting to all that you have experienced throughout your life.

Carla takes us on a journey of discovery—an adventure for the whole self to dive deeply into! Her background, in both her studies and her many years of exploration and work in the field, uniquely positions her to share this adventure in a way that provides us grounding in the history of cultures that dance around the globe, and then leads us through a body-based emotional and spiritual meditative experience that is truly transformational.

I am amazed at the level of detail and precision that Carla gives us in these pages. When you open the door of page 1, I know that you too will be awed by each page as it unfolds its treasures for you to embrace. In addition to the deeply powerful words that will fill your mind and heart, the practical ideas and suggestions are the golden nuggets in the treasure chest! Carla's descriptions and instructions are clear, concise, and easily understandable, and having the videos is incredibly helpful in "seeing" what the daily movements look like. However you choose to take this 365 day journey—whether it be each day one at a time from the beginning of the year through to the end, whether you start in the middle of a year, whether you jump in here, there, and everywhere as the Spirit calls you, or if you join together with others and make this a group journey—you WILL be inspired in ways that will surprise you. I wanted to find one of those nuggets to share with you—one example of something specific that particularly touched me personally—but I simply cannot! I have always been drawn to the many cultural and spiritual expressions of dance and have studied most of them over many years. This book is like I have fallen into the pot of gold at the end of the rainbow, and everything is there in one place that I can delight in and explore to my heart's content. What an amazing gift to receive.

Whatever your personal understanding of The Divine is, this book engages in an inclusive and deeply personal way, while also connecting you back to people from another time, to others on this journey in the present, and to those who will be in your future. This book draws from a plethora of spiritual and religious traditions, and I am sure you, like me, will have many "aha" moments as you learn, laugh, and dance your way through each day.

In addition to the incredible personal benefits of taking this journey of discovery with Carla, I believe this is an important book for our times. As we engage and understand globally, we are called to action—to be and do what we each personally can to create a world that is kinder, more compassionate, and caring to each and every Soul on the planet. I am grateful to have Carla as a colleague and member of the Sacred Dance Guild (www.sacreddanceguild.org)—an organization that has been dedicated to advocating and celebrating dance as an expression of the sacred since 1958. As the president of this organization, I wholeheartedly embrace the words in our statement "*One People, One Planet and One Heart in the Dance of Life.*" Carla's book underlines this in a bold, meaningful, and timely way.

I suggest you take a deep breath and dance in with the whole of who you are! You will be changed.

Wendy Morrell, President, Sacred Dance Guild

ACKNOWLEDGMENTS

I HAVE HAD A love of sacred dance for as long as I can remember, but I didn't know why. I've realized over the course of my life through dancing, meditating, teaching, and choreographing that sacred dance is key to well-being, healing, and wholeness. With that knowledge, my purpose is to offer this modality to as many people as possible so that we can elevate ourselves, and thereby change the way we are in relation to each other and the Universe. Sacred Dance Meditation offers a focus on nonmaterial matters that often gets neglected at the expense of perpetuating or causing harm unknowingly.

In the Spirit of love and compassion, I offer you these meditations and hope you'll share them with others in your communities.

A special word of appreciation goes to Cherie Hill, who worked tirelessly to demonstrate the choreography for this book. Please realize the suggested videos aren't professionally done; they are meant to help you visualize what the sacred dances look like in practice. I'd also like to thank reviewers who helped with drafts of the work, providing clarity and support when I needed it most. Of course, I am very grateful for the editors at North Atlantic Books for their dedication to ensuring you have this book to help you continue moving on your spiritual path.

Thank you for engaging with Sacred Dance Meditation as a spiritual Practice.

INTRODUCTION

DANCE IS THE AGE-OLD and timeless connection to Spirit, or the Creative Force in the Universe. Many religious Practices consider deities, gurus, or others as spiritual leaders, yet I believe they are all manifestations of that Creative Force. In this daily reader I use Spirit, Divine, Universe, Cosmos, Higher Self, Realized Self, and other terms interchangeably to refer to the Creative Force that I believe we all embody and that orders the Universe.

Peoples of the world have always danced before the gods and G-d, in celebrations, in rituals, during change, and during times of despair. Dance's ability to work in tandem with spiritual growth, healing, and recovery is truly magnificent. Just by watching dance, people participate in the healing process. The commonality of these dances is that they were accessible for people in need of love, support, hope, and, most important, connection to their Higher Power. In this book I honor all spiritual traditions and the myriad related or unrelated Practices that you might be doing. In combination with those Practices or standing alone, many of the sacred dances from ancient history and from around the globe can benefit you.

This book is meant for advanced spiritual seekers—those who have already been involved with spirituality in some way, have read about spirituality, have been initiated into a group through rituals, and have asked about the meaning of life and want to know more. I assume readers are well versed in the chakra system, the mystical and magickal kabbalah, and concepts that explain the third eye. Readers can find resources at www.cswalter.org as they relate to this book, or they can search the internet about these topics.

If you've gotten a little contented in your Practice or hit a plateau or just want to find new connections, this book is just for that.

Historically, some sacred dance cultures were nearly extinguished, although the antagonism against them has gradually changed. I don't delve into that history here but have instead amplified certain sacred dances and beliefs integral to human thriving and spiritual development. In this book, I refer in the past tense to cultures and use the word *ancient* because the cultures are being discussed historically; this is not to negate people from those cultures who practice today or the Practices themselves. Also note that my presentation of sacred dance is factually supported but hew to any archeological or historical theories. Lastly, there are more sacred dances than I can write about in the confines of this work.

The sacred dances you'll read about here are reconstructed from research and generally date from before colonialism. I tried to reinstate the sacred and give it agency, as you will find many peoples around the world are re-creating their dances to honor their ancestors. I also wanted to avoid perpetuating the Western whitewash of history that favors a Eurocentric and masculine outlook. As such, the book has taken me several years to complete. The meditations are suitable for anyone who wants to avoid assumptions about indigenous peoples and embody a way of being that honors the sacred and incorporates the mind. While writing this book I learned that, often, the paths of sacred dance and the formulation of peoples' intentions converged—around creation, Cosmos, and celebrations.

This daily reader is arranged on a Gregorian calendar year, but you can begin at any time. Within each month, an ancient culture whose religious and spiritual history drew sustenance from sacred dance provides the basis for expanding your enlightenment and achieving your intentions. Each month has several Entry Points, typically at the beginning of a seven-day week, where a new Sacred Dance Meditation is introduced, and sequential segments of the choreography are introduced throughout that given week. Your dance journey begins in winter, where you travel to ancient Egypt, the expansive African continent, and then Native America and Mesoamerica. In spring, I take you to Austronesia, Iberia, and then Tibet. In summer, I bring you to Greece, India, and Asia. I end the year with Andean and Israeli dance and a series of personal reflections on the sacred dances to explore the Season of Light.

Each month, I present dance meditations that allow us to remember Spirit and make new moves toward it and toward one another. Dance not only heals our innermost being but also contributes to healing the earth. I have deliberately selected these dances because I want to help us develop deep communicative channels and flows through dance for spiritual growth, healing, and recovery.

When it's appropriate, you can invite others to join you and thereby create or expand a sense of fellowship. Regardless, you will have a connectedness to Spirit with you all day, so that you listen, hear, act, and speak from the amplified messages carried within the body temple. Or at the very least, your heart and Soul will lead your interactions as Sacred Dance Meditation becomes central in your life.

Sacred Dance Meditation Practice

I recommend you perform Sacred Dance Meditation in a designated space, which you could call your Sacred Dance Studio. All you need is a space large enough to move around in and, if you like, a way to play live or prerecorded music. Music is unnecessary but not prohibited. Your studio could be in your home or business, indoors or outdoors, as you prefer.

When beginning each dance, your posture should be erect but not rigid. Stand up straight, lengthen your spine, and press the shoulders into their proper place. Bring awareness to your neck, back, shoulders, and waist, and notice how they connect to your hips and legs. Finally, feel your feet, arms, and hands. They are energized. The posture will be referred to as the Sacred Dance Posture throughout the book. Take a moment to center and connect to your Inner Mystic Dancer before you begin.

Every day set aside about twenty minutes to fully get into the practice. Wear comfortable clothing and soft-soled shoes, or go barefooted. I like to have a few choices in Sacred Dance Attire. I don't mix them in with my regular clothes, so they become special and sacred clothing while I'm in my sacred space.

At the beginning of each entry, you will find directions for the daily sacred dance. Review them, and perform the movements a few times until you get the hang of them. Keep your dance simple, and don't worry about perfection. The idea is to feel and connect to Spirit. Then read "Meditation and Practice." Focusing on the reading, your Spirit, and the Divine within you, perform the dance as long as you'd like. Have a journal handy to make notes since many of the Sacred Dance Meditations offer you moments to reflect and jot down ideas.

Keep in mind that Sacred Dance Meditation is a cumulative practice—you advance in depth and connection with time and repetition. At some point, sacred dance will evoke a spiritual response with your Inner Mystic Dancer—the Spirit within that guides and leads you. You should expect to feel calm, enlightened, and enabled to move forward in your Light. Throughout the day, incorporate one dance movement to remind you of your connection to Spirit and to humanity.

New Moves, New Ideas

THE ANCIENT EGYPTIAN DANCE TRADITIONS

Many writers and theorists acknowledge that humans originated from the region we now call Egypt, or earth's motherland. Depictions of Sacred Dance Meditation in ancient Egypt, dating back to about 4000 BCE, show sacred dancers with upraised arms reaching to the heavens. During this period, dance was an art form included in worship, which was understood as a private relationship between Spirit and Self.

The ancient Egyptians believed that people were composed of a physical body and a multifaceted spiritual being. Parts of Spirit Being included the Shadow, the Life Force, the Soul, and the Divine Name. Most important to this view was that human knowledge and emotion originated from the heart, not the mind. We also learn from the Egyptians that Spirit and the heart were considered more important than the body.

Directly tied to this complicated worldview was the ancient Egyptian practice of several forms of sacred dance. Both men and women participated in Sacred Dance Meditation, which was done for many rituals and celebrations and directed toward the heavens and the gods—who lived below the earth at times. For funerals and transitions from life to death, a ritual dance expressed grief, and dancers placed their hands on their heads or made the ka gesture by holding up both of their arms. In temple rituals, dancers summoned the highest sacred aspects of human beings and consoled people who were suffering. Together, sacred dance and music provided meaning and gave people a way to overcome suffering. Sacred Dance Meditations elevated each Spirit that participated or watched.

Sacred dances ushered in or celebrated rebirth in all its forms, especially in relation to ringing in the New Year. The New Year meant a Nile River flood was imminent. At the southern border of Egypt, ecstatic celebrations greeted the new water with its promise of prosperity. Sacred dance was part of cyclical and seasonal change, as well as calling on the Divine. Sacred dance prepared people for moments of radical change, beginnings, and endings. Correspondingly, in this month I focus on New Year Celebration Dances, in anticipation of manifesting a glorious New Year and in visioning prosperity and spiritual guidance.

PREPARATION

For this month's Sacred Dance Meditations, you'll want to gather incense, or a scent-producing gadget, for your Sacred Dance Studio. Get into your Sacred Dance Attire so that you're comfortable and can move around easily. If you'd like to, you can embellish your Sacred Dance Attire with cowrie-shell necklaces. Invite others to join you if this is an option. Drums and handheld percussive instruments, such as rattles, tambourines, bells, and cymbals, are excellent for this week's work. Live music is great, but you can also use music found online.

Please visit www.cswalter.org/sacreddancemeditations for video demonstrations. They are not intended to be step-by-step instructions but are meant to give you a view of the sacred dance.

JANUARY 1–7
Shadows (Entry Point)

My Shadows: The Grace of Powerlessness

Light, shining in the shadows, is a natural part of creation and life, guiding us to evolve into balanced, healthy, whole, and humble spiritual beings.

January 1: Awareness of My Shadow

SACRED DANCE

Stand facing east in your Sacred Dance Posture and in your chosen Sacred Dance Attire. Place your left palm, turned outward, at the small of your back with fingers pointing down, and hold your right palm open and turned upward in front of you. Pull your elbows in toward your torso. Begin to walk in a circle, moving clockwise. Exaggeratedly lift your right leg, as if you're stepping over a pile of wood logs onto a bed of rustic redwood mulch. As you place your leg down, land first on the ball of your foot, and roll down on your heel. Repeat this process with the left leg and foot. Make as large a circle as is comfortable for you and possible within the space; move to the beat of the music, if you have it, and try to match your breath to the rhythm. Take large steps in each direction: to the south, then west, then north, and then returning to your original eastern-facing position. As you move around the circle, note your physical shadow and the effort it takes to be aware of it relative to the light in the center of the space.

MEDITATION AND PRACTICE

The past year, along with years before it, has moved on. Yet some issues from the past may still linger on. Often, we think of shadows as where darkness dwells. They're scary places harboring all manner of creatures real or not! Our ancestors didn't hold this view but embraced the shadows for what could be created from them. The ancient Egyptians believed that our Shadow held spiritual solutions for living and creativity. Shadows give rise to Light! From the shadows we often emerge to find new awareness and growth.

What kinds of events, behaviors, histories are casting shadows over you? For example, do you have regrets? Are you worried about the future? Do you procrastinate or move too quickly? Are you concerned about your finances? Do these shadows arise from your mind, your body, or your heart center? Which of them would you like to change? Write about two or three shadows in your journal, and explain why you choose them.

January 2: The Shadow and The Spirit

SACRED DANCE

We build upon yesterday's Sacred Dance Meditation by adding an arm movement. Hold your right hand and arm close to your body, and turn the upward-facing palm toward the left. Move the left hand to the front of the right hand and move it in a counterclockwise circle, palm facing outward. As you did yesterday, move your body in a clockwise circle, being mindful of the motions. Dance to the rhythm of your breath, in through your nose and out through your nose, or to the music, or both. After dancing a few circles and becoming more aware of your Higher Self, note that the circle on the floor and the one made by your left hand move in opposite directions. See if this feels natural. The area you are working with is the heart chakra, the location of serenity, love, and the Higher Self. When you're ready, return to the Sacred Dance Posture, facing east.

MEDITATION AND PRACTICE

The ancient Egyptians saw the Shadow as an essential, inseparable, and representative part of the whole being, representing comfort and protection. It showed all sides of a person, reflective of the Soul and Self. To exist, the Shadow needed Light. A person's Shadow was always present in life and the afterlife and always held information about the person it represented.

The Shadow has a great deal to offer your Spirit, and vice versa. Creation happens in the Shadow, usually wordlessly but with an inner drive for something—to fill a void, to contribute—which is positive, always. These drives lie dormant or ignored, deep in your Shadow self. Without words or thought, allow your Spirit, through Sacred Dance Meditation, to express, intend, and bring forth your heart's desires.

What are some of your heart's deepest desires? For example, do you desire a closer relationship with the Divine? Or to keep the knowledge of your true nature in the front of your mind in all situations? To change how people act? Or simply to be able to respond differently to challenging situations? Or to accept prosperity in your life? If you manifested your deepest desires, who would be affected? Write responses down in your journal.

January 3: Shadow Protection

SACRED DANCE

Today we build on yesterday's dance by tilting the head side to side. As you move around the circle, with each step, tilt your head to the same side of your body as the foot you're stepping on. This may take a bit of practice! Dance to the rhythm of your breath, in through your nose and out through your nose, or to the music, or both. Add a phrase or passage that holds spiritual significance for you if you wish. After dancing a few circles and becoming more away of your Higher Self, note the shadows in the circle on the floor and the shadows in front of you. Also consider how your head movement affects your balance and the location of your awareness of your Shadow. When you're ready, return to the Sacred Dance Posture, facing east, and bring your awareness back to your heart center.

MEDITATION AND PRACTICE

One ancient Egyptian creation story concerns Atum, a deity of the Sun. He mated with his Shadow, which created Shu (air) and Tefnut (moisture). They in turn created the Universe, earth, and other gods.

Humans were looked upon as creators, and their Souls, like those of the gods, were eternal. The idea of death was cyclical, having nothing to do with an end of life but rather a rejoining with the eternally Spiritual realms.

When it's understood that creation comes from the Shadow, fear of shadows seems silly. Ancient Egyptians considered the Shadow as protection against pain until we're ready for that new creation within. Sometimes we can't get past an event without healing and self-reflection, until we're prepared to receive more Light or until we have just had enough—grief, addiction, poverty, codependency, selfishness, or such—before we can move on. We can be grateful for the Shadow and its protection of our Spirit. Our movement can synchronize with the rate by which the Shadow's protection is revealed, the Light transferred, and new growth emerges.

January 4: Creative Ideas from My Shadow

SACRED DANCE

Connect with your Inner Mystic Dancer while pausing a few moments to transition into your Sacred Dance Posture. Begin by repeating the dance you learned yesterday. After you become comfortable with the movements, pause and momentarily shift your torso slightly to the right; then repeat on the left. Resume the circular walking, and intersperse the hold-and-shift motions as they feel right to you. Now consider how your torso movement affects your balance and your awareness of your Shadow.

MEDITATION AND PRACTICE

Sacred Dance for the ancient Egyptians was essential to creation and communion with the gods. Priests and priestess danced east to west across symbols of the Cosmos placed in the temple spaces. The goddess Hathor was the mistress of sacred dance, and divine dwarfs praised her and other goddesses and gods in a "dance of the gods."

So often we look for a grand presentation or a grand miracle, but, for many, small nuances underlie creative shifts. The money, the relationship, the accident, the drama of life causes us to seek protection in the Shadow. And yet, from these incidents sparks of new life begin to form. Get up, move up, go up, step sideways, tilt away, dance a new dance. Everything negative holds a spark of the divine in it, even if it only causes us to take notice. The ancient Egyptians knew this intuitively. But we don't always think this way, especially if we have hurts, pains, and beliefs that don't support who we are. Now that we have come to understand that our Shadow is part of our Spirit, there is no need to run from it. Actually, it's a Higher Source we can rely on, to propel us forward. What ideas, inspirations, and creative endeavors are resting in your Shadow? How can you bring them into your Light? Start with your deepest desires to help you identify them. Make some notes in your notebook.

January 5: Dreams from My Shadow

SACRED DANCE

Review what we've covered so far this week and begin your dance. After completing the torso shift you integrated yesterday, move your chin around in a circle, right to left and forward and back. As you continue dancing, consider how your neck movement affects your balance and observe your focus. Repeat the dance movement until you're doing it without thinking, just getting into a flow or trance. When you're ready, return to the Sacred Dance Posture, facing east, and bring your awareness to your throat chakra.

MEDITATION AND PRACTICE

The ancient Egyptians believed their gods talked directly to them through dreams, giving them faith, courage, direction, and protection. They expected to stay connected with the Higher Self, even during sleep. Dreams were essential for living and discovering the next right step to manifest their heart's desires. Sacred dance brought forth the relationship with Higher Powers so that during sleep the dance meditation continued.

Today, some give less credence to dreams and what they can teach us. But the Shadow displays information to us in our dream life. Some believe we live two lives, the one of daytime "real life" and the one we enter when we sleep. Whatever our beliefs, dreams do influence us during the day, while our day life influences our dreams. To benefit from this, we loosen our reliance on thinking, understanding that we can know in the body.

What can you realize from pausing, shifting, reimagining, looking, and considering as you dance sacredly? If you saw yourself from a different vantage point, what would you see? What would you do if you weren't afraid, knowing that you couldn't make a mistake? Write some ideas in your journal.

January 6: Using My Shadow for Growth

SACRED DANCE

Instead of dancing to the right, as you've done the last few days, today you will move left. The left palm faces outward and upward, and the right hand creates circles in front of your heart center. Repeat the dance meditation until you're doing it automatically, feeling a flow or trance. When you're ready, return to the Sacred Dance Posture, facing east, and bring your awareness to your chakras.

MEDITATION AND PRACTICE

One's Shadow was responsible for evoking healing, change, recovery, and growth. Ancient Egyptian goddess Hathor, the symbol of life-giving energy and abundance, therefore encouraged people to engage with it. Sacred dance was a large part of meditation, which Hathor dwelt within. People came to her in gratitude for what they had and with their deepest desires and petitions. She was the queen of sacred dance, igniting the Spirit with joy, through which Sacred Dance Meditation delivered ancient Egyptians to their Highest Good and awareness.

As uncoordinated as it may feel, turning in an opposite or different direction can offer new insights and much needed support for healing and recovery, the ability to make relationships satisfying and loving, and a change of our own fundamental story we tell ourselves. Note that the shadow moves with you and, depending on the light, shows itself differently. As light is applied from alternative directions, it increases or diminishes. Through the metaphor of shadows, you can learn to view the environment differently, think about a situation differently, or understand your desires from a different perspective. Write down one belief about yourself that you think is negative. Trace this belief back to where it came from, and see it differently by recrafting the story around it. Be aware of the story as it drives your actions and behaviors today.

January 7: Totally New Perspective

SACRED DANCE

Today you will do the Shadow dance in both directions. Start on your right, and move in that direction several times; then switch to the left as you arrive at east. Repeat the dance an equal number of times on each side, and then move left for one rotation and right for the next. Mix the pattern as you wish. Repeat the pattern you select until you're doing it without thinking about the movements, feeling a flow or trance. When you're ready, return to the Sacred Dance Posture, facing east, and bring your awareness to your chakras.

MEDITATION AND PRACTICE

Hathor dripped with abundance, wearing gold and silver, and created and sustained an empire of turquoise. Her demeanor radiated confidence, and her body and Spirit projected only good health. She ruled trade markets and manifested abundance for ancient Egyptians. On a spiritual level, the goddess embodied the natural reflection of the Shadow and the Spirit. Ahead of her, Atum was the first to take the Shadow and reflect the Spirit. He was the god of creation, which meant he ruled and made manifest beauty and courage. Atum wore exquisite crowns and headdresses, which he imagined out of his Shadow. Both Hathor and Atum used Sacred Dance Meditation to propel them forward.

After dancing the last six days, you might have a totally new perspective of yourself and your Shadow. Engaging with it can facilitate your growth, creativity, and recovery. You use your new perspectives to work with your Shadow in relationship with yourself first, and then with others, and extract Good from the darkness and bring it into the Light.

You have power to change by turning to your Inner Mystic Dancer, working with your dreams, and knowing that out of the darkness only light can come. When you interact with other people at any time, let them see you from the inside out, and be mindful of their Shadow *and* their Light. In this way you practice compassion and remain humble—not being better or less than anyone—since you know we're all in this human condition.

JANUARY 8–14
My Life Force (Entry Point)

My Life Force: The Essence of Tiny and Expansive

The ancient Egyptians believed in a Life Force, described as the holder of tiny things and the producer of miracles, the fabric of the stars and the gods. It is the source of order, sustenance, and abundance and accounts for the reliability of spiritual, mystical, and natural laws.

January 8: Order

SACRED DANCE

While standing or sitting, inhale deeply into the lower abdomen, then exhale slowly by pressing the lower abdomen to release all the air. Take five deep breaths this way. Reach your arms outward and up toward the sky on the last inhale. Gently bend your arms at the elbows so your forearms still point toward the sky and your upper arms are parallel to the earth. Gently cup your palms so they face the sky. Straighten your right wrist so your hand faces the floor, and begin rotating your wrists in opposite directions. When you're ready, return to the Sacred Dance Posture, facing east, and bring your awareness to your chakras.

MEDITATION AND PRACTICE

In ancient Egyptian lore, human and spiritual existence began with the creation of Earth and the rest of the Universe out of darkness and swirling chaos. It was utterly silent since the water was completely still. Out of this watery silence a primordial hill rose on which Atum stood and considered how lonely he was. Through magick, he mated with his own Shadow and brought forth Shu and Tefnut. The two offspring engaged in a sacred dance in which Shu supplied principles of life while Tefnut developed the principles of order.

A Life Force runs through your body, mind, and Spirit—consciousness, if you prefer. Throughout your life the Life Force has sustained and driven you. Sometimes that force has pushed toward the Good. At other times, you seemingly have had no control over your own life, as if driven by an unknown force or events that "happened" to you.

Reflecting on personal powerlessness and acceptance, you can acknowledge this Life Force as an aid in bringing manageability to your life. You are powerless over the rising and setting of the sun, for example, but not over your choices. Ponder the Life Force that stretches back to the beginning of time and its existence forward light years away. Use your imagination. Feel that same Life Force inside you. Imagine you can feel it at the molecular level. What can you say to the Life Force that will enable you to foster a manageable life? What are some phenomena that you absolutely cannot change? Make some notes if you like.

January 9: Receiving My Life Force

SACRED DANCE

Begin by practicing yesterday's dance. As you rotate your hands in opposite directions and come to a natural resting point, circle your chin counterclockwise side to side, imagining you're crafting a small circle above your heart. See if you can alternate the chin circle with each change of direction of your hands, so that when the left hand is flexed, the chin moves counterclockwise, and when the right hand is flexed, the chin moves clockwise. You may find that crafting a heart circle with your chin is easier in one direction than the other or not. Repeat the entire dance eight times. When you're ready, return to the Sacred Dance Posture, facing east, and bring your awareness to your solar plexus chakra.

MEDITATION AND PRACTICE

In the ancient Hymn to Amen-Ra, Ra was revered as the "Lord of truth, father of the gods, maker of men, creator of all animals, Lord of things that are, creator of the staff of life";* Ra encompassed nearly all of creation, was the provider and sustainer of Life Forces for humans and the gods and goddesses, and stood for all the invisible forces that explained the vast seen world. Every day he was born as the sun rose and died as it set. Each new day he saw creation with fresh new eyes but brought understanding and wisdom from the former life of yesterday. He was the giver of good and the remover of deception. He danced a sacred dance with the heavens and the underworld.

Life Forces travel throughout the Universe, including to our solar system. It takes several light years for the Life Force to arrive here on planet Earth. None of the energy is lost, as it cannot be created or destroyed—only transformed. Tap into the knowledge and power of that Life Force now. Imagine it traveling down through the galaxies, entering the solar system, and moving into Earth's atmosphere, before it moves down through the Earth and out the other side to circle back into the solar system and out into the galaxies. Capture some of that energy in your palms and imagine it concentrating right around your heart. It's creative, healing energy—the

---

* Hymn to Amen-Ra, quoted in E. A. Wallis Budge, *The Literature of the Ancient Egyptians* (London: Aldine House, 1914; Project Gutenberg, 2005), chap. 12, https://www.gutenberg.org/ebooks/15932.

kind of energy the Egyptians knew how to receive and harness to build structures and civilizations while staying in touch with their Inner Mystic Dancer.

January 10: Honoring Life Forces of My Surroundings

SACRED DANCE

Begin by practicing yesterday's dance. While keeping your chin moving, after alternating left and right with your hands twice, bring your hands together so the palms touch, with fingers elongated and held closely together in front of your heart, and then move them upward to rest at your forehead, between your eyes. Your elbows should be outstretched so that your forearms are parallel to the floor. Now, shift your torso laterally to the left and then to the right, keeping your palms together. Repeat the movement until it feels almost natural. Return to your Sacred Dance Posture.

MEDITATION AND PRACTICE

The ancient Egyptians revered the goddess Ma'at, who oversaw truth, justice, and the cosmic order. Born the moment Ra spoke the world into creation, Ma'at ordered the galaxies and the seasons. Her Sacred Dance Meditation of harmony and balance infused the creation and caused the world to run rationally according to purpose. When in alignment with Ma'at's Spirit, ancient Egyptians thought people would live abundantly here and in the eternal peace in the afterlife. If people refused to live by the principles of Ma'at, then they brought on their own consequences. The Egyptians believed strongly that every individual was responsible for his or her own life and people needed to live with other people and the earth in mind.

Do you know that everything in your surroundings has a Life Force? Some beings are embodied and terrestrial, but others are unseen and extraterrestrial. Don't feel alarmed at the idea of an unseen Life Force. We experience that type of force, such as gravity, all the time. Unseen Life Forces hold the planets, stars, and universes in place. They set the Earth on its course and make the sun rise and set, move the oceans, and keep the moon in orbit. The ancient Egyptians believed in the unseen—terrestrial, celestial, and extraterrestrial.

The more we use science as a tool of inquiry, the more we find Life Forces that shape reality. Your Inner Mystic Dancer is aware of this already, however, since it relies on deep intuitive knowing rather than on fact and "scientific proof." Humility guides every dance and allows for new information to shape the experience as the dancer travels through the embodied journey. What are your beliefs about Unseen Forces? What do you consider to be your life's "harmony?" Write down some ideas.

January 11: Honoring Life Forces of Spiritual Laws

SACRED DANCE

Engage your Sacred Dance Posture, and begin with the dance components you have already learned this week. As you shift your torso laterally, pause and contract and expand your muscles, and continue to hold your hands up to the middle of your forehead. The muscle movement essentially exaggerates your lateral shift. Feel the depth of your abdominal muscles and how they connect to the breath. Repeat several times, and then return to your Sacred Dance Posture.

MEDITATION AND PRACTICE

In accordance with Ma'at, Egyptians envisioned a formula for human behavior that obeyed the will of the gods. The goal was to bring in a universal order and harmony of things so that life would be pleasant now and in death. The work of ancient Egyptian astronomers also showcased this cosmic balance. They charted Earth's orbit by observing the paths of the stars and planets. They also realized that these orbits were harmonious. The principle of honoring harmony was adopted into their daily lives, which in turn led to the spiritual laws.

According to spiritual laws, we create "angels" by what we think, do, and say. We can create negative or positive angels through our thoughts, and those angels remain on our plane of creation. And, of course, Buddhists and others often emphasize the principle of karma, which is a spiritual law that indicates that every action—thought is action, by the way—produces an outcome. Spiritual laws govern all Life Forces, seen and unseen.

Spiritual laws are as real as observable reality, and through them we create our reality. It's a known fact that Life Forces obey spiritual laws. For example, one spiritual law states you're one with the Divine. That means it's inside, not outside in some form. You and everything in the Universe have a vibrational energy. You know that there are some people you like being around and others you don't. Think about why. Some laws explain why you may be in certain patterns that you need to get out of. Repeated losses and repeated negativity are patterns, as are repeated successes and repeated joy.

You can also consider spiritual laws that pertain to how you treat your neighbor or people you resent, self-centeredness, honesty with people or a default into people-pleasing, how you think about yourself, and how you react when you're not getting your way. Spiritual laws, which are unchanging, internalize in your abdominal core, as they connect with your Life Force.

Jot down a few spiritual laws that you are aware of and want to amplify and have a more central role in your life. No matter where you are on your spiritual path, there is always something more to refine.

January 12: Honoring Life Forces of Mystic Reliability

SACRED DANCE

What do we think of our feet? Not much, until we stub a toe or break a tiny bone! However, our feet are very complex, as they relate to all parts of the body (think reflexology). We rely on our feet unconsciously to move us. Begin today's dance by assuming your Sacred Dance Posture, standing in a comfortable position with your feet shoulder-length apart. Notice how the floor or the ground feels as you stand there. Shifting your weight onto your left foot, gently lift the heel of your right foot so that the ball of your foot and your toes stay on the floor. Press your ankle forward. Lower, and repeat with the left foot. You will notice a natural rise and fall. Repeat several times, and then return to your Sacred Dance Posture.

MEDITATION AND PRACTICE

Ancient Egyptians believed in magick, using it to restore harmony and balance, to harness Life Forces that can make miracles happen, or to know deeply within the Spirit that all was harmonious within the Divine Order. The mystics of the day were able to use the Life Forces and spiritual laws to create environments that sustained healthy human and godly endeavors. In their daily Sacred Dance Meditations, they rested in the awareness that any human being could be a mystic.

The Rabbi David Cooper and present-day mystics confirm this truth: what you say and think comes to pass, even if you don't think about your thoughts and words or if you don't believe it.

Mystic reliability is being aware without being concerned or focusing directly on how you affect Life Forces, attend to spiritual laws, and are an example for others. Using magick, manifesting miracles, and being humble are key to this practice. You must know without directly knowing; you must cultivate change inside without expecting. You must not take credit. You must stand in readiness for receipt of mystical awareness when it comes through. Mystics aren't the same today as they were yesterday or last year or at birth, and they will be different tomorrow and next year. Energy flows through mystics, and they take assignments as they are given. They believe that love is the basis for everything and that helping humans to realize they are pure love is central to their calling. In this way they are reliable.

Are you a mystic? Make some notes.

January 13: Honoring Life Forces of Natural Laws

SACRED DANCE

Please embody the dance we have done through the week by repeating it several times. Let your Spirit guide the beauty of the dance. Continuing from yesterday's focus on our feet, now, flex the right foot, and shift back to the center, then flex the left foot. You'll notice a natural bend of the knee on the standing leg. Repeat the moves several times, and you'll notice a rhythm emerging from your body and Spirit as you move from a pointed foot to a flexed one. Return to center, and focus on your Inner Mystic Dancer as you move.

MEDITATION AND PRACTICE

Ma'at, the ancient Egyptian goddess of truth and justice, was concerned with natural laws. She often manifested as an ostrich feather, which was placed on scales that could detect minute imbalances. Fair and equitable treatment of humans was considered a Divine right, and Ma'at measured this in one's behavior. The Egyptians believed that before passing to the afterlife their hearts would be weighed against them with the feather as the indicator. If the individual lived a good life, following the rules of Ma'at and treating others well, their heart would be lighter than her feather. But, if not, they would have a heavy heart, full of guilt and shame that needed to be destroyed, and so they wouldn't enjoy bliss in the next life. The laws of Ma'at are called the Forty-Two Negative Confessions, known today as the Forty-Two Ideals, and they were revealed in *The Egyptian Book of the Dead*, or *The Papyrus of Ani*. The laws state that we treat each other with certain manners, being very aware of the implication of how we use Life Forces. The certain indelible ethical, spiritual, mystical, and natural laws are manifest because of the chaos in the world. Balance needs to be struck at all times and in all encounters, with the idea that a code of ethics governs all.

Do you speak and act truthfully and justly with every being? Do you believe deeply that all Life Forces are subject to truth and justice? Do you believe in outdated systems that were given to you, or do you know your own truth and justice? Do you think you're better than any human? Write down some notes in your journal.

January 14: Revel in the Unseen Life Forces

SACRED DANCE

Perform the Life Force dance today in its entirety, beginning with what you learned on January 8, remembering your Sacred Dance Posture. Be in tune with the Universe and the earth, and notice your breath and your surroundings. Be aware of your feet, and see with your third eye. Feel free to move about the Sacred Dance Studio you have created as you do this dance meditation.

MEDITATION AND PRACTICE

Order is in the Universe, the world, and all of us and is subject to unchanging laws. We can't always see the Life Forces in our surroundings. But we can be aware of our nature as mystics. Importantly, because of order we know there are no coincidences. By cultivating our consciousness of these truths and applying them justly to ourselves and our interactions with seen and unseen beings, we create positive angels and contribute to our healing and wholeness.

Make some notes about this topic if you're inclined.

Today, meditate on this idea: I am a humble human being in the world, and I am responsible for being aware of my existence on many levels. Although people dance at their own pace, learning as they go, I know that I can expand my connections with the unseen Life Forces, and it's important for me to do so.

※ ※ ※

JANUARY 15–21

What Is a Soul? (Entry Point)

My Soul: The Location of Spiritual Experiences

Soul is the recipient of the spiritual experience and conscious contact that brings new awareness and enlightenment. It's the I Am, the Atman, the location of the place of cocreation, the spark that is a part of the eternal Light that shines through Universes and dwells in beings.

January 15: My Soul

SACRED DANCE

Please take a seated position, with your legs tucked under you in whatever way is comfortable. (If this is difficult for you, please instead use a chair that allows your torso to move and your ankles to cross.) Feel your connection to the floor or chair. Imagine the Light coming into the crown of your head and flowing through your torso and down through the earth. Place your hands, palm-down, on your lap. Circle your torso counterclockwise around that beam of Light, and note that the Light enlarges with the size of the circle you create. Close your eyes, and repeat this dance for a few repetitions, making large and small circles. Imagine the upward-reaching spirals you're creating. When you're ready, open your eyes and return to the present.

MEDITATION AND PRACTICE

When Atum created human beings, the act was considered magick. It manifested as the human Soul, a Life Force that existed in people. Ancient Egyptians believed that the human Soul, ib, was one's physical heart, as well as the essence of the individual. The Shuyet was the Shadow of the Soul. For the ancient Egyptians, one's Soul was the person's distinguishing characteristic and lived during and after life. This was what was weighed against the weight of Ma'at's feather.

Pure eternal Spirit is your essence and true nature, which is formless and consistent. It shines on all, across the planets and around the Universes. When talking about being connected, think of another's Spirit and your Spirit as One. There is no separateness. The Soul, meanwhile, is the essence of an individual. It's the self, the ego, the "I." Spiritual experiences move the Soul and change the way you interact with yourself and others. These are those awe-producing experiences that make you change course or change the way you perceive yourself in relation to the Universe. They often first come about with events that seem negative, like loss of a loved one, a natural disaster, an admission of addiction, or an encounter of a miracle. Write down one or two of your spiritual experiences.

January 16: Ministering to Your Soul

SACRED DANCE

Begin by repeating what you learned in yesterday's dance. After circling the Light a few times, come to rest in the center. Bring your hands together, palms facing each other as they rest in front of your forehead. Press your palms together so that your forearms are parallel to the earth. Make sure you engage your upper arms too, through your shoulders and across your chest. Now, move your palms so that your fingertips point in front of you, and then return them to pointing upward, tracing a disc in front of you. Notice that your torso will go with you, naturally almost. Repeat this pattern, with your eyes closed, all the while keeping your focus on the Light running through you. What do you hear? What do you "see"? After repeating this several times, bring your palms to rest directly in front of your heart chakra. Take a deep breath or two. Place your palms facedown on your lap. Open your eyes to return to the present.

MEDITATION AND PRACTICE

Ancient Egyptians knew there was more than what could be seen with the physical eyes. They knew Souls needed to be ministered to and Souls had to minister to others. The sacred dance included the awareness of the Soul's need for Spirit, which they brought into the temples and in everyday activity while remaining connected to the Universe. In so doing, the Soul and its Shadow received necessary encouragement from the Spirit.

Spirit is what and who you are. It ministers to your Soul, helping you in various ways. Sacred Dance Meditation is one of those ways. Envisioning good outcomes is another. Remembering the Light is crucially important to ministering to your Soul.

Just as you must sustain your physical body every day, you must do the same for your Soul. Every day you must direct your will appropriately to help yourself to a better life. You must allow Spirit to guide your thinking and acting. You must send positive thoughts out for other Souls. You need to recognize the power you have. It is real! You are given the ability and responsibility to engage with and remember the Light, to celebrate it, and allow it to lead and guide you and others. This Practice has been handed down through the ancient Egyptians and has come through many spiritual Practices over time. How are you connecting through Practices that minister to your Soul? How are you ministering to others?

January 17: Let Spirit Lead

SACRED DANCE

Repeat yesterday's dance several times until you're comfortable with the flow. Then, move from a seated position to a kneeling one. Place your palms facedown on the floor next to you. Note the Light in the palms, and send it into the earth. Next, extend your legs in front of you, and realize the Light that exudes from the soles of your feet. Keep your awareness on the Light radiating through your torso, and roll over onto your abdomen so that your third eye is facing downward, projecting Light continually. Your forearms support you, palms flat and fingertips extended. Bring your legs and ankles together and press up to a kneeling position, bringing your palms together at your heart chakra. Repeat this dance until you have been able to do it in a seamless flow. Your eyes may be open or closed. Remember to breathe as you arrive at each new position.

One Soul principle found in the ancient Egyptian world is that different levels of awareness of the Soul exist; they drive our thoughts, emotions, and experiences to help us remember the spark of the Divine. A steady progression upward through these levels of Soul is required to draw more Light into our reality and connect to Spirit. The result is that the conditioning of Western society—driven by meeting expectations of others, earning money, feeling inadequate, or some other outward dictate—is placed in the appropriate perspective.

Your Spirit, the Inner Mystic Dancer, is leading you, whether you are standing, sitting, kneeling, or lying down. Aim to be aware of your thinking and your reactions to life situations, and let Spirit lead. This is a challenge since it is the norm in this society to let your mind drive you. Connect the Soul to Spirit and let it guide, let them merge. Set the ego aside so the Spirit can infuse your consciousness.

January 18: Soul Becomes Spirit

Repeat yesterday's dance several times until you're comfortable with the flow. Today, begin from the kneeling position, with palms pressed together in front of your chest at the heart chakra. Lift your right knee in front of you, and sweep your leg around you, keeping the tips of your toes on the ground, creating a semicircle from the front of your body to the side. Put some pressure on this foot for a moment, and use your hips to press your abdomen forward, placing your gaze in that direction as well. Then, make the same sweeping gesture from the side of your body back to the front, and return to the kneeling position. Repeat these motions on the left. Repeat the dance several times until you're able to keep balance. Keeping the Sacred Dance Posture and palms pressing together is important for this.

The Soul is pure; the Soul is our essence. Knowledge emanates through our different levels of awareness from earthly existence through different levels of our being. In ancient Egyptian parlance, these levels include the *ba*, which describes one's personality, consciousness, character, and likes and dislikes; the *ka*, which is the spark of the human essence that leaves the human body at physical death; and the *jb*, the heart. The ka is pure Soul, and the Soul is always connected to Spirit. The Soul knows nothing of separateness, with no secular versus spiritual distinction.

Celebrate the life you have. It is very helpful to realize the timelessness of your Spirit and that your personality doesn't matter. We can evolve and grow while we are on this plane. As you gaze toward the light, would you like to alter your personality or ways of being to be more useful? Are there any semicircular pathways you can apply to changes you want to make? For example, do you need to connect your daily comprehension with your awareness of the power of your thoughts more strongly? What would you like to change in yourself today or over the next year? Write answers in your journal.

January 19: Soul Circles

SACRED DANCE

Start combining the dances from the previous days, and practice them until they flow together. After you have completed the semicircle on the floor with your right foot, push up to a standing position, and keep your legs shoulder-width apart. Face the right, slightly, with your palms pressed together and forearms parallel to the floor. In a sweeping motion, trace a semicircle on the floor with the ball of the left foot, and shift your torso in the direction of the left side of your body. Repeat on the right side. Repeat these moves, left and right, keeping the palms pressed together.

MEDITATION AND PRACTICE

Creation is a result of energy shifts. Existing long before the Common Era, gods and goddesses through the course of time spawned or created offspring and worlds. We've read about how being shocked out of an existing inert state is needed for creation—the generation and celebration of Spirituality entering a new vessel. In creation stories of the ancient Egyptians, the complexities of the Soul are such that the Spiritual planes we reside on correspond to the shifts our Souls make when they encounter the creativity or shock needed to propel them forward. We call these moments of clarity, spiritual awakenings, revelations, and resurrected consciousnesses.

On the physical plane, the inkling of the higher realms pierces our consciousness. As the Soul is activated in the circles described, we advance in our understanding until we reach the highest planes of awareness. Because we are in the celebratory phase of the year, we express gratitude for our ability to know where our Soul is and whence it came through its evolution and awakening in this current life.

Where are you now? On what plane do you exist? What moments of clarity can you attribute to your Soul's reach for the Light? Are you receptive to situations that cause you to create mental offspring? Do you take your cocreative abilities seriously? Have you created worlds you would like to erase? Or found yourself on new planes of awareness that you wanted to leave? How do you embrace what you have learned and created, while continuing to spiral up? Note where you've been, where you are, and where you're going, using the concept of Soul circles to guide you.

January 20: A Soul-Fulfilled Tree

SACRED DANCE

Today, we'll add on to yesterday's dance. In your standing position, continue switching back and forth between the left and the right side. After the torso shift to the right and left, as you arrive at each directional change and sweep your leg to the side, shift your weight back onto the heel of your foot. Then use the heel to create the semicircle as your return to center. You will notice that your standing knee will bend and your pelvis automatically adjusts to allow the heel to execute the choreography. Try to keep the pelvic area from protruding backward; instead, focus on keeping the center of your body in alignment with the earth. As you make these motions, press your arms upward and open in a semicircle in front of you, and keep the palms facing outward, keeping the tension in them so they have energy. Bring the palms back to the heart center when you arrive at center.

MEDITATION AND PRACTICE

Human bodies conceptualized as trees of life are Spirit with branches reaching to the heavens and roots going into the earth. This tree of life is a mirror image of the Cosmos, which we know is continuing to grow and expand.

As above, so below, as the saying goes. If the Universe continues to grow and develop—though it may be beyond our comprehension—it must stand to reason that a Soul-filled awareness will allow you to step up to new planes. On this plane, the earth is the incubation place for all seeds. With careful attention to the seedlings, growth occurs. Water, light, enriched soil, and space are some of the needs of a growing and expanding tree. Without them, a tree stagnates and dies. Likewise, the human can be represented as a tree expanding through Soul-fulfilling nurturing. What do you need to do today to nurture the expansion of your Soul? Is there any resistance? One requirement is the belief that your Soul is real; it's not made up or some trick. The Soul resides in the Light of the spiritual realms, which is as real as the ground. In this celebration of the New Year, what ways can you tune in with the reality of Soul needing fulfillment and nurturing? What can grow and expand in you this year? Note these intentions in your journal. Be mindful of the fact that what you think comes into creation, and ensure that you're talking about intentions now, not someday.

Jan 21: Soul Buoyancy

SACRED DANCE

Perform what you've learned of this week's dance so far. To draw this week's choreography to a conclusion, when your hands are together in front of your heart center, shift your weight onto your left foot, and gently place your right foot, with the top of the foot facing the floor, slightly behind you so that you may lower down on your right knee. Then, bring your left foot in so that you're on both knees. Lower yourself to rest on your heels and knees. Try to keep your Sacred Dance Posture as you flow through to the kneeling position. Gently lower your hands to your lap, palms down, as if they were floating on wind. After a breath, place the palms on the floor in front of you. Slide them forward with the arms slightly bent to take you to a prone position where you face the floor. Roll over onto your back and up to a seated cross-legged position. Return your palms to your heart center, and, after a breath, rest them on your lap.

Use a chair if kneeling is difficult. You may lean forward, return to vertical, and then arch backward to your level of comfort. Return to center, lowering your hands to rest on your lap. Cross your ankles, and breathe.

Engage with the dance freely, repeating it several times and attempting to leave your thoughts aside as you let the Soul guide. Let your Inner Mystic Dancer be your focus.

MEDITATION AND PRACTICE

The ancient Egyptians believed in the unchanging aspects of the Spirit, which endure through time and space; they also believed that a Soul, when loosed from a human body, could transmigrate, or direct itself into other bodies at will. Metaphorically or literally, Souls were and continue to be conceived of as buoyant, meaning they are active, moving, and able to direct their actions and the actions of the body and mind. The headiness of consciousness isn't exclusively within the realms of thought as we know it today.

You have the power to activate your Soul's buoyancy. You can think of it as a rebirth, a removing of blinders, or the achievement of wisdom. The point is to allow your Soul the buoyancy it needs to be unlimited in the earth's sphere. Whether you fully embrace the ideas of reincarnation and transmigration is immaterial. They both occur, and you can think of that in relation to your own life. Think of the times when you were a different person, like before you chose to change beliefs or behaviors, like getting over being shy or eliminating a habit that no longer served you. When you completed those changes, you transmigrated, and the Soul came with you. Contemplate transmigrations you have had that you can recall now. Note that your Soul buoyancy is required to move you forward through each of those lives and relationships.

※ ※ ※

Soul Supporters (Entry Point)

My Divine Names, My Divine Directions

What we say about ourselves matters. It dictates who we are.
What we allow others to call us also shapes reality.

January 22: What We Call Ourselves

SACRED DANCE

Standing in the Sacred Dance Posture, notice your hands and what they're doing. With your arms gently draped by your sides, palms facing behind you, focus your attention on your hands, expanding and contracting the fingers a couple times. Then, slightly cup the hands so they face the ceiling as you bring your elbows to rest at your waist. Bring the cupped palms together above your forehead. Without moving your head, you should be able to see the wrists when you use only your eyes to look up. Keeping your palms and arms in the position, use your eyes to look to the left and then to the right. Have a pleasant expression on your face, but keep the lips pressed together when smiling. Now notice your neck. Where is your chin? Pull it in if it's protruding, and place it on a plane parallel to the floor. Keeping the palms and arms steady and your eyes looking left and right, shift your neck to the left and right. Add an eye blink between each look left or right and neck shift.

MEDITATION AND PRACTICE

Internal Soul circling and spiraling upward are needed for understanding, remembering, and growing who we are and who we want to be.

At the same time, we remember that we are timeless and that we have transmigrated. The Soul is always pure in all places. Yet, we are human beings and need the interaction of others. Our Soul supporters can be embodied or disembodied. Embodied supporters are those we feel a sacred bond with, those who are of like mind in terms of our directional leanings. Disembodied entities can provide the Soul much support. In the ancient Egyptian teachings, numerous gods led the people through life and death. The human-spiritual distinction didn't exist.

However important connections with disembodied entities are for the Soul, we also need to dance with Souls clothed in a body. What ways can you increase your sense of physical community with other dance meditators? Is a dance meditation group near you? Perhaps you could attend online opportunities or retreats. Write a few ideas for committing to engage with Soul supporters on a daily, monthly, and quarterly basis.

January 23: I Call Myself

SACRED DANCE

Review and perform the January 22 choreography until you are comfortable with it. After eight repetitions, return to the center point and hold the position. Keeping your torso in place and palms pressed together where you can see them by looking up with your eyes gently, pivot onto your heels and face the right side. Your upper body faces one plane, while the lower body faces another. The feet should be with positioned with the right foot slightly in front of the left. As you gaze toward the direction your upper body faces, walk forward in small steps, exaggerating your heel-ball-toe movement. Take two steps forward, beginning with the left heel. On the third step forward with the left heel, rest on it gently, and turn the left toes to the left by twisting the heel into the floor and back. Then, starting with the left foot, move backward, again with small steps, emphasizing the toe-ball-heel movement for three steps. On a left step backward, bring the feet together, and gently rise on the balls of both feet. Return your lower body to the point in the same plane as the torso, facing forward. Repeat on the left. Notice your knees will bend slightly through the dance.

MEDITATION AND PRACTICE

In ancient Egypt, people were very careful about what names they gave others and themselves. Names were associated with different aspects of Soul and Spirit; they sometimes incorporated human and animalistic traits, especially for deities and gods, and constituted one's identity for the present and eternity.

Many cultures have associations with birth names given to children, with names applied upon achievement of a rite of passage, and with names characteristic of actions or temperament. For example, a woman is named after her grand aunt, a man is a warrior after successfully completing tests, and someone is called Picky because he's a picky eater. Some of these names and labels are based on our personas, deep beliefs we hold about ourselves. These beliefs might box us in.

Do you call yourself a hero or rescuer? Are you a martyr? A victim? What name would you give your personality? How much of you is what *you* have determined for yourself, versus what you've been *told* about yourself? What do you want to change about what you believe about yourself, or what has changed recently? What is your given name, personality, and character? Note these in your journal.

January 24: Your Name, Your Meaning

SACRED DANCE

Align gently with your Inner Mystic Dancer, and slip into your Sacred Dance Posture. Review yesterday's dance until you're comfortable with it. Returning to the center, flower open your forearms to shoulder level with palms facing up. Your palms are on the same plane now, and you should be able to see them in your peripheral vision. With the pleasant expression on your face, eyes looking left and right, and a slight shift in your neck on the chin plane, circle the left palm upward four times to create an invisible spiral with your fingertips. With the right foot, twist the heel so your toes point to the opposite side of the raised left arm, and bring it back to center.

Then spiral up the right palm before twisting the left heel and bring-ing it back to center. With your eyes only, follow the direction of your palms. Your palms should be raised now so that your arms are almost completely outstretched but in the same plane as your head. Turn your cupped palms downward toward the floor, and bring them down to rest at your sides while retaining the cupped position.

MEDITATION AND PRACTICE

We dance toward who we want to be and attract our deepest desires. This often means we emerge from old behaviors, labels, and charac-teristics imposed upon us. Have you ever changed while everyone in your environment continues to treat you the same, while family and friends might only see you as you were, not as you are? Perhaps you can only see yourself as that too. Ask Spirit to enlarge you mind and imagination and connect it to your Spirit and Light. Say, "I imagine it, and it comes into reality. Thinking and imagining is the first step toward any metamorphosis. I imagine it manifested now. And it's so."

The key is to evolve (or transmigrate, if you will) and develop an internal vision of what you want to become. Do you want to move from being a victim to a leader? From a martyr to a cocre-ator? From being a taker to a giver? These abilities are evident in ancient Egyptian Sacred Dance Meditation Practices and are avail-able to you today. Review your heart's desires. Do you need help in achieving them? If so, what kind? What will you name yourself when those desires materialize?

January 25: What's Your Story?

SACRED DANCE

Align gently with your Inner Mystic Dancer, and slip into your Sacred Dance Posture. Review the previous day's choreography until you're comfortable with it. Today you start with your cupped palms at your sides. Raise your arms so that your palms face outward away from the sides of your body, with a slight bend in the elbow. Spiral in place, first left and then right. As you return to center you'll add a heel twist with the opposite foot. Place the ball of the left foot directly behind the right, step on it, and turn to your left. Repeat that three times, facing your left, then behind you, then to the right of you. After the third one you will face forward in the original position. Transfer the weight on to the left foot, and twist your right heel. With the right foot, use the ball of the foot to step behind the left foot, and complete a spiral to the right. Do that three times, one for each direction. When you return to the forward-facing position, place the weight on the right foot, and execute a heel twist with the left. Do this several times, remembering to keep the energy in the arms and palms as you twirl. Spotting will help you keep from getting dizzy!

MEDITATION AND PRACTICE

History can be the stuff of myths, and the present contains miracles, the awareness of unseen dimensions. They happen every day. History, written based on a point of view, can have a window into last week or into the last century or millennium. The death of a loved one, an addiction, a government coup, colonialism, the inheritance of an empire, birth into a social class, the attachment of gender values to the body—all form histories that can define us. They can keep us down, benefitting others, or we can overcome them. What is your history, your people's history? What cultural stories keep you in bondage or keep you in your place? Name them and write them down in your journal. Determine if you want to keep those stories or if you don't. Please be active in the decision process, for it will create tectonic shifts in your being and reality. Are you a creature of fate, or do you cocreate your experiences?

As humans, we are cocreators with the Divine. Affirmations, denials, mantras, and Sacred Dance Meditation—we use all to align our Inner Mystic Dancer with the Divine within and without.

January 26: Name Your Soul

SACRED DANCE

Today you will combine the choreography from the last four days to create a square on the floor. As you always do, remember your Sacred Dance Posture, and let your Inner Mystic Dancer lead. Your initial position is the first corner of your square. Keeping your upper body facing forward, use the heel-ball-toe walk to your right with small steps, then twist the left heel. Bring the torso to face forward, and flower the arms so that the forearms are at shoulder height with palms cupped toward the ceiling. Spiral up the left palm, twist the right heel, and bring the foot back to center. Spiral up the right palm, twist the left heel, and bring it back to center. Move the arms so that the palms face out and the arms are in line with the shoulders. Place the left foot behind the right, and twirl to the left. That will be the first of four ninety-degree turns; continue twirling to the left so that after facing the left, you'll face behind you, then to the right, and back to the starting place. Make four such circles. Then twist the right foot, and twirl to the right, mirroring the movements when twirling to the left for four circles. Bring both feet to center, and bring the palms back to their cupped position slightly above your forehead. Shift the neck and eyes, blinking and keeping a pleasant countenance. Repeat these moves until you have created a square on the floor, with twirling at each corner.

MEDITATION AND PRACTICE

Disrupt the story, disrupt the status quo, make something happen, pray, or chant, but whatever action you take, you move the energy. Moving energy is a simile for transmigration. Ancient Egyptians knew this. What is the energy in your life's history? What kind of energy does your Soul have? Think of the pure timelessness of the Soul, and if you haven't already, give your Soul a name. You may wish to select one from the myriad deity names available; if you want to seize the attributes, they carry within you and your life. Review some names that resonate with you, and then write a few names down in your journal.

The point is to recognize and revere the power of words and other forms of communication that form and inform the Life Forces around you. Words are powerful. What we tell ourselves creates and dictates who we are, who we will become. Your Inner Mystic Dancer needs a name that you can call on to bring the reality of cocreation to your being.

January 27: Cocreate or Re-Create Your Story

SACRED DANCE

Now you will take your sacred dance in the opposite direction. Your initial position is the first corner of your square. Keeping your upper body facing forward, use the heel-ball-toe walk to your left with small steps, and twist the right heel. Face the torso forward, and flower the arms so the forearms are at shoulder height, palms cupped toward the ceiling. Spiral up the right palm, twist the left heel, and bring the foot back to center. Spiral up the left palm, twist the right heel, and bring it back to center. Move the arms so the palms face out and the arms are in line with the shoulders. Place the right foot behind the left, and twirl to the right. That will be the first of four ninety-degree turns; continue twirling to the right so that after facing the right, you'll face behind you, then to the left, and back to the starting point. Make four such circles. Then twist the left foot, and twirl to the left, mirroring the movements when twirling to the right for four circles. Bring both feet to center, and bring the palms back to their cupped position slightly above your forehead. Shift the neck and eyes, blinking and keeping a pleasant countenance. Repeat these moves until you have created a square on the floor, with twirling at each corner.

MEDITATION AND PRACTICE

The Law of Attraction states that what a person thinks determines what he or she attracts. Going after something or wishing for it delays its manifestation. Whatever your story has been to this point, what would you like for it to be? In an ideal world, what would your life look like? What would you tell people about your family, history, or culture? What privileges do you have in your story? What imagery can you leverage? Importantly, what empathy or compassion can you show to characters in your story? How does that impact your dance? What ways can you reframe your story and characters, events, and feelings to shape you into a new reality that allows you to cocreate with your Inner Mystic Dancer? Spend some time reflecting and writing today. Knowing the truth is not enough; doing the truth is manifestation.

As you write, remind yourself that you have the freedom and the responsibility to recast your story so that it serves you, without fabricating the truth. Words have power. Imagination is the source of cocreation and manifestation, no matter what the heart's desire is. Allow your Inner Mystic Dancer to lead you to the story you want.

January 28: Claim Direction as Divinely Named

SACRED DANCE

Please review the sacred dance choreography from this week so that you are comfortable with it. Today you are moving in both directions. When you have completed the square in both directions, twirl into the center of the square you created by stepping backward and turning to the left, then twirl to the right. Repeat this a few times in each direction, remembering to spot so you won't get dizzy. With the final twirl to the right, return to the position with the palms touching, just above your forehead and your eyes looking upward. Hold this position for a few beats.

MEDITATION AND PRACTICE

The Ancient Egyptians used the constellations and the stories of gods to determine their course, actions in the world, and rightful place in the Universe. Each of the attributes of humanity and the animal worlds were called upon, with many of them imagined to be god- or goddess-like and possessing the power to make change. Did the people have doubts about themselves or engage in beliefs that led them to feel secure?

As we go through life, we must recognize the need for self-confidence, practice, and discipline, to know that dimensions operate on different planes and that we must understand our Divine direction. We are to constantly spiral upward, turn new corners, and lay claim to our Good. This is the essence of cocreation and a Divine right for all humanity, for the good of all.

When you reach a corner or a plateau, myriad planes intersect it, and when you spiral around the intersections energy vortexes are created. The vortexes are powerful. At each of these moments it's the perfect time to imagine the story you want to bring into reality and to connect your Inner Mystic Dancer with that unseen energy and the Light of the Universe. Celebrate as you twirl, and let go! Release any negativity, limitation, doubt. Know who you are, how special you are, and the magnitude of the love you're showered with through the Divine.

January 29: Name Your Ancestors

SACRED DANCE

Invoke your Inner Mystic Dancer, and, if you're inclined, wear some Sacred Dance Attire. You will dance today in all the fullness of Spirit, creating vortexes of energy at the corners of your sacred square, as well as in the center. Play music if you like, invite others into your space, and perhaps teach them the dance. Or if they've been with you through the week, simply dance together. Try to dance without thinking about it too much and until you feel as though you have achieved a level of trance or distance from the cares of the world. Think of your new directions and new story—what you want to cocreate—and the Beings that will help you achieve your heart's desires. To conclude, slow your twirl, wind up in the center of your square, and lower your arms to your sides.

MEDITATION AND PRACTICE

In ancient Egyptian cultures, as in many others, ancestors were believed to be in the present. Ancestors are known to help make life easier, soothe situations, and guide us to Good, in this life and in transmigrations. In any story, no matter how it's been absorbed by you, ancestors reside in the history, those people who did something remarkable, incredible, or heroic. Some have said that because we are all connected in humanity, all who have passed through the gates of life are our ancestors, whether they lived last week or in the last millennia. Whom do you identify as your ancestors from your family tree or from the spiritual tree? Please write down in your journal the names of six or seven folks whom you respect and would want to lean on, talk to, or learn from, especially as you have developed a new story about your Soul. Alongside their names, please write what traits and attributes they possess that attract you and why.

We are unlimited, and unlimited resources wait to aid us in our storytelling to ourselves about ourselves. The cocreative process requires that we ask, that we align, and that we allow energy to initiate us into the higher realms of consciousness.

January 30: Embody Your Name, Direction, and Story

SACRED DANCE

You will dance today in all the fullness of Spirit, creating vortexes of energy at the corners of your sacred square and in the center. Play music if you're open to that, and invite others into your space. Teach them the dance if you like, or if they've been with you through the week, simply dance together. Try to dance without thinking about it too much and until you feel as though you have achieved a level of trance or distance from the cares of the world. Think of your new directions and new story, what you want to cocreate, and the beings that will help you to achieve your heart's desires. To conclude, slow your twirl, finish in the center of your square, and lower your arms to your sides.

MEDITATION AND PRACTICE

The power of change must be linked with the power of silence. In re-creating and reframing your story, you must silence your old way of thinking and practice new ways of seeing so that new grooves are drawn in your consciousness. For example, when someone asks you a question about your family, you'll have a different response—one more positive, more uplifting, and one that creates the field of reality you desire. When you're thinking about your cultural history, focusing on the strengths displayed in that history and claiming as your ancestors any being that has graced the Universe is so powerful! With these changes you will want to discern with whom to share your heart's desires. In ancient Egyptian rituals, we learn that if something is to materialize it may be wise to keep a spiritual silence. The expression exists that one shouldn't cast pearls before inappropriate beings. So, take care to keep your intentions and cocreations in a dear place as you grow in the new name you have for your Inner Mystic Dancer. You may want to write a few notes in your journal about your feelings, embodied directions, and awareness.

You could say the following to yourself: *I invite the power of silence to encompass and empower me as I remember my heart's desires, my Divine name, and the way my story unfolds from today forward. Thank you for the ability to change directions, to use every resource available to me, and to design a world for the good of all.*

January 31: Closing the Ancient Egyptian Dance Entry Points

SACRED DANCE

Dance the dances from the previous weeks. Try to develop a sense of detachment from the earth and any of your physicality. Be mindful of the physical, but try to lead with the Inner Mystic Dancer as you do the dances.

MEDITATION AND PRACTICE

Reflect on the following: *Change and growth are part of celebrations of Spirit. As I transition into the upcoming days, I know that endless hope and endless resources exist, and all of them cheer for my good, the earth's good, and the good of the Universe. My work with the ancient Egyptians has ended, for now. However, they are with me as ancestors and cocreators. I am aware that there are celebrations I can see and those I can't. I am very grateful to be able to harness the power of change; learn, revisit, and apply new principles; and celebrate every aspect of my being.*

FEBRUARY

Getting Grounded

AFRICAN DANCE TRADITIONS

February's meditations draw from ancient African dances. Of course, Africa is an enormous continent with many different cultures and landscapes, ranging from desert to rain forest. Many have aspects of sacred dance in common. For example, African dances are typically earth-centered and are used to relate to ancestors and deities. The earth is the focal point in sacred dances, which is one reason why sacred African dancers bend toward the earth and flatten their feet against it. The stances are usually wide and solid. The people embrace gravity, as it pulls them down toward the earth.

There are three distinct sacred dance postures in African dance: an upright position, an inclination from the hip area, and a position in which the torso parallels the floor. Regardless of the postures, sacred dancers respond to percussion and give messages through their movement. They see the space they dance in as marking spiritual points. Furthermore, no separation exists between dance and music in African cultures—they are one and the same.

Just as dance and movement are inseparable, sacred movement is essential to life and living. Sacred dance is a key aspect of community, celebration, and festivals. Dancing sacredly is thought to bring prosperity, and for these ancients, no line separates sacred from secular: everything is sacred. African sacred dance follows lines and circles and is done in groups. Dancers believe in spiritual power in the circle or sphere.

Intensification is another aspect of sacred mystical African dance. Resulting from repetition, it can cause out-of-body experiences, euphoric feelings, possession, and exhaustion. Also, the ancient Africans had no sense of marking time, which aided the intensification. The sacred dance naturally completes after achieving the desired results.

PREPARATION

For sacred mystical African dances, you'll want to have percussive instruments: bells, tambourines, shakers, drums, whistles, and the like. You can place many of these on your ankles and wrists to create the percussive rhythms to accompany your movements. Or you may work with a drummer if you know one. African dances are usually done in community, so you may want to invite others to dance with you. You may dance alone and imagine the ancestors and others who are embodied all over the earth engaged in this sacred dance.

Prepare a fragrance of your choice, such as frankincense and myrrh, that will linger with you in memory and in the physical space you dance in throughout the day; lighting a candle while dimming other lights is a good practice. If possible, place the candle in the center of the area you will move around in.

Center your breathing by taking a deep breath through your nose as you feel your lungs and belly expand. Through your nose, exhale all the air from your lungs and belly. Repeat three times. Relax.

Please visit www.cswalter.org/sacreddancemeditations for video demonstrations. They are not intended to be step-by-step instructions but are meant to give you a view of the sacred dance.

FEBRUARY 1–7
Getting Grounded (Entry Point)

Getting Grounded: My Linkage to the Earth's Nourishment

In our lives we walk on the earth, drive on it, fly over it. But the earth is a place of stability for our Souls, where we find healing and comfort. Earth is also a formidable force with many forces acting upon it. This week we embrace the wonder of the earth and how it provides a true north for humanity.

February 1: Anchors to the Earth

SACRED DANCE

Stand with your hips and knees bent slightly. Stand on the right foot, tap the ball of the left foot as you move the left leg toward the right foot, then slide the left foot back to its original position and stand on it. Tap the ball of your right foot as you slide it closer toward the left foot. You should notice a natural swing to your arms. Focus your gaze downward to the floor. Your torso will also naturally swing a bit from side to side. Give yourself the freedom to walk forward and back and side to side. Stay on the balls of your feet and develop a pattern for yourself, as your Spirit guides you. You'll find that this dance works well with drums or percussive instruments should you choose to use them. If not, you'll find that you create your own rhythm. Try to move your feet as fast as you can once you get the hang of it. This will be called *fast feet*.

MEDITATION AND PRACTICE

This week we focus on sacred dance Practices from the central region of Africa, including what we know today as Cameroon and Chad. The Sao civilization lived in this part of the continent, near the Chari River, from about the sixth century BCE to around the sixteenth century. Rhythm in movement and in sound made work lighter, whether that was internal self-reconstruction or concentration on perfection of the mundane tasks of daily life. People danced sacredly, meditated on the connection they had with the gods, revered the earth, and contemplated the Universe and their place in it.

What we do on earth anchors us. Internal anchors include beliefs, practices, ideas, or thought patterns, including how we talk to ourselves, how we regard people, and how we think about ourselves relative to the earth. Sometimes, internal anchors limit us because we don't notice we're even affected by them. External anchors are created by where we live, whom we interact with, and how we structure our routines. Routines can be very comforting, or they can become mechanical, without any thought or feeling.

While you know Mother Nature is beyond your control, depletion of the supply of the earth's bounty isn't. Be ever mindful and courageous enough to voice the truth to others that we should look upon the earth as a member of our family and a receptacle for all our manifestations.

February 2: Positives and Negatives

SACRED DANCE

Yesterday, you may have noticed your shoulders getting into the action while you moved your feet. So today, with the knees slightly bent and leaning forward a bit, with the feet planted squarely on the floor, toes spread out, contract your abdomen and roll your shoulders forward and then backward as you open your abdomen. The accent is on the shoulders moving backward. You want to think of this as a connected move. Do this shoulder dance slowly a few times and then fast as many times, then slowly again. Create a rhythm for yourself. Sway the body to the left and right, moving your head in the same direction as your body. Rest your palms on your thighs, and let them gently and naturally slide up and down your thighs with the moves. Lean forward, and rise back up to the slightly bent-forward stance as part of the pattern as well.

MEDITATION AND PRACTICE

The concerns for health, wealth, and procreation were at the core of several African religions. As such, Africans developed institutions for healing, commerce, and the general well-being of humanity here on Earth and with the ancestors. Ancient African cultures, especially the

Bantu people of Central Africa, viewed duality and polarity—male/female, right/wrong, good/bad, etc.—as essential in the cocreation and universal order. The Bantu people thought of life as resting on the premise of being and becoming. After the process of becoming had taken hold, it was then that one received a Life Force. That set people up to be able to change and engage in forward motion. In the origin myth, importantly, the Life Force was the organizer of chaos. The Life Force was considered to be the first aspect of creation.

Ancient Africans really reveled in the notion of opposites but lived in a sense of the need to be able to synthesize contradictions as well as to be peaceful and cooperative. They didn't like strife or strain. They also saw men and women as equals and weren't judgmental of good or evil. Rather, their beliefs were based on the idea of the utility of complementary natures: both sides of a duality were needed and important to maintain a world of calm and remain outside of chaos.

Within many cultures, feminine and masculine principles are considered equal and aren't gender-based because both are needed. In the same vein, the cultures avoid making hard distinctions between the two aspects of a duality or labeling one good or the other bad. Each exists because of its opposite interacting with it in harmony. Inside everything is a balance between masculine and feminine in different degrees.

What are three "feminine" and three "masculine" situations in your life today? Write them down in your journal, and try not to judge them as good or bad.

February 3: Isolation and Syncopation

SACRED DANCE

Today we add pelvic motions to yesterday's dance. Lean forward slightly, with the knees bent, and place your weight on the balls of your feet with your toes spread out. Contract your abdomen and roll your pelvic area forward, then backward as you open your abdomen. Add fast feet from February 1 and yesterday's shoulder dance. After you have gotten the hang of this, walk forward and back a few times. Keep your knees slightly bent, and exaggerate your forward bend from the hips. Now, lean your torso to the left, and take a few fast-feet moves to the left. You'll almost be walking in place, along with keeping the pelvic tilt. Take it to the right again while walking in place. Keep this rhythm going until you can feel the isolation and the syncopation in your body.

MEDITATION AND PRACTICE

Manifesting the upwardly spiraling Spiritual Awakening is the goal, and being grounded is a requirement. When we have spiraled upward even the tiniest bit, we often find ourselves isolated because there are fewer of us as we dance the path toward the Ultimate Reality. We must leave people behind in many instances, though they are still here with us physically in some cases. We may feel isolated as well when changing old beliefs and still honoring those who have taught and cared for us. Our work is not for the faint of heart, nor for those who fear isolation as a result of knowing and growing. Isolation brings authenticity in the transition from one vibration to another.

At the same time, syncopation, or disruption, purposely enhances a flow or draws in a meaning. In our work, we use it to ground us in the idea that we can purposefully attract higher experiences by utilizing the unusual, by harnessing multiple aspects of Practices to move us forward and upward on the Spiritual Path. Isolation can be chosen and not imposed, and syncopation can feed beauty into it. We can take this ancient learning from the Sao peoples, who knew the power of combining syncopation and isolation for manifestation, and bring it to our Practice here and now. Both are required as the Life Force guides your Inner Mystic Dancer.

Have you been isolated or isolating? Sometimes this shows up as shunning a group because you no longer subscribe to its beliefs or choosing to avoid going out or talking to people. Isolation could also happen when your life is so overbooked with activities that you don't take time to be with yourself—that is, you don't have to be alone to feel isolated. What kinds of syncopative events can you identify that have pushed you either into or out of isolation? Such events are when you were forced to take an action or ask for guidance or help. Write about isolation and syncopation, and put down an example or two, from recent or older past, in each category.

February 4: Call and Response

SACRED DANCE

Refresh yourself on the dances done the past few days. Imagine you hear someone drumming near you; add a quick jump to face that drummer, and continue with the dances you've learned. Imagine you hear another drummer nearby, and jump toward him or her. Add your shoulder and pelvic isolations at the landing of each jump. Keep jumping to face these drummers, taking small jumps to the right, casting your arms out in front of you as if gathering a sweet aroma, until you return to the original position. Make sure to land on the balls of your feet after each jump.

MEDITATION AND PRACTICE

Call from the Spirit and response to it, very important aspects of Sacred Dance Meditation, come to us from the Central African peoples. The relationship between living on the ground and connecting to the Supreme through ancestors has influenced cultures all over the globe. Through dance and music, which were considered inseparable among ancient Africans, the call from Spirit (music) and a response to it by people (dance) show that Being is always connected. Community, family, extended family, tribes, and so on were integral to call and response within Sacred Dance Meditation in ancient Africa. Unification through the response to the call from Spirit produced an intimacy only achievable through Sacred Dance Meditation to heighten the spiritual experience.

Remember that we are being called by the Divine and are responding in our various ways as we muddle through the physicality of the earthly existence and tap into the isolation and syncopation needed to engage with the upward spiral. Part of this call and response, though, coupled with isolation and syncopation, necessarily requires living in communities.

What calls from Spirit have you heard lately?

February 5: Our Original Goodness

––––––––––––––––––– SACRED DANCE –––––––––––––––––––

Begin by practicing yesterday's dance. After you jump in response to the drum, walk toward it, and imagine the drummer is playing for you alone. You add pelvic and shoulder abdominal isolation. At the end of each jump, walk out to a curved arch on the floor to the left, and walk back. Then walk out to a curved arch on the floor to the right. Turn a bit to the left and then walk it back again. You're making a pattern on the floor that looks like spirals from a central point.

––––––––––––––––––– MEDITATION AND PRACTICE –––––––––––––––––––

Western culture sometimes brings with it the concept of original sin or the belief that a human is otherwise born with less-than-desirable tendencies. These perceptions are not found among the ancient African beliefs of the Sao people; rather, they believed in original goodness and that, although evil exists, it can be brought against oneself by the way one treats others. Humans, in community and individually, have a choice in how their lives are conducted. In Western culture is an emphasis on the individual and a seeming neglect of community. Ancient African cultures focused more on the community.

We are all connected in some form in community. If we consider that the Soul is pure and we understand that humans are endowed with free will, then we should embrace our original goodness. We can therefore come to believe in and definitively know our inner value. With isolation and syncopation and with the ability to hear Spirit's call and respond to it, we gradually replace deeply rooted old and outdated beliefs and awaken to manifest our deeply desired life.

As you dance today, think the following: *The ebb and flow of my spiral carries me forward more than it takes me backward. I need to realize that I am pure and originally good, and so are all people. Some may act in ways that seem to deny this truth, and so might I from time to time, or I've been that way in the past. For sure, none of us is perfect, though we must try our best. When my Spirit receives more information, I adjust into new awareness.*

February 6: Feeling the Earth's Community

SACRED DANCE

Choose one or two people you'd like to engage with on the spiritual plane today. As you practice today's dance meditation, incorporating what you've learned this week, carry the thought of them with you to the edge of the spiral and offer them up as they are. As you return, envision them transformed as pure. You will want to repeat the sacred dance of the spiral and create a small circle on the floor.

MEDITATION AND PRACTICE

Many ancient Central Africans marked, adorned, scarred, tattooed, or masked the body during rites of passage, celebrations, funerary services, worship—really, in all aspects of community life—to point out connections to the Cosmos and spirits. These masks, marks, and adornments connected the individuals and communities in their physical journey. During communal Sacred Dance Meditations, the spiritual was embodied through masks, along with other special and purposeful clothing, with the human element concealed. These adornments helped bring the reality of the Supreme Being and Deities to the earth and community and allowed participants to embrace the reality that earthly life is ordered and accompanied by Higher Intellectuals and Beings.

Increasingly in our day-to-day lives we must actively seek community connections. In community, we wear figurative masks all the time to hide who we are or to keep our beliefs hidden. We mask our personalities, and spirits hide us and guard us while simultaneously serving us. What about what we wear and how we view clothing and accessories—or tattoos and piercings—of others? The key is to not judge.

Take on a figurative mask or point of view, adorn yourself with fabrics and jewels, use body markings and piercings if you choose to, and so on. That will put your Inner Mystic Dancer into a sustained higher state, ready to help make our community a better place and keep yourself consciously connected to the Supreme Being. What are your reactions to the idea that tattoos and piercings show the world a commitment to attain a higher realization?

February 7: Loving the Earth

SACRED DANCE

Today would be a great day to invite others from your community to this Sacred Mystical Dance if schedules and space permit, either physically or live on social media. Regardless, please bring the spiritual community you're involved with into your immediate consciousness and invite them to the sacred circle. Perform the sacred dance from this week until you reach a trancelike state, which you will know you're in from moments of feeling release and escape. After you have attained this state, write a few reflections in your journal.

MEDITATION AND PRACTICE

Getting grounded means being in community and understanding that the earth is in relationship with people and the Divine. Both sustain us. It's especially important to show love and respect for the earth, to recognize it has an invisible Life Force. Consider that the earth is a sphere, a set of circles in a fractal pattern of its own, embedded in the larger fractal circular pattern of the Universe. It's the manifestation of thought and the receipt of the feminine principle.

You might have certain opinions and feelings about the state of the earth, its origins, and our relationship to it. Or you may consider yourself and community in isolation, not impacting anyone else. And, if you think humans are tainted from birth, there's no way to fully change the Soul. So, review what you think about tattoos, or yin and yang, and calls from Spirit and your response. Think about what you can bring to make life a little lighter.

※ ※ ※

FEBRUARY 8–14
Stability in Turbulence (Entry Point)

Spiritual Storms: Remaining Steady

We live in a Universe constantly changing, never stagnating. Storms are a manifestation of change, cues to new opportunities on the horizon, and a part of perfection. The human tendency is to ask why things happen. We sometimes never will know why, but some things happen because it's what happened.

February 8: Why Things Happen

SACRED DANCE

This week's dance will call back to last week's. With the knees slightly bent and leaning forward a bit, with the feet planted squarely on the floor and toes spread out so you can feel each one, contract your abdomen and roll your shoulders forward and then backward as you open your abdomen. The accent is on the shoulders moving *forward*. Do this slowly a few times, then fast for as many times, then slowly again. Create a rhythm for yourself, such as three fast, then one slow, and three fast. After this, return to the Sacred Dance Posture.

MEDITATION AND PRACTICE

Ethiopia and Somalia are the Horn of Africa countries where human beings began around 100,000 BCE. The ancient Egyptians called the area, in English translation, G-d's Land, or the Land of Punt, at about 2500 BCE. It was rich and beautiful, having a plethora of earthly products such as gold, spices, herbs, and fragrant agriculture. It supplied the world, sitting across the Red Sea from Arabia. The region was led by queens, including the Queen of Sheba, who were open to various beliefs in multiplicities of deities.

The Oromo tribe of ancient Somali believed that after death individuals existed in Spirit form, and the tribe didn't believe in suffering after death. If one fell short in life, he or she had consequences while still alive. The Oromo visited the Galma mountain, where they'd perform a ritual dance called *dalaga* to achieve a trance state, which often culminated in possession by a higher Spirit. The *eskista* dance, or the Dance of the Shoulders, was performed by the ancient Ethiopians.

Since the beginning of time, people have been questioning the meaning of life. Why do things happen the way they do? Why am I here? Who is G-d? What happens to us when we die? The answers are unsatisfying because really, we only have theories. Sometimes we become apathetic, which can be worse because life then becomes something to be endured rather than enjoyed. What questions do you seek answers for? What have you stopped asking about?

February 9: Dealing with Death

SACRED DANCE

If you have neck problems, you'll want to adjust the intensity of the moves in today's dance. First, roll your head to the left a few times, then in an opposite circle to the right. Then roll your head forward and backward. Stand with your feet firmly planted on the ground, knees slightly bent. Create a rhythmic pattern for this move as you did yesterday, like a set of four to the left and a set of four to the right, and make sure you pause in between sets. Be aware that the moves will make you dizzy! Keep your eyes open, as that tends to help until you get the exercise into your muscle memory.

MEDITATION AND PRACTICE

The ancient Ethiopian people considered the internal essence of the person as eternal. At the same time, they believed that all who pass from life to death dwell with the living. In their belief system, no one suffered in any way after they left the human body, and their religious and spiritual Practices supported the notion of original goodness. This set of beliefs supported the notion that the Divine was within people. Sacred dance played a key role in all these beliefs, transitions, and rites of passage.

In the West, little attention is given to dealing with death until it hits. Elisabeth Kübler-Ross and David Kessler wrote extensively on the theory of the five stages of grief we go through when dealing with death. These stages have often been applied to other situations—divorce, changing jobs, moving our residences, getting married—anything life changing that causes grief. Grief is the result of loss, even if the loss results in a positive change. Without dealing with grief or death, we lock into patterns of behavior that blunt feeling and prevent us from being in community and growing toward our Divine Nature.

What do you believe will happen to you when you reach the end of your life? Do you believe the answer drives all of spirituality? Make some notes.

February 10: Dealing with Disappointments

SACRED DANCE

Stand with the feet shoulder-width apart with your weight forward on the front of your feet. Do a few toe-taps on each side, letting the arms swing naturally about eight times on each side. Next, make short jumps, landing with knees bent. Set a rhythm so that your jumps are interspersed with the toe-taps. Then take a small jump to the right with your body angled out to the right, and next take a small jump to the left with your body angled out to the left. Make sure to look where you're going! Return to the Sacred Dance Posture when you're done.

MEDITATION AND PRACTICE

Living on earth brings many events beyond human control; as we know, the earth has its own Life Force. To deal with that, ancient Ethiopians learned to appeal to the gods, deities, ancestors, and each other to continue life with lack of rain, crop infestations, disease, and all manner of disappointments. Furthermore, the ancient Ethiopians had technological innovations to abate some of the disasters, as they spiraled upward through their connection with Spirit. Disappointment was nevertheless part of the process.

When the earth produces an earthquake, volcanic eruption, tsunami, tornado, hurricane, famine, or other disaster, we don't expect it. When our loved ones leave the earth before we're ready, we're taken aback because we did not get to spend more time with them. Disease, political disruption, and unforeseen life events can be debilitating and problematic. Many situations leave us disappointed.

What disappointments do you clearly recall or are happening to you right now? What were your expectations? What do you expect from yourself? Do you believe that having no expectations can alleviate disappointment and provide stability?

February 11: Self-Deception

SACRED DANCE

Today, combine the pieces of the sacred dance from the last few days. Let's roll the shoulders, roll the head, and do the small jumps. Stand with your feet firmly planted at shoulder width. Do a pattern of three quick shoulder rolls, then one slowly. Now roll the head three times to the right, with a pause, then three to the left, with a pause. Jump three times to the right and angle to the right; next, roll the head twice to the right, and pause. Jump three times to the left and angle to the left; roll the head twice to the left, and pause. Do the same pattern a couple times. Jump to the center of your starting place, and roll the shoulders with a patterned rhythm. Return to the Sacred Dance Posture when you're done.

MEDITATION AND PRACTICE

Peoples of the Horn of Africa enjoyed knowing the Divine and the certainty of the spiritual realms; they were prosperous, wise in matters of life and death, and connected to the world at large. Still, people feared being tricked. They were warned about wandering too far from the path and the tribe. That voice of caution helped steer the course and ensure prosperity for the community, which in turn ensured it for the individual.

We fool ourselves into believing certain things are false, and we refuse to believe other things are true. Self-deception—when we live in denial or lie to ourselves—comes out our thoughts and beliefs, behaviors, emotional reactions, relationships, and how we treat the earth. If we are driven by something outside of our awareness or consciousness, it can be problematic. Sometimes we deny aspects or events of the world that threaten our self-image. When we grieve, self-deception can fall away so that we can see the true Self. But often if we sense that our character was built on falsehood, sometimes we add more self-deception; otherwise, admitting the truth is too painful. We go back to daily routines, buy stuff, and conform.

Can you accept that your life is supposed to be directed internally by Source but is instead often overridden by delusions? How can you honor internal guidance instead of conforming to delusions? How can inner guidance help you find stability?

February 12: Longing Souls

SACRED DANCE

Kneel, if you are able, on top of kneepads or a cloth, so you can protect your knees and slide them across the floor. If you are unable to kneel, repeat the dance from last week. With the knees at shoulder width, move them toward each other and then away from each other. Then move your body to the left. Roll the head slowly, being mindful of your limits and avoiding injury, and then roll the shoulders. Now move your body to the right, roll the head slowly, then roll the shoulders. Try to develop a pattern and rhythm, and move in a circle. Nod your head as you stand up and return to a toe-tap side to side.

MEDITATION AND PRACTICE

The ancient Ethiopians knew that their Spirits were not their bodies; the temporary life of a body carried the Spirit. They dealt with changes in life by using Sacred Dance Meditation to soothe, celebrate, and expand their horizons. They mastered the art of looking within for answers, looking to Spirit when they longed for connection.

So, let us look within. It's important for us to acknowledge our longing for love, assurance, comfort, relief, and knowing. A longing Soul either does not know its Higher Power, wants more connection to It, or feels the absence of Spirit. With a longing Soul, we seek to be satisfied with knowing we are on the path.

Sometimes, especially during grief, change, and instability, we turn to the external—work, family, romance, sex, money, food, drink, drugs, and everything else the world has to offer—to try to fill the longing. We long to know why things happen, why we're here, and what we need to do to make our lives better. The worldly answers always seem to leave us unfulfilled, and so we're back to longing again.

What are you longing for? What has been a lifelong longing for you? How are you satisfying it? Write these questions and your answers in your journal.

February 13: Filling Our Longing

SACRED DANCE

Review and repeat the elements of the dance meditations in the order presented this week until you feel a sense of stability from them.

MEDITATION AND PRACTICE

Ancient Ethiopians aligned themselves with Good, looked within for Soul satisfaction, sought to avoid self-deception, and positioned their lives according to Earth and the planets. They carried out these practices in community, under the guidance of Spirit and the deities and ancestors, moving up through unseen worlds through dance meditation. To be sure, imperfection existed—people doubted what they knew—but they desired to see clearly. So they were able to draw into themselves and their community the power they needed to acknowledge and fulfill their Souls' longings.

In our human form we dance meditatively, and we receive power from turning to our Inner Selves and realizing this is where creation occurs. We call on faith and love as we traverse our experiences, and we know that we are sane when we can be authentic and honest with ourselves and those around us, which provides for a community that deals with their limitations while receiving abundance and cocreated Good.

February 14: Know Where to Turn

──────────── SACRED DANCE ────────────

Today repeat the Sacred Dance Meditations given this week and add your own improvisational rhythms and pauses, head rolls, shoulder rolls, small jumps, and toe taps until you feel you've reached a trancelike state.

──────────── MEDITATION AND PRACTICE ────────────

With Earth's changing trade winds, currents, and seasons, the ancient Ethiopians turned to their Source for stability. In transitions from birth to death and loss to gain, doing so was part of the daily communing. Occasions for change were celebrated, welcomed, and required. Although the people experienced sadness and grief and were not always model human beings, their Practices nevertheless show us that humanity exists in relation to each other and to the Universe. This understanding restores sanity, recognition of love, and the awareness of the spiritually foundational nature of our lives.

In your journal write down some ways you may have been acting from a place of instability. How has your Inner Mystic Dancer, which connects to the Divine through time and space, helped you realize where to turn? Write down some thoughts in your journal.

────────── ❊ ❊ ❊ ──────────

FEBRUARY 15–21
The Body Temple (Entry Point)

Do you see the trees?

The earth's trees feed us, and we feed them. Sometimes we can think of the earth as the base of a universal tree, where creations manifest, including the spiritual seeker.

February 15: Turning Over the Will

SACRED DANCE

Stand facing eastward with feet shoulder-width apart, knees slightly bent. To begin the sacred dance for this week you will bob forward with your upper body, like a small contraction, ever so slight and hard to notice. Move the upper body forward in three small bobs or contractions forward, and then return to the preparation position. Repeat the three contractions forward, and return to center.

MEDITATION AND PRACTICE

The Maasai warriors of Kenya engaged with the sacred *adamu* dance, and the Kikuyu people of Tanzania engaged with sacred *kilumi* and *ngoma* dances. They performed these meditative dances in lines and circles at healing and rainmaking ceremonies. These ancient Africans believed the role of humanity was to find a life of harmony on earth to receive and expand the supernatural experience. They recognized Spiritual Forces, acknowledging they were involved in daily events. For many believers, ancestral spirits were thought to influence the living. Beliefs in magick and a tree of life were also important.

The cosmological significance of a human body symbolized as a tree epitomizes an ideal of our relationship to the Universe. Other Practices consider the human body as a temple, where the indwelling Spirit leads and guides us. In this Practice, we are admonished to allow the Spirit's will to be aligned with the human will. Victory manifests through the alignment of power with the Spirit's will to overcome all barriers and limitations.

What do you know of your will in relation to the Creator's will for you? Are they the same? What obstacles are in your way?

February 16: Inventory

SACRED DANCE

Stand with feet shoulder-width apart and the knees slightly bent. Today you will slightly bend the knees as if you're going to sit down in a chair but stop short. The slight bend is quick, as if you suddenly realize you can't sit down right now. Do three of these slight knee bends in a quick rhythm, and then return to the center. Repeat several times.

MEDITATION AND PRACTICE

Much of the celebration in sacred dance in ancient Kenya resulted from taking inventory. The people appealed to their Higher Powers and looked within to explain what was happening. Did the community have enough food and clothing, housing, and other material goods, and would there be enough to set aside a reserve for when the seasons changed? These questions underlay many activities. Each person likely took stock of what they were doing and how they were being in relation to each other. Were their human traits and tendencies overriding the good of all? Were the principles of the Divine more important to them than self?

Apology was a very real part of the inventory process, whereby faults, internal and external, were noted. Change and recognition were celebrated and sought, to bring out the light and make assets outweigh liabilities.

The principles of willingness and humility underlay the very essence of who we are. We couple that with the practices of honesty, fearlessness, and love. They aid in assessing what's happening inside us in relation to the Supreme Force in the Universe. This is difficult in today's world, where self-promotion, accumulation of wealth, and the comparison of what's inside us with the outside images of others are all normal.

Take an inventory of yourself: What are your assets and liabilities when it comes to your interactions with yourself and with others? Are you a clear channel for the light to flow through you?

February 17: Admit Your Faults

SACRED DANCE

Stand with your feet shoulder-length apart and knees slightly bent. Jut the chin forward and back so the head moves very slightly. The shoulders will move forward and up a bit. Do this motion three times in quick succession, then return to your center.

Ancient Kenyans practiced the art of reconciliation and sacrifice, aiming to ensure their assets outweighed their liabilities. People admitted their liabilities in a ritual ceremony and gave gifts to demonstrate the degree of sincerity. Through admission and giving, the individual expected to find relief—from deities, ancestors, and Divine Spirit—which would then transmit throughout the community.

We find great relief and can stand more fully in the Light when we admit our shortcomings and failures. We all have challenges, no matter where we are on our evolutionary path. Some are spiritually smug, and some still consume too much, so the need to reveal is always there.

What limiting behaviors and thinking do you need to share to find relief? Can you find a trustworthy healer to confide in? Will you seek to free yourself to enjoy the principles of open-mindedness, acceptance, prudence, and serenity in your life and community? Take a few notes, and make a list of people you may turn to, including healers and community members, and get all of yourself out in the open.

February 18: Ask for Willingness

Let's put it together today. Rhythmically bob the upper body forward, and then return to the standing position. Bob the knees as you do so, and jut your chin and move the shoulders forward. Deepen the movements so you bend from the waist and your upper body is moving forward toward the earth. Bend forward once, return to standing, then do three juts with the chin and shoulders.

In ancient Africa, individuals sought cosmic, mystical, and spiritual control over life through incantations to draw from the power of G-d and other deities. Like any attribute, the desire for control can lead to negative outcomes. Being aware of the misuse of power was important, so it was necessary to give one's will to the entities behind mystical and sacred powers. People believed that error came from their actions and that things could be corrected through reconciliation, restoration, and peace-making. Offerings and gifts were given to restore spiritual and cosmic harmony. They sometimes also served as an outward expression of one's willingness to change and grow. Application of will is a faculty of the Soul, which can be used to move forward an idea or desire, beneficial or not.

You are responsible for applying your will appropriately. And if you have a difficult time doing so, then it's important to ask for willingness to do so. How willing are you to use your will to control your way of being in the world? To allow the Spirit to lead you and your decisions and attitudes? If fear of losing yourself is in the way, are you willing to ask for willingness to apply your assets to reverse your liabilities? Make a list of what you'd like to change—about your life, your dance, your destiny—but need to be willing first. How can you apply the correct use of your will to do so? Do you believe that what you do and think have affected you and the world? What about the Cosmos? Make some notes in your journal.

February 19: Remove My Shortcomings . . . Please

SACRED DANCE

Repeat the dance as you performed it yesterday until you can do it without thinking too much. Then add a jump after you return to the standing position. The jump can be high if you'd like, or you can keep it low. Jump three times, then return to the beginning of the sacred dance. Repeat as you'd like.

MEDITATION AND PRACTICE

Ancient southeastern African spiritual Practices drew on the love and kindness of G-d, deities, and ancestors, assuming no separation between human beings and the Higher Power, to shape the individual and the community. Whereas human will had the acknowledged capacity for destruction, the community also recognized it could be used for the positively creative. To commune with the Divine, people understood the importance of allowing for new thoughts and ways of seeing. The African Practices were transmitted by oral stories and parables, which were an essential part of internalizing, hearing, and acting from the Spirit.

Being ready to have our shortcomings—fears, anxieties, and lack of faith—removed helps us to use our body temple in the appropriate manner. Through self-compassion and knowledge of the Light, we use kindness to access strength to change, to honor the internal Spirit that inhabits our body temple.

Identify the deities, ancestors, or chants and mantras that will help you focus, and incorporate them into this sacred dance. You will use them tomorrow, so it's a good idea to jot the names and mantras down today.

February 20: Becoming Apologetic

SACRED DANCE

Refer to the list of names or chants and mantras you wrote yesterday. Begin practicing the dance moves you've learned up to this point, performing each in a pattern of threes, returning to the center between each move. Add a chant, an ancestor's or deity's name, names for the Lord of the Universe, or mantras as you dance through the phrase. Call out on exhaling and with the rhythm of the dance.

MEDITATION AND PRACTICE

It wasn't enough to become willing to commit to change; one had to acknowledge the people who were harmed. In ancient African sacred dance, with the entire tribe present—the living and the ancestors, all the deities, and so on—people acknowledged that actions harmed or soothed like a ripple in a pond by a thrown stone. Everyone and everything were viewed as connected and inhabited by the Life Force. The Soul of the individual needed to be strong and healthy. Foods, ceremonies, healing, and every aspect of life were geared toward recognizing the sacred body temple housing the pure Soul. This aided the community and the earth to maintain harmonious balance. Using chants and mantras was common, and with it, people were able to identify and acknowledge those who received the shortsighted impact of the use of one's will. Favorable ancient traits included forgiveness, calmness, brother- or sisterhood, thoroughness, responsibility, tolerance, and objectivity.

We sometimes rub our fellow travelers the wrong way. Write down names of a few people you've hurt. Knowing what you know now about your Soul, would you be willing to make amends to these folks? Why or why not? Now, write down the names of some people you've helped, along with how and why. Reflect on what you find.

February 21: An Apology

SACRED DANCE

Put it all together today, including the chanting, and get into a trance.

MEDITATION AND PRACTICE

Ancient Africans knew the value of apology to make change and to go in sacred directions. As was shown through "Meditation and Practice" earlier this week, gathering community to join the sacred dance, engaging with the Life Force, and being received within the body temple were expected activities. The goal was to focus on the inner truth and how that connected with the Supreme Being and to disconnect from old ways of being that no longer served the Highest Good of all. An apology requires directly acknowledging the event that caused harm, making restitution, and committing to sustained change without any expectation of praise or gain.

Spiritual power is released during this apologetic process. In other words, patterns and underlying themes in our lives are revealed when we engage this process. It focuses only on you and airs what you have done. So often we want to justify what we've done or blame the person we're apologizing to. The apology is for you, for your healing and growth. After you admit the action you took or the behavior that caused the problem, admit that you caused suffering. Next, say what you are doing to implement sustained changes of your attitudes and behaviors. And you should not expect to be forgiven. Change—revision of points of view, beliefs, ways of being, etc.—necessarily involves people, communities, organizations, and the self. Said differently, the apologetic process and the process of change require us to choose a new way of relating, a new self-opinion, and a new approach to being who we are. It's not easy because such a change will unmask our authentic selves—it's risky to show others ourselves as spiritual being. With apology, we must decide what to do differently, how to become, or what to evolve our lives into. We align our will with that of the Divine.

Do people, cultures, institutions, or aspects of your life warrant an apology? Have you acted, spoken, or thought in ways that aren't reflective of your authentic being? Do you need to apologize to yourself? Please reflect and write.

❋ ❋ ❋

FEBRUARY 22–28
Bearing Fruit (Entry Point)

The earth is a metaphor for wholeness; bearing fruit comes from practice.

Gratitude begets gratitude. With gratitude on the tongue, in the mind, and in the heart, more is manifest for the spiritual seeker. It's the mantra of all mantras, and any practice requires diligence.

February 22: Daily Diligence

SACRED DANCE

Fast footwork governs this week's sacred dance. With the knees slightly bent and your weight on the balls of your feet, tap the left ball of the foot ten times, and then do a tiny jump to shift your weight to the left foot so you can tap the right ball of the foot ten times. Repeat on each side a few times, and begin to reduce the taps by even numbers—eight, six, four, two—on each side. Then tap and hop imperceptibly from one foot to another. Vary your rhythm of the hops and taps so that you have three on the right, then one on the left; then switch so that you have four on the left and then two on the right. If you have them, wear percussive instruments on your ankles, wrists, and waist. Let your arms and torso move naturally.

MEDITATION AND PRACTICE

Ancient Yoruba culture, located in what is today Nigeria, flourished from around 500 BCE to 200 CE. Yoruba philosophy stems from the sacred powers of wise aged women. Women are associated not only with wisdom but also with the keen ability to lead fair and equitable trading and selling of goods and services, governed by the higher awareness of the good of all. The sacred dance masquerades are an important feature of Yoruba spirituality. Like other sacred dances in Africa, the *gelede* dance draws on ancestors as a collective and vital force. In addition, gelede taps into the sacred powers of mothers to bring up social and spiritual matters, helping to shape society in constructive ways.

Yoruba religious Practice encompasses several practical methods of growth and spiritual attainment for each person. It's necessary for multiple perspectives to come together in our daily Practice. One perspective is that we are what we eat. We could extend that to include we are what we read, listen to, think about, watch, buy, sell; we are where we live and who we surround ourselves with. In other words, we have choices and must align them with our will.

Turning off awareness and letting other people or institutions dictate what we will do or think is easy. It's entirely different when we see the world from above so that we can manifest it here below. Our ancestors and elder's ancestors know this. Being present every day affords us many benefits, like the opportunity for small course corrections, letting go of expected outcomes, making apologies, and refraining from judgments. It is important during this process to be aware of self-deception and be willing to live in Truth and Light.

Today, consider at each moment what you align to your will. What is difficult about being aware through this process? How do you react to the idea of being utterly present and constantly awakened? What impact does this have on your community and its reach? How can you harness this feminine energy? Make some notes in your journal.

February 23: Manifestations of the Spirit

SACRED DANCE

Revisit yesterday's tap-and-hop sequence. Once you're moving in a rhythm, lean your torso forward while you tap the balls of the feet. Keep your hips loose and your knees slightly bent. When you shift your weight from one foot to the other, come upright, and clap your hands or thighs. Bring your feet as close to each other as you can during the tapping.

MEDITATION AND PRACTICE

Yoruba tradition emphasizes a progressive ascent toward the Divine, or Divine's desire to make life on earth, with Oduduwa being a location of ultimate compassion. Oduduwa, the power of the womb that brings form into existence, represents omnipotence, and affects and reconstructs the physical reality at will, is the principle that created the physical reality.

Gaining initiation and stability with Oduduwa is an intentionally directed spiritual aspiration for human beings, requiring daily diligence. We can arrive at this awakening and manifestation of the Spirit by daily seeking the will of the Divine as it relates for the good of all. Each day we awaken knowing we want to remain in conscious contact with the Higher Power. And by doing so we can easily see manifestations of the Spirit in our community, providing a salve to the earth's planetary wounds. The manifestations of the Spirit take daily practice, and, when effective, act alike a magnet to bring Souls to you. It's therefore important to attract by your behavior, rather than preach from your speech.

Yoruba religious Practice, while intricate, encompasses several practical methods of growth and spiritual attainment. It uses will and knowledge from the point of view of "above," internally, and from "below," externally, with the goal of making individual and collective life aligned with Spirit. It's necessary for multiple perspectives to come together in our daily Practice.

February 24: Being Whole on Earth

SACRED DANCE

Yesterday you added clapping to the tap-and-hop sequence. Today let's add arm movement after your clapping. Here you will simply extend your arms up and out away from your body when you return to the standing position.

MEDITATION AND PRACTICE

In the Yoruba Tradition, *ashe* is the Life Force emanating from Olorun, the Supreme Unfathomable Being. Olorun, also called the Mystery of Source, is beyond human comprehension. Olorun created Olodumare to run the Universe. Olodumare, who is like the G-d of the Heavens, contained every potential form of Being that could be manifested. Ashe leads to manifestations of the Spirit. An interesting aspect of the Yoruba tradition is that it makes room for spiritual changes in Light. It avers that we each dance a spiral, explaining the Universe we can see, in order to be whole, creative, awake Spirit Beings. In our unique vessels we must make room for change, revision, apology, and new knowledge as we receive new information along the path. Yoruba tradition is adaptable and makes room for spiritual changes: for example, Obatala, the Spirit Entity that was originally tasked with molding creation, got drunk, and the task of creation was reassigned to Oduduwa. Being a whole human encompassed the entirety of existence, and the gelede dance reflected this.

Being a whole human means being awake to interactions between ourselves and others and to the fact that some answers are not revealed to us. We can still be whole humans, being where we are on the spiral path, without knowing the Source of the Source. Reflect on and jot down your beliefs and feelings about being whole. What will you say to someone who asks you about how to be whole while in the vessel of the body?

February 25: Staying Grounded While in Flight

SACRED DANCE

Begin by turning around in a circle in place. Practice turning to the left and right a few times, spinning on the ball of your foot, and try to get all the way around in one sweep, keeping your arms at your sides. At the conclusion of each turn, add the rhythmic sequence from yesterday's dance, keeping your torso slightly bent forward, and see if you can lean a little forward on the turn as well. Keep your knees slightly bent. As you turn, look at a spot on the ground until you must turn your head to come full circle. This is called spotting. If you find a spot to focus on, or perform a longer sequence of ball-of-the-foot taps in between the turns, you won't get as dizzy!

MEDITATION AND PRACTICE

As above, so below, as the saying goes. A tree is a wonderful image for spiritual growth and practice because it keeps us grounded while we are in flight. The tree roots reach below the earth while the branches reach toward the heavens. We are Spirit, and our consciousness is in contact with our Higher Power while we dance here on the ground. Like all people since the beginning of time, we must attend to our spiritual *and* physical needs. We can show manifestations of the Spirit by carefully and mindfully aligning daily spiritual diligence with daily physical practices. That means eating healthy foods, drinking good water, spending adequate and safe time in the sunshine, conducting our life's work in moderation, sleeping, recreating, resting, and dancing. Before drinking or eating anything, practice thanking the Universe for it. Thank your Inner Mystic Dancer for bringing every nutrient to its full use while it travels through your cells. Slow down, and enjoy what has been provided.

Gently and lovingly refuse all invitations from any source to consume harmful substances or to consume more than your reasonable share. Put together a moderate schedule so you can prioritize your body temple's nurturing to maximize your manifestations of the Spirit. Write a plan in your journal. If you need to seek professionals—physical therapists, trainers, recovery-clinic practitioners, grief-clinic practitioners, acupuncturists, nutritionists, or what have you—in this process of change, please include that as well.

The body is the home, the dwelling, the temple of my Spirit, as Yoruba tradition points out. A healthy body allows us to be of maximum service to our communities and an example for others who are being drawn to an awakening.

February 26: Provoking Spiritual Experiences

SACRED DANCE

Just as you did as a child, today take low jumps and land with your feet a little wider than shoulder length, like doing a jumping jack. Jump and land with feet apart, then jump back to feet together. Jump out again, jump together. Then, clap hands before the jumps, spin in one direction when the feet are in the wide position, then jump with the feet together. Clap your thighs when you spin. Keep your knees slightly bent, and bend slightly forward in the jump and the turn from the hips. You're looking at the floor during this sequence. Stay on the balls of your feet, and always land with bent knees!

MEDITATION AND PRACTICE

It was customary that community members participated in provocative ceremonies in the days of ancient West Africa. Many of the ceremonies marked periods of change, pled for change, or expressed gratitude for abundance. Others had the sole purpose of bringing about spiritual experiences. In our current world, we can bring these practices to the forefront to take care of and rejuvenate our communities, our earth, and ourselves. They help us remain attuned to our Divine purposes.

Tasks take our attention—work, focus on self, daily chores, and a thousand and one other distractions from Spirit. For this reason, it's good to set aside time regularly to ensure alignment of your priorities with what you do each day.

You may wish to create a provoking spiritual-experiences practice plan that considers a personal schedule of planned quarterly retreats, spiritual ceremonies, and personal reflection time, along with daily Practices; this can help you provoke those spiritual experiences and continue your ascent. Attending a few Dance in the Spirit dance meditation retreats each year is very important. How will you place yourself in position to be elevated? Write down plans to increase your spiritual experiences.

February 27: Encouraging Souls on the Path

SACRED DANCE

We're going to swing our arms today in big, slow, easy windmill motions like you did as a child. The dance will want you to alternate arms. You'll gaze over the shoulder of the swinging hand, so the head turns to the same direction as the swing. Once you have this rhythm to your liking, put the weight on the foot opposite to the swinging arm, and add three or more ball-of-the-foot taps with your other foot as your arm swings. Keep your knees slightly bent, and bend forward from the waist slightly.

MEDITATION AND PRACTICE

You'll meet Souls along the way as you travel the spiral path. In ancient western Africa, Souls seemed more visible, as folks dwelled in communities and tribes without the veils of modern technology and isolating structures and practices. They were still filled with human emotions, confused at times by events and how to make life more palatable. We have those same considerations today, and there are no easy or certain answers to some questions. Often we cannot find the right words, or our reactions prevent us from supporting others. But just being there for them, holding them, smiling, and giving an affirmation can soothe, encourage, and lead them. Such loving behaviors toward your fellow travelers are the most powerful influences we have.

Reflect on these thoughts: *It's not always about me, and, actually, helping others is the key to a lot of my complaints. If I am not helping them directly, I help with thinking and prayers. My Inner Mystic Dancer encourages others just by being there. I will be able to affect the course of the earth in doing so.*

February 28: Express Gratitude

SACRED DANCE

Let's put the whole dance together today. Alternately tap the ball of each foot. When the feet are together, do a small jump to get the feet at about shoulder width. Remember to add claps. Keep your knees and waist slightly bent. Shift the weight from one foot to the other and swing the arms. Add in your 360-degree spins between foot taps, then add your arm swings, gazing over your shoulder each time. Improvise, and allow the dance to take you.

MEDITATION AND PRACTICE

In ancient west Africa, people embraced not taking things for granted, which is partly why the community celebrated rites of passage and appealed to the ancestors and gods for help. Let us be grateful for polarities so that we can find a sacred middle ground.

Make it a part of your practice to express gratitude. Praise others, give credit to them, and find ways to put others ahead of yourself. Thank Spirit for multiple paths and the spiraling, seeing each issue that arises as an opportunity to improve the earth and our fellow travelers.

What I focus on multiplies; what I speak or think influences my family, friends, community, and the earth itself. Much of the focus is an internal one, not intended to magically change my external circumstances. While not falling into denial or acceptance of unacceptable behavior as I am being clearly authentic, manifesting Spirit, provoking spiritual experiences, and being a magnet for others, I express gratitude for all my blessings, realized and yet to come. I also express gratitude for appropriate reactions and clarity to see what I need to, in moving upward on the path. I encourage others when I have gratitude, and it can be infectious, eliminating unnecessary criticism, needless judgments, anxieties, fears, and depression.

February 29: Open Earth

In a leap year, this day is open for you to expand your focus on getting grounded. Engage with the ideas and guidance found in the moves of the bearing-fruit gelede dance. There is no need for new awareness if none comes. It's okay to simply sit quietly in reflection and thank the earth for all its blessings to humanity.

MARCH

Leaping to Life

MESOAMERICA AND INDIGENOUS AMERICAN DANCE TRADITIONS

Mesoamerica is thought to be a cradle of civilization. Located on an isthmus bridging southern North America with South America, it encompasses the geographic spaces from what we know today as southcentral Mexico to the Isthmus of Tehuantepec.

Mesoamerican peoples' ritual dances were based on the movement of the stars and the cardinal directions. They believed that sacred dance and music came to them from the gods as gifts and thought their gods therefore felt honored when the people danced. They believed rigorous foot-stomping fertilized the earth as if it were a form of raindrops. Both men and women danced, but only in groups of their same genders. Traditionally, sacred dance was performed in large open spaces outside the temples. Statuettes carved during these early times depict dancing as early as 1500 BCE.

The Olmecs, who inhabited what is now Veracruz and Tabasco, Mexico, were the first known Mesoamerican culture and civilization, which some believe lived on earth around 5100 BCE. They are often considered a mother culture to later Mesoamerican cultures. Led by shamans who acted as healers, priests, interpreters, and diviners, the Olmecs believed in three tiers of existence: the earth, the underworld, and the sky. Sky was home to most of their gods. The physical world was held in place by the four cardinal points and natural boundaries such as rivers, the ocean, and mountains.

They believed people are imbued with an animal Spirit. They worshipped the jaguar, believing it to be a supernatural force that inhabited humans, represented ancestors, and was itself a god. Sun-worshipping was also prevalent.

Succeeding the Olmecs were the Mayans, who thought the Universe was structured with thirteen levels of heaven and nine underworld gradations. Because deities were powerful, Mayans conducted ritual ceremonies and made offerings to appease and petition them. Between the heavens and the underworlds was the tangible world where people lived. The four cardinal directions characterized each of the heavens and underworlds, in addition to the earth itself. And these in turn were connected to a different energetic color.

At the center of Maya spiritual rituals was honoring and remembering ancestors, who Mayans believed traveled between the worlds for the living, carrying requests to grant prayers and petitions. Shamans played a key role in Mayan spirituality. Some used hallucinogens to expand their experiences and commune with the forces. For the Mayans, dance was formulaic and included the essence of psychic and spiritual restructuring, change, and transformation. They held that sacred dance does the work of transformation and change, which is facilitated by the star god.

Mexicas were an indigenous people of the Valley of Mexico who were the rulers of the Aztec Empire. Mexica sacred dance has been characterized as thought and concentration in motion, a movement meditation. These people believed sacred dance movements were prayers that generated cosmic energy in the Universe. Concentration on the dance movement channeled an offering to the gods from the dancer and conveyed the dancer's deepest desires and prayers. Sacred Dance Meditation during this time represented an eternal search for integration and harmony within the body, mind, and Spirit. It was a philosophy, a way of life, a method for being awake and present, and a means to communicate their sense of what mattered most. The Mexica were drawn to the spiritual and natural aspects of the dance.

This rich culture of Mesoamerican and indigenous North American sacred dance is presented here to show the depth of what these peoples offer us from a spiritual-growth perspective. It's not in any way to diminish or ignore the path that many indigenous peoples were forced to follow because of colonization.

PREPARATION

For sacred mystical Mesoamerican dances, you might want to wear colorful outfits; regardless, they should be comfortable. Be barefoot for these meditations if you're able. If not, wear shoes or socks that will enable you to feel and grip the floor. If you're inspired to dance to the rhythm of indigenous instruments, such as ankle rattles, hollowed log drums, conch-shell trumpets, bamboo flutes, and clay whistles, which are designed to imitate the sounds of nature, get these ahead of time and store them in your space. Or you may work with prerecorded music of your choice. Mesoamerican dances are usually done in community, so you may want to invite others to dance with you, but it's not required. You may dance alone and imagine the ancestors and embodied people all over the earth engaged in this sacred dance.

Prepare a fragrance of your choice—homemade sweet grasses, resins, or incenses of sage, lavender, and copal are excellent—that will linger with you in memory and in the dance area. Walking with a homemade smudge bundle is a good practice here. Burning sweet grass reconnects you to the earth at this time of the year. The smoke emitted invites spring and attracts new life and growth. State your intentions as you prepare the space. If you do use smudging, make sure you face each direction and walk clockwise near the corners of the room.

Center yourself by taking a deep breath through your nose as you feel your lungs and belly expand. Through your nose, exhale all the air from your lungs and belly. Repeat three times. Relax your jaw and face.

Please visit www.cswalter.org/sacreddancemeditations for video demonstrations. They are not intended to be step-by-step instructions but are meant to give you a view of the sacred dance.

MARCH 1–7
View of Earth from Space (Entry Point)

Climb up the sacred tree.

From the top of a sacred tree you can see to the ends of the Universe, across time and space.

March 1: Tree of Life

SACRED DANCE

This week, we practice the jaguar dance, as performed by the Olmecs. Start out standing in the Sacred Dance Posture, and tap the left foot behind the right foot, then shift to tap the right foot behind the left. Get a patterned rhythm going, then bend your knees slightly when you shift back and forth. Dance left and right a little faster, adding a bit of a hop as you shift from one foot to the other. Try to keep that tap directly behind the front foot.

MEDITATION AND PRACTICE

The Olmecs, who came into existence at about 5100 BCE, are credited with conceptualizing the world tree. World trees depict cultural understanding of the makeup of life, change, and emerging anew. The Olmecs and other pre-Columbian Mesoamerican peoples used world trees to display cosmologies and show their understanding of Life Forces, where they came from, and what the Universe held for them. Theirs displayed the four cardinal directions and a symbolic axis, which connected the underworld, the sky, deities, and the terrestrial world. The tree depicts a snake in the form of a double helix, like DNA, and an all-seeing eye, as well as branches reaching upward to the Cosmos and downward into the seas. It may also depict Africans visiting and inhabiting Mesoamerica, giving rise to cultures and peoples that would follow. Depictions of the Olmec world tree have been found in Olmec art and mythology and in those of other peoples of the region.

The Olmec civilization was very advanced, leading in gigantic temple-making and representational sculpture, agriculture, art, and education. In spiritual matters, they were able to comprehend the Universe with their world tree, bringing forth prosperity and change. This comprehension led them to have the single-mindedness to move forward. It takes a great deal of strength to go from one place to another, to leap forward or to leap into life. It doesn't have to be a physical leap, and often the leaps are internal, emotional, mental, and spiritual. Whether internal or external or a combination of both, it almost takes superpower to make small changes in human behavior.

Adorn your space with supportive world trees, iconic metaphors, statues, or photos of reassuring intuitive messengers. Today or this week, adorn your space with reminders of completed leaps of faith and with supportive messages, statues, charms, images, and such to encourage and strengthen your continued movement toward your Highest Good. Hold the realization of your ability to dance sacredly into the reality you seek.

March 2: Shamans

SACRED DANCE

Bend forward from the waist as you hop sideways from one foot to the other, moving your body slightly backward with each hop. After you've hopped backward a few times, arise, and bend a bit backward as you hop slightly forward, and then tap the alternate foot behind the other. Gaze in the direction of your bend, so that when you bend forward you look at the ground and when you bend backward you look at the sky.

MEDITATION AND PRACTICE

The Olmecs were one of the first human civilizations that adapted shamanic rituals, and, according to lore, they were ancestors of the jaguar. The Supreme Being was a jaguar who could sustain and thrive on land and in water. The jaguar was all-powerful over the earth, the heavens, the underworld, and in between. Because of this worship, the Olmecs developed the jaguar dance.

The jaguar in Olmec culture was the Spirit companion of shamans. A shaman, a class of priest, acted as an intermediary between people and the Spirit realms. The Olmec rituals reinforced the concepts of the Cosmos. In them, the shaman sacrificed blood to the jaguar, wore masks, danced and chanted mantras, cracked whips to imitate the sound of thunder, and accessed trance states through rhythms from percussive instruments. A were-jaguar (half man and half jaguar) was a shaman who transformed into jaguar Spirit via ritual by crossing of the threshold between the seen and unseen worlds. The transformation was brought on by a series of rituals, which could incorporate singing or chanting to the jaguar deity.

Shamans are the healers, conveyers, and carriers of our messages between the worlds. If we look at shamans from an extraterrestrial perspective, an alternative plane such as the world tree, we see them touching Souls, uniting them whether human or not, incarnate or not, and shape-shifting to mold and embody all life to leap into existence. They heal us, divine for us, mediate, assume the needed roles, and give us a spark to leap we need when we need it most. Have you any shamans in your life? Who are they? If you haven't any shamans you can identify, what will you do to attract them to you? Today or this week, seek out the guidance of a shaman.

March 3: Animal Totems

SACRED DANCE

Add your arm movements today by sweeping them beside and slightly behind you toward the sky when you bend forward, and in front of you toward the ground as you bend back. When moving forward, if you're standing on your right leg, your right arm should be extended away from you, and your left arm should be across your midsection. If you're standing on your left leg, your left arm should be extended away from you, and your right arm should be across your midsection. When moving backward, your arms should be raised so that your whole body resembles the letter *W*. Tilt your torso naturally with each movement left and right.

MEDITATION AND PRACTICE

The Olmecs and those who succeeded them believed that humans could take on the characteristics of animals. They demonstrated that by wearing costumes of a given animal, including the deer, eagle, jaguar, and so on. Animal wisdom comes to us without our asking, and each animal, it's said, knows more than humans do. According to Olmec traditions, animals guided the sacred path, led humans to desirous lives, and protected them from harm.

The jaguar was known for its ability to help humans shape-shift; it could bring sanity to chaos and give the people power to fight off unwanted circumstances. The eagle could see, heal, renew, and bring courage, and both the jaguar and the eagle brought the Divine to humanity. The deer is the manifestation of peace, compassion, grace, and fearlessness. The tradition of studying animal totems reaches back to the ancient Mesoamerican peoples and persists in our present day. From ancient traditions we learn they desired to *be* the animal. Sacred dance always brought those animals into the center of the temple and into the spiritual seeker.

Are you drawn to any animals or creatures, or are they drawn to you or your living space? These animal spirits may be teaching and guiding you to leap into a different appreciation for the Unseen Forces they harness for you. The spirits of animals can help us move forward if we are open to them. Note your animal guides. Today as you dance, imagine you're half human and half your strongest animal guide. Use what they are telling you to spring forward to your next plateau.

March 4: Medicine Wheel

SACRED DANCE

Visualize a large circle on the ground as you dance today, turning to the left with the arms swinging, torso bending, and feet hopping.

Your feet come close together, but getting the foot to tap right behind you is a bit challenging! Move in the same way to the right, and then alternate in each direction. Get as low as you'd like when you bend forward, and bend backward as far as is comfortable. Make sure you keep breathing!

MEDITATION AND PRACTICE

The Olmecs used a Medicine Wheel both for spiritual guidance and as a sophisticated circular calendar. A Medicine Wheel is the center of a culture's worldview and spirituality and has many facets. Generally, it sets out cardinal directions, Cosmos relations, and sometimes a creation story. For the Olmecs, from whom we likely have adapted our calendar, each cardinal direction represented values and beliefs. The calendar also reflected aspects of the human self, the seasons, family, life's stages, and creation, helping the Olmecs understand who they were in relation to the world.

The Olmecs were skilled at creating advanced calendars and tracking time and had intimate knowledge of mathematics and astronomy. Their use of technology allowed the Olmecs to build pyramids and temples and carve very large, sometimes-helmeted heads that aligned with celestial calculations. The heads reached nearly ten feet tall and wide.

Their celestial-navigation symbols and formulas, and accurate drawings of constellations, support mathematical formulas used nowadays for navigation. Because of their sophistication, it's said that they were in communication with other beings on different worlds; some believe the Medicine Wheel originated with the Olmecs.

Many peoples across the globe and through history benefited from the Olmecs, including the Mayan and Aztec peoples, who adapted their own Medicine Wheels. Though the wheel does not move, when we dance upon it, we move—spiritually and emotionally. The Medicine Wheel gives us a sense of place, location, history, and destination. It is a wonderful way to draw a story, to set times and dates, to orient ourselves to true north. Sketch a Medicine Wheel for your use, marking sacred days, secular days, solstices, equinoxes, birthdays of importance, your beliefs about the origins of our civilizations, and the cardinal directions using your Sacred Dance Studio as a north orientation. No one needs to see it, so feel free to go all out. Drawing and painting skills are not required; only your thoughts and important moments are. In your Sacred Dance Studio, set some stones and markings on the floor to help you work.

March 5: Prosperity

SACRED DANCE

We'll add a little twist to the step today by spinning around with the dance and moving along the imaginary circle on the ground. Spin to your left, and move on the circle to your left; spin to your right, and move on the circle to your right. You might find yourself hopping on one foot as you spin. Take it easy because it's easy to get dizzy. The way to avoid dizziness is to focus on a point as you make your turns.

MEDITATION AND PRACTICE

The Olmecs were delivered to a veritable promised land where they could thrive, expand, and prosper—a region near the current Gulf of Mexico. There, they grew crops and could accumulate an agricultural surplus. Within easy reach were fruit and nut trees, fishing, and so on. The Olmecs traded with their neighbors with goods such as serpentine, mica, rubber, pottery, feathers, and polished mirrors of ilmenite and magnetite. Precious stones like obsidian, jade, and quartz were often used to create sculptures of supernatural animal spirits or to create ritual craft items.

Absolute signs of prosperity can be seen in the architectural grandeur of Olmec religious centers, buildings with four colossal heads at certain places along the north and south, which seemingly guard the region. It is thought that the heads as they are placed are in relation to the Medicine Wheel.

Effort is often accompanied by prosperity, and one such effort is faith. The effort, and risk, of investing knowledge and intuition into the unknown can prove rewarding. Although we all want to prosper financially, physically, mentally, and spiritually, action needed to materialize prosperity may feel overwhelming. Like the Olmecs, the answer is simple. Follow the stars where they lead, with faith, and let your intuition be your compass. The land of milk and honey, the promised land, waits. It's both an internal connection to Spirit and an outer manifestation of the Good the Divine wants you to have. All that is needed is the asking—and doing the footwork.

March 6: Abundance

SACRED DANCE

Today we continue with the jaguar dance. Begin by pausing to remember the Mesoamericans who have contributed so much to our way of life today. Feel their presence. If you're using shells, bells, rattles, or other percussive instruments, please spend a moment setting a rhythm with them. Review the dance given so far this week if needed. Now, hop and tap as you've learned this week, with forward and backward bends to the left three times and then to the right three times. Then, with the right foot, tap one heel in front, followed by two quick tip-of-the-toe taps behind, then a flat-footed tap to the side and then to the front to shift your weight. Practice this a few times on the right, then do the same on the left. You should begin to notice a transformation.

MEDITATION AND PRACTICE

The Olmecs enjoyed abundance of material, spiritual, mental, emotional, physical, and communal well-being. One might say they had the favor of the unseen in the land of milk and honey. They did not suffer limitations; without limitations one can leap forward mightily. These principles are still guiding today's world. All that was needed was for them to focus and hold whatever abundance looked like in their hearts, knowing it was for the good of all.

Sometimes it helps to ask the Divine Spirit to show us what abundance looks like and open ourselves to receive those images. Once the information is firmly placed into our Spirit, we can tap into the wellspring without hesitation. What does abundance look like to you, and how do you continually cultivate it? Do you believe abundance exists in your life right now? To know that you're blessed now is a mighty key. Imagine abundance here, now, immediately for yourself and others, the earth, the community. What is your heart's desire? Hold the image in your mind and Spirit; assume it's real now. Know it to be true now, not at some vague point in the future. Think of this sacred community of the Olmecs, who knew no limits and manifested abundance to the point that we can continue to learn from them some five thousand years later. Watch for signposts as you continue forward and follow your path to abundance.

March 7: Sharing

SACRED DANCE

Today we continue with the jaguar dance. Again, bring your awareness to the Mesoamerican ancestors as you engage in the dance you've learned this week. Repeat the dance until you find a trance, and feel transformed from being a shaman to the were-jaguar, accompanied by your animal totems.

MEDITATION AND PRACTICE

The Olmecs shared their abundance with their neighbors and within their community, in their families, and with the gods. Sharing seems foreign in our society that focuses on earning from a young age. Yet we all know that tremendous abundance and prosperity is of no use if we're alone with it all. Through sharing the good received, we are transformed. Those who share receive abundance and do not focus on what they lack; they are connected to the Source. With sharing, more abundance and prosperity are directed to the sharer because he or she knows lack or limitation doesn't exist and all comes from the Source. By giving we receive, said Saint Francis.

What kind of sharing practice do you have? Do you give time, talent, or treasure without any regard for return or reciprocity? If you do, can you increase it? If you don't, can you plan to do so? Of course, all this sharing must be in support of your well-being—do not become codependent in your giving and sharing.

Of course, the Olmecs are no longer a civilization we can see. They did what they were called to do while here in the body. Sharing resources, being prosperous, and manifesting abundance do not exonerate anyone from physical laws. But we know that ancestors are with us, including the Olmecs, helping us leap forward through transformation.

Say to yourself, *My mind, body, and Soul have been renewed.*

MARCH 8–14
Leaping to Life (Entry Point)

Shed your protective layer until it's time to shed it again.

After a while we move out of one house and into another.

For this week's dance, you may wish to use a horn or similar instrument to clear the vibratory channels. A percussive hand instrument is also recommended. In your Sacred Dance Studio, visibly mark the cardinal directions in your space: east, south, west, and north.

March 8: The Assumption of Other Spirits

SACRED DANCE

Each day this week you will begin by facing east and either calling vocally the sacred Spirits of the east or using your horn to do so. Repeat in clockwise fashion, pausing at each direction. As you return to the east, allow the silence to fill the space. Place your horn aside, and vigorously shake the handheld percussive instruments. Stand with your right hand and your instrument in front of your heart chakra, with the forearm parallel to the floor, and your left forearm behind your back resting on the small of the back. Pause as if you're hearing someone calling your name in the distance, and gently gaze to the sky. Then take small jumps facing south, west, north, and back to east, pressing your arms close to your body and alternating their positions with each turn to the right. Be deliberate, and hold your hands in fists.

MEDITATION AND PRACTICE

For the pre-Columbian Mayans, *dance* was a sacred word that meant offering or sacrifice. Dance created, and was used in, sacred spaces and temples; bridged earth and other worlds; and rescued Souls from Xibalba, the Mayan underworld. To accomplish supernatural tasks, Mayan people wore clothing and masks that represented their *wayob*, or Soul companion, which they became when entering a trance dance.

Often, the Maya worked with sacred implements such as staffs, spears, rattles, scepters, and even live snakes as dance aids. Contrary to modern representation, Maya regarded snakes as highly evolved messengers, in tune with the Life Force. Therefore, they represented past, origins, and the human code, what we consider now to be our DNA. In Mayan culture, snakes bridged lunar and solar relations, between the elements of water and fire. Snakes symbolized alternation, change, transformation, and eternity, Divine communication personified. They could be a sign of healing from being reborn, as in turning over a new way of acting. Serpents are also seen at the base of world trees, symbolizing prosperity, protection, and abundance. Mayans also believed in a cosmic light serpent that traverses the Universe. What can be learned from the Mayan culture that can help us leap forward into uncharted spiritual life?

Each serpent is useful in bringing us the assumption of Spirits. Feathered serpents are powerful images and have appeared in many ancient sacred dances. If you are turned off by popular religious characterizations of serpents, you could briefly study them to see if changing perspective benefits your leap into a new life.

March 9: Healing Practices

SACRED DANCE

Familiarize yourself with the moves from yesterday, and prepare your space and body. When you return to facing east, add two jumps in place, and then kick forward with your right foot, do two jumps in place and kick forward with your left. Keep your forearms parallel to the floor, like you're resting them on a ledge. Now jump to the south, west, and north, and repeat the pattern in each direction. Afterward, repeat the pattern in a counterclockwise rotation. Mix your turns from clockwise to counterclockwise, with two jumps and a kick in between each rotation. Please be deliberate with your directions.

MEDITATION AND PRACTICE

The world tree is a very important motif in the Mayan mythology, specifically depicting the Mayan view of the Cosmos and creation. According to Mayan beliefs, the sacred tree of life originated in the underworld, grew through the earth, and then rose into the heavens. By this course, the tree gave birth to life on this planet and ordered the Universe. The Mayans held the tree of life to be a vertical axis, complete with the serpent, connecting the three cosmic realms. Mayans believed that the ceiba tree was an actual manifestation of the sacred world tree. Ceiba trees were frequently grown in Mayan cities and are placed at the center of Mayan villages.

The medicinal and healing qualities of the tree are considered sacred in Mayan culture. A qualified shaman uses prayer, divination, and guidance from spiritual guardians—who communicate through dreams—to make holistic remedies developed from sacred trees to cure, purify, or cleanse a person. Nothing separates the Spirit and well-being, according to these Practices.

A healing Practice is probably available to suit every Soul. Yet any Practice must include a way of being, as we take our health and well-being as a Divine right. That means prioritizing rest, relaxation, retreats, and fellowship instead of making money.

We must also mind our thoughts, affirming the good, denying the untruths about ourselves and others, and refusing to own an illness. How often we hear people identify themselves with their ailments, saying, "my pain" instead of, "the pain I feel"! This binds it to the psyche and makes seeing it as a separate, inanimate thing difficult.

Do you spend time dancing in the Light? Or do you give in to being immobile? Do you know deeply that the body is a temple capable of miracles being energized by the Divine? Do you seek the best foods, the best healers, and the best thinking all the time?

March 10: Immaterial Things

SACRED DANCE

Please warm up, and prepare yourself today as you have been for the sacred dance this week. Then, please review the movements. After doing the small jumps and kicks and being comfortable with the turning jumps, now we add large arm swings like windmills as you turn. When you turn to the right, swing your left arm out to the side, placing the right arm behind you at the small of your back. You will exert a bit of force when you move your arms, as they are not carried by gravity; they are directed and positioned deliberately by you.

MEDITATION AND PRACTICE

Art and architecture—temples, pyramids, palaces, stone motifs, masks—were often created to give homage to the immaterial. People were engaged in metaphysical study of life and death, emotions, and change. Change has always been a constant reminder of the immaterial and impermanent nature of human life and the desire for the presence of Spirit. Ancient Maya believed in the cyclical phenomenon that we call time. The people observed, documented, and inscribed on calendars hundreds of cycles and celestial changes. The Maya shaman interpreted these cycles in terms of explanations of past events and predictions of future challenges. They were not really hooked into past, present, and future as it's considered in today's culture.

For the Maya, every physical object has Soul, and every Soul thrives in an embodied physical. This means that, for the Maya, the world was abuzz and alive because every object, animate or not, has a Soul. Immaterial is in the material, and they both form a whole, a symbiosis that cannot be embraced fully. Body and Soul, material and spiritual, tangible and intangible, need and complement each other.

This thinking refutes the idea that immateriality is to be feared or debated over whether it is important. It just is, like you are. How can you think of everything having a Soul and the embodied nature of such a thought at the same time? How does that impact your ability to leap forward? What arguments do you escape from?

March 11: The View from the Temple

SACRED DANCE

Today we're going to tap, swing the legs, and move the arms across the body. Step on the right foot; allow the left leg to swing in front of you, and bring the right arm across the front of your body, with the left arm going behind. Step on the left foot; swing the right leg in front, and the left arm comes across the front of your body, right arm behind you. Your hands are still in fists. You move deliberately; a hard stop with a bit of a hold pose and a head nod goes in between the left and the right leg swings.

MEDITATION AND PRACTICE

The Tikal in Guatemala is one of the largest and earliest Maya pyramids. All the pyramids located there were created in veneration of the cosmic blueprint design replicating Pleiades, a nearby star cluster, which is said to be the home of their star god ancestors. The Pleiades has been characterized as a passageway or luminous chord between the earth and sky. In the Mayan understanding of human life, the Divine indwelling and human consciousness originated from the connections between the stars and intelligent life there, which provided codes of Light hidden deep within human cells. These codes lent early Maya civilizations an inherent knowledge of the laws of nature, sacred geometry, astronomy, and generation of energy. The Maya believed their arrival on the earth was the origin of human existence from outer space. They looked to the sky for guidance and direction, assurance and stability.

The sky can help us chart our course, physically and metaphorically, and help us retain our humility and realize our human frailty. Sometimes these realizations will allow us to leap forward from judgment, fear, blame, shame, grief, and any number of mental constraints. Similarly, we can have gratitude for what we have, what we have learned, and what we know that guides us to be better human beings in the service of the Divine. What have you learned lately that has caused you to reevaluate your position in the Cosmos? Is your heart open and receptive to new ideas that may help your Inner Mystic Dancer?

March 12: Time and Eternity

──────────────── SACRED DANCE ────────────────

Begin by reviewing yesterday's dance moves. Move from east, to the south, to the west, to the north, then move in the opposite direction. See if you can speed up the moves while keeping the hold pose and adding a bit of energy to the leg swing so that the knee bends and the foot is flexed.

──────────── MEDITATION AND PRACTICE ────────────

In the Maya civilization, the calendar was based on the moon's cycles. Each "moonth" was twenty-eight days, which is the same length of a woman's menstrual cycle, generally. They tracked how the moon and sun traveled across the sky; these orbital trajectories, and planting seasons, marked the days and the years. The calendar was simply based on human relationship to the Universe. They let their bodies and their communities be in sync with the natural rhythms of solstices, equinoxes, and seasons. There was no such notion as hurrying. Living in the present was their directive; that meant that eternity was available to them spiritually, especially when knowing their spiritual home was with the star gods. They "spent time" in such a way that honored the Divine and their Inner Mystic Dancer.

Do you live in an area where you can see the night sky? If not, plan to visit a place where you can see the stars at night. Do you know the times of the moon changes? The time of sunrise and sunset? The dates of the equinoxes and solstices? Please develop a calendar of these events so that they are readily available to you. You can visit this link to get started: www.timeanddate.com/moon/phases/. Begin to use them in your daily Practice of dancing in Spirit.

Today, contemplate your relationship to time: *Being driven by the Western notion of time robs me of serenity and inhibits my ability to commune with my Self. Having too many commitments and working too much or overtaxing myself will end up in disappointment. If I am driven by the lash of the clock or if I escape facing myself by being bored or scared of what I will see inside myself, let me find a way out—a door, a window, a crevice—that will let me out of the box of time and open me into the space of eternity. Cutting my activity down to reasonable bites is the main objective of moving toward Spiritual time that lands me in Eternity, now.*

March 13: Cross Circles and Labyrinths

SACRED DANCE

Please prepare your Sacred Dance Attire, gather your instruments, and assume your Sacred Dance Posture. Please warm up. Now, let's put all the dances from this week together.

MEDITATION AND PRACTICE

Cross circles are large-scale artworks etched in fields, which depict sacred images such as star formations, trees of life, geometric fractal patterns, and so on. They were devised to count the days, the seasons, and the solstices. Some believe these were created by alien beings and have attempted to place them within Mayan belief systems. In what is today known as Zacatecas, Mexico, we find the Mesoamerican ceremonial site of Altavista, where a cross circle also serves as a labyrinth. The labyrinth, which is squared with the four cardinal directions, is comprised of long corridors, with curves and walking passages. Strikingly, the eastern area of a corridor and the nearby hill of Picacho Pelón are in alignment during the summer solstice. Moreover, the ceremonial center and its orientation are part of a sacred geometrical connection with three other centers within Mesoamerica.

In our current culture, labyrinths are used for meditation, contemplation, and peaceful relaxation. Using them to stay in the present while realizing the universal, larger sense of elapsed time can really be a powerful way to find our relationship to the universe. When we know we are but a speck in the Universe and simultaneously own our power and devise systems to navigate life, we have the sustained knowledge of who we are and what is important.

What are you contemplating today? How long have you been doing so? Are any sacred sites near you that you could visit to help you understand who you are in relation to other civilizations? Or help you to draw on their wisdom in your life's path?

In meditation today, think about the following: *Every day that I can be in a cross circle with other human beings and walk a meditative path, I am experiencing great leaps forward in my life. Civilizations and humankind before me have taken herculean and heroic efforts to do impossible things, perhaps miracles. But miracles often happen out of necessity. The ability to achieve the kinds of outcomes the Maya people achieved seems so vast and unimaginable. I can experience the labyrinth of sacred remembrance and draw on this knowledge, courage, and certainty that lies within my own inner being. I can be authentic, whole, and fulfilled. I know the powers of the Universe are accessible to me.*

March 14: Extraterrestrials

SACRED DANCE

After getting into the Sacred Dance Attire and warming up as you've done each day this week, please find your Sacred Dance Posture and set into motion all your musical instruments. Complete the dance in its entire splendor, as you have learned it this week.

MEDITATION AND PRACTICE

We know that the Mesoamerican Mayan people believed in extraterrestrials and cosmic life and worshipped star gods, as these have been depicted on their petroglyphs, art, and ceramics and in their ceremonial spaces. They believed that the people of the earth were brought here by another intelligent life form in space through an intergalactic highway.

Teotihuacán, the "City of the Gods," is the location of the Pyramid of the Sun, a significant pyramid that works in tandem with the orbit of the earth and marks the calendrical spaces on the cross circle and labyrinth at Altavista. It's currently unknown how this and other similar structures were built. Can we be open-minded to the fact that just because we can't see something doesn't mean it isn't there?

Ask yourself, *When I am confronted by evidence of the unbelievable, do I have difficulty reconciling the reality of what I see with what I've been taught? Am I open-minded and nonegotistical about what others believe? When was the last time I took a concerted effort to learn about another faith or Practice? We get through this life being unable to seriously and concretely answer questions about why we are here, where we come from, and, importantly, where we are going. Instead, I gently leap forward to being okay with not knowing and adopt nonjudgmental and flexible stances.*

MARCH 15–21
Calling on Positioning (Entry Point)

Color me purple—just don't color me gray.

Colors represent the levels of Spirit and the resonance I seek.

March 15: Geomancy

SACRED DANCE

This week, we learn an ancient Aztec Quetzalcóatl dance, in honor of the feathered serpent god. Aztec dancers would wear colorful costumes and use percussion instruments, conch-shell trumpets, bamboo flutes, and clay whistles designed to imitate the sounds of nature. You may do so as well. Standing in place and holding your percussive instruments, get a beat going at a reasonable pace, one that is right for you. Once you are comfortable with it, shift your weight side to side from one foot to the other with the beat. The movements are simple and low impact. Knees are slightly bent, and you're moving at a medium pace. After you have shifted left and right for a few minutes, move forward and then backward, keeping the percussive music going.

MEDITATION AND PRACTICE

The Toltecs lived in the area we know today as Hidalgo, Mexico, between 800 CE and 1100 CE. Toltec theology rested upon Quet-zalcóatl, the feathered serpent, which later became the central figure of the Aztecs or Mexicas, their successors. Life was considered endangered in the Aztec cosmos, but the Mexicas developed a way of life to arrange for the challenges life presented them. There was no sense of future or past, only the present, and this led to permeability of situations, as well as to no distinctions between Divine and human nature. That meant simultaneous existence of human nature with the Divine being, power, person, or animal.

Aztec sacred dance, done at sacred locations, was focus in motion. The dancer's concentration on the movements could channel an offering to a god or center on earthly prayers. The sacred Quetzalcóatl Pyramid, an area where dance was performed, is both a solar clock and calendar. It represents a pre-Columbian application of geomancy, useful to position sacred dance and to know the goals of the spiritual work.

Geomancy is the art of placing or arranging buildings or other sites based on knowledge about living in harmony with the earth. It's about finding the most appropriate locations for human activities and structures that automatically involve Spirit, indirectly obliging landscapes and ecosystems to create abundance. This ancient Practice includes sensing and channeling energy to increase innate abilities to feel, shape, and transmit life energy. Some say geomantic arrangements can affect interspecies communication with not only animals but also tree spirits and landscape angels to tap into their memories and guidance. What is the sense of geomancy that you have within the places you reside and frequent? Are you in touch with this energy? If so, what is your experience of it? If not, would you be open to practicing connecting with the place?

March 16: Sacred Temples

SACRED DANCE

You will now add head movement to yesterday's moves. When you move forward, slightly bow your forehead; when you move backward, slightly raise your forehead. After doing that a few times, shift your weight from the left foot to the right, keeping your percussive instruments going. With the right foot, step forward, then cross over with the left foot in front of the right, then step back with the right, then place the weight on both feet. Do a few shifts from left to right in place. Then repeat on the left side by stepping forward with the left foot and crossing over with the right; step backward on the left foot, and then return the right foot to center. Repeat this a few times, and return to the weight-shifting from left to right and walking forward and backward with head movements.

MEDITATION AND PRACTICE

The Quetzalcóatl Pyramid is one of many pre-Columbian sacred temples, which were located near the water and had seen and unseen gates and portals. Their three-dimensional shape was intended to attract energy into the space, and they were placed strategically in sacred geometric relationships to other temples on the earth. They were always oriented to the Tropic of Cancer or Capricorn and anchored to the four cardinal directions. Energy was connected to the temples and recharged with sacred dances. Only the highest good was sought for the earth, its inhabitants, and the supernatural beings. Do you have a sacred temple you attend to regularly?

Many of us have affinities for sacred spaces, temples, churches, and community centers, which are scattered throughout the landscapes of our lives. We would benefit greatly by transforming our homes and offices into sacred temples. Their various elements and spaces connect us to the earth and Cosmos. The author Freddy Silva is currently urging this return to the sacred, making it accessible to us, and drawing on ancient wisdom of the Mesoamerican people. Connecting to the elements of earth, water, fire, and wind or air, and to Spirit, is key to our leaping forward. It is also very necessary to be aware of our geomantic relationship to the rest of the Universe as we create sacred temples.

March 17: Gateways and Portals

SACRED DANCE

Today we will repeat shifting the weight from the left foot to the right, with your percussive instruments giving you a beat. Walk forward and backward a few times as you've done already. Now, take a step forward with the left foot, move the right foot close to your ankle and then away before placing it down. Then step on the right foot, and move your left foot close to your ankle and then away before placing it down. You will feel as though you are creating a semi-circle in the air before you put your foot down, slowing your steps. Do this on the left and then the right, moving forward evenly on both feet, then shift your weight from left to right with the rhythm. Repeat this moving backward. Note that your knees always need to be slightly bent.

MEDITATION AND PRACTICE

In many ancient cultures with sacred dance, sacred temples were understood to have portals or star gates leading to other worlds. Entering through them allowed one to directly communicate with sacred spirits without any medium, shaman, priest, or anointed human.

The physical manifestation of passages into the domains of the Universe is almost always coupled with progression through spiritual gateways. But these are not mutually exclusive, and you don't need a portal to necessarily find a spiritual gateway. Gateways sometimes are visible, with the planetary motions required to access the portals. From a figurative perspective, gateways relate to stages of movement when we spiral upward in our awareness and influence others and ourselves. We go from awareness to enlightenment, traveling through different aspects of time and space while we are here on earth and dancing through many portals to arrive at gateways along the way.

You can check your own progress along the path of awareness by remembering where you started dancing on your spiritual path. And you can establish gateways and portals in many locations to remind you that you're not here on earth alone, with no direction or guidance. Try to mark a doorpost or archway in your home or office, or anywhere you frequent, that you're sure will remain intact. These are reminders of the miracles, changes, and stages of growth that you have experienced. In your daily Practice, dance through the portals you have established, and remember the gateways of change that have brought you to where you are. Could those gateways be loss or gain of a loved one? The realization that the leaders of your chosen faith are human? The loss of or a change in a career or position? The acquisition of a material object? Being bored? There are so many gateways, if only we look for them, that help us remember and accept exactly where we are and imagine where we'd like to go.

March 18: Sacred Crystals, Sacred Geometry—Fire

SACRED DANCE

Today, start by shifting the weight from the left to the right foot as we have done all week. Move forward and backward, adding your head movements. Go with the crossover step on the right, move forward and backward, take a crossover step to the left, then move forward and backward. Then, standing in place, slightly bend your knees and bounce up and down in place. Lift the right foot, tap the toe on the floor in front, side, and back motions, timed to the sounds of your percussive instruments. Bring the foot back to center, shift the weight, then tap the left-foot toe on the floor in front, side, and back motions, timed to the sounds of your percussive instruments holding the beat. Now, shift the weight to the left and right feet, while standing in place, and then repeat the toe taps on both sides, first right, then left.

Sacred geometry, or the use of sacred shapes, has been a part of almost every ancient culture, many of which built their sacred sites and cities in adherence to it. These shapes include the Platonic solids—tetrahedron (fire), cube (earth), octahedron (air), icosahedron (water), and dodecahedron (universe). Importantly, we realize there are spiritual relationships between the Life Force and sacred stones and crystals with certain geometric shapes.

Fire energy is known as Kundalini energy and is found only in human beings. Kundalini is said to rest quietly at the base of our spines within a pyramidal geometric encasing. Once awakened, this energy pushes human beings toward spiritual freedom and enlightenment. As a fire element, it's connected with our deep intentions and drives, and we use this elemental energy to achieve our goals.

Many valuable resources on healing and spiritual advancement with crystals and stones are available. Search for tetrahedral crystals. Gather some that you're attracted to. Then perform a prayer over them, asking for them to be energized to lead you forward in the Highest Good for yourself and those around you. Then set an intention to be mindful of their energy. Leave them in a place where you can return to them in the coming days. We know for certain that the Aztecs used such techniques to enhance their sacred experiences.

Using sacred-geometry crystals in your home or office brings the energy of the Divine into your space. Dance meditations with sacred geometry crystals in your space are also very healing, connecting your mind, body, and Spirit with sacred, spiritual energy.

March 19: Water

Our moves today will be heel and ball-of-the-foot taps on the left and right. Have your knees slightly bent, and repeat the shifting the weight from the left and the right foot. Now, tap the heel and then the ball of the right foot, directly in front of you. So, it's heel, ball, heel, ball, etc., and repeat this eight times. Shift the weight, and repeat on the left eight times. Walk forward and backward, using your head movements.

MEDITATION AND PRACTICE

Turquoise crystal, associated with the healing energy of water, has been discovered in ceremonial masks and battle gear of the Aztecs. It's said that Quetzalcóatl taught them the art of cutting and polishing turquoise; it was considered sacred by Mesoamericans and those cultures that followed in their footsteps and was used as a powerful tool for creating a connection between heaven and earth. In crystal healing, turquoise crystal is associated with personal protection; on a cellular level, its healing power promotes an energetic flow of love.

Water sustains the planet, makes up most of our bodies, is the origin of abundance in life, and is a conduit for energy. We can charge water, even that within our bodies, with intentional vibrational thought energy and blowing into the water. It's conductive to electricity and sensitive to the emanations of our consciousness, including subtle levels of energy that science is only at the edge of being able to measure. With that in mind and with invoking the power found in turquoise crystals, we begin to give shape to our directions. Write some intentions for yourself, the people close to you, and your community. If you have any turquoise, bring that into your immediate area. Fill a large glass bowl with water, and bring that into proximity to the crystal. Ask that the water be energized and pull from the ethers, using your hands to wave over the top of the bowl. Think about what you'd like to manifest in the world as a way for you and others to leap forward. Always include words that allow for all to realize their Highest Good.

While we realize the power and healing properties of water and turquoise crystal, remember that areas of the globe lack water, and people have very little. When we set intentions for our own lives, it's well to remember we are all connected, and always remember the availability of water as a gift.

March 20: Spring (Vernal) Equinox—Air

SACRED DANCE

As you assume your Sacred Dance Posture and get your instruments, remember today is a change of season. Enjoy dancing in the rays of sunshine, even if it's cloudy or rainy where you are. Note of the first day of spring as many living organisms leap to life! Dance in your space today in free form, and celebrate your circumstances, whatever they may be. As you dance, verbally express gratitude for what you have and what you don't.

MEDITATION AND PRACTICE

Twice each year the earth's equator dances with the sun directly above it. On days like this, today, the daytime and nighttime lengths all over the world are the same. It's a wonderful reminder of our physical connectedness through time and space. Peoples from the sacred dance cultures talked about in this book all acknowledged the importance of the way the earth interacts with the sun. The relationship marks changes in seasons, times for carrying out obligations, and celebrations of praise and gratitude.

Etheric energy can be considered the space between things, events, and changes and the provocation of intention into reality. When we breathe, at certain moments we neither exhale nor inhale; they are pauses between actions. When we dance, at certain moments we aren't moving. Between celebrations of manifestations, whether large or small, is often unseen growth or new ways of thinking and behaving.

What growth have you seen in yourself leading up to this equinox? What is springing to life before you? Do you have any new intentions you'd like to add, or would you like to revise existing ones? Write them down to put them into the Universe, carried by ether to the heavens so that they can manifest.

Imagine that your desires are fulfilled today. Thinking they will manifest in the future keeps them from manifesting sooner. See them in your life today, and see how they will support the Highest Good of you and those around you. Bring your intentions into your crystals if you have them.

March 21: Embodying the Temple—Earth

SACRED DANCE

Let's put the week's dance all together today, complete with your music and percussive instruments. Remember where you are in relative position, as you get into a trance doing the Quetzalcóatl dance.

MEDITATION AND PRACTICE

Earth provides a stable environment from which all life with the other elements spring. Earth, sometimes referred to as Gaia or Mother Earth, is feminine and receives, incubates, and nourishes the "seeds" of intentions, which in turn are granted to us as gifts and fulfilled abundance. The yield from the earth element springs from both substance and intuition. It's the bringing into the physical what has been conceived of in the Spirit, cultivated by love and fed with actions and thinking. Earth acts as a container for all the other elements of air, water, and fire.

According to the Aztecs, all life on this planet was created by the interplay and relationships between the four elements. Each element is under the direction of a particular deity:

- Fire—eastward, spirituality, male energy, light (Huehueteotl)

- Water—southward, emotions, child energy, willpower (Tlaloc)

- Air—northward, mental, elder-wisdom energy, movement transformations (Ehecatl)

- Earth—westward, physical, integration, female energy (Tlalnantzin)

Earth energy is needed as both a place of production and a necessary ingredient for life. It's the key to our existence, renewal, grounding, and hope. Deep within the earth lies fire, surrounding it is air, and most of the globe is covered with water. Mother Earth and her energy allow life to exist, integrating all the elemental energy in each human being.

❀ ❀ ❀

MARCH 22–31
Transitions (Entry Point)

Which way is north?

Know which way to turn for Divine intervention.

March 22: Cardinal Direction—East

SACRED DANCE

For this week's eagle dance, a drum in the background or handheld or worn percussive instruments producing a constant, even beat can help to set the tone for the sacred space. If you have access to feathers and feel inclined, wearing them along your arms and around your waist could bring in the Spirit of the dance.

Begin by marching slowly in place, moving forward in a line, and then turning to the right to make a circle. Repeat these motions, then turn to the left to make a circle. Bring your knees high as you march, often to hip level or higher, holding it for a beat and then lowering. Repeat with the other leg. Afterward, return to the standing position. You should exert yourself when doing these movements.

MEDITATION AND PRACTICE

Many Indigenous American tribes performed the eagle dance when there was a need for Divine intervention, particularly during spring when water was crucial to planting. This eagle dance was particularly associated with the Jemez and Tesuque Pueblos in modern New Mexico, where it's still performed every spring. Male and female dancers celebrated this sacred dance, both wearing headdresses that contained yellow beaks and feathers from eagles. The dancers circled each other as they imitated an eagle's movement.

The eagle stands for spiritual protection, strength, courage, and wisdom. Additionally, the eagle is thought to have supernatural powers to transport prayers to the gods through its ability to move between heaven and earth. As a Medicine Wheel totem animal, the eagle represents the ability to see broad truths that we cannot see from our normal perspective; often, these are shown to us through transitions. Transitions are therefore key factors in spiritual growth. Like knowing where we are, it's important to know what direction we are going. In indigenous cultures of North America, eagles are associated with the east, which represents the spring season. East is the direction from which light shines on the earth daily. Observing sunrise is very sacred, and we rarely take time for it. Facing east each day reminds us of the importance of the light as it transitions us from various types of darkness. It brings new beginnings and renewal and answers questions by shedding light upon them, giving rise to new vision.

When you see an eagle soaring, you're being guided to progress spiritually and to complete a transition. When you are unsure, turning eastward can bring stability to soar high and see clearly. Are you soaring? Would you like to? What action is needed? Please make some notes in your journal.

March 23: Cardinal Direction—West

SACRED DANCE

Repeat what you learned in yesterday's dance, and as you do, move your arms slightly forward and away from your sides, up over your head with the notion of soaring. Raise your arms in gradations, marking positions in space, not in one movement. You may find the positions at the level of the waist, the shoulder, and the ear.

MEDITATION AND PRACTICE

The cardinal direction of west coincides with autumn, or the harvest season, when we reap the harvest both metaphorically and, in times past, actually. The main point here is to understand that we can plant seeds in the spring—faith, love, harmony, compassion, prosperity—in our minds, bodies, and Souls. Light and hope shine on these, so in autumn, we can reap the harvest of mental abundance: freedom from worry and anxiety and the knowledge that we are all connected and all affect each other. We hope this will sustain us until the next planting.

Spending time in the west, represented by the color black because it signifies the womb and is full of feminine energy, we cultivate all we can imagine. It's a return to the womb of creation. You begin to conceive what you want to give birth to, bring into being, or release in the spring. Stillness and quiet, like the nighttime, take precedence in the womb, a powerful place full of creative potential. Give yourself permission to enter the womb as needed to renew and nurture new potential within yourself.

When we trace the path of the setting sun, our eyes are left looking upon the physical manifestations, changed attitudes, healed relationships, or healed and released emotional pain. We also understand the oft-used phrase that "this too shall pass" and realize no duality matters.

March 24: Cardinal Direction—North

SACRED DANCE

March in place as you did earlier this week, then add the arm movements as you did yesterday. Today, keep the arms moving and do not lower them below your waist. Alternate the arms so that one is higher than the other and the marching is working with the rhythm. Move the arms in synchrony with the steps. The emphasis of the march is down, and there is a slight bounce to the movement.

MEDITATION AND PRACTICE

As represented on the sacred Medicine Wheel, the cardinal direction of north is associated with winter and wisdom. North represents shedding earthly physicality and completing the transition to Spirit. North is considered the location of wisdom, where one has earned knowledge, compassion, and holistic thinking after a lifetime of experiences. The grandparents and elders, both those in physical form and those whose energy we draw from Spirit, reside in the north. The north is the place to share wisdom with others and to seek guidance. Because of this, one finds majestic beauty in the north. The north represents healing, rest, recovery, and renewal, where things are held solidly in place until winter passes. Of course, anyone who pays attention during a winter hike will see how much life and motion there actually is during this time.

Transitions are not blips in time; they occur over time. As we transition from one state to another, we are healed, fulfilled, challenged, and rendered better than before. We honor the north by being open to illumination, curiosity, discovery, understanding, and compassion. At this location we are deliberately engaged mentally while adhering to our Inner Mystic Dancer's intuition. This is a place of integration, where knowledge leaves the mind to be absorbed by the body.

What may need this kind of integration in your world? Where can you use this energy of understanding? Are you able to offer your wisdom, or do you need to seek wisdom? In what situations, locations, places, or organizations can you give and receive it? Please contemplate how you can give back and receive as you or others transition from one phase to another, through stages of recovery, grief, healing, or simply learning how to be.

March 25: Cardinal Direction—South

SACRED DANCE

Today, let's repeat yesterday's moves but with a bit more energy. After you have gotten the rhythm down and are comfortable with synchronizing the arm movements and marching, increase the pace somewhat. See if you can enter a trance as you make these moves in place, forward in a line, then following a circular pattern on your floor. Use the space you have.

MEDITATION AND PRACTICE

The southern cardinal direction is associated with summer, faith, trust, and harmony. For our indigenous ancestors, Sacred dance ceremonies such as the sun dance were often held during the summer to help groups of people return to harmony; this dance is still practiced today. During the sun dance, the participants typically abstained from eating. Among some Indigenous American peoples, including the Sioux, dancers suspended themselves from long poles with ropes attached to pins that pierced the skin, enduring the pain until they lost consciousness. Dancers set intentions of healing, world renewal, and thanksgiving. People prayed for knowing their place in the Universe, or healing for friends or relatives, while the sun dance healed every being, as well as the earth.

Indigenous American people believe that if the sun dance isn't performed every year, the earth, a thriving being herself, will lose touch with the creative power of the Universe and will no longer be able to regenerate. The sun dance is performed every month during the full moon and annually in an extended three- or four-day cere-mony during July.

We honor this cardinal direction by practicing empathy, trust, faith, inclusion, love, and emotional balance. We also honor the childlike freedom and energy that we still embody during summer. Although some may associate negative memories with summer, we can still grab the promise represented by it. Summer represents serenity, growth, fire, passion, fertility, happiness, and peace. It's a time of relaxation, fecundity, leisure, and lounging. Interestingly, we can have summer anytime we face south by recalling and embracing these feelings and imaginings.

Would you like to dance during the full moon each month?

March 26: Direction—Above

SACRED DANCE

Repeat yesterday's moves and increase the energy while keeping your rhythm. Work at your pace. Today, when you've completed a circular pattern on the floor, march in place six or eight times, then, turn counterclockwise 360 degrees. Repeat in the clockwise direction and then march in place. Make sure you move your arms!

MEDITATION AND PRACTICE

As we've learned this month, many Mesoamerican and Indigenous American people revere the sky gods, stars, planets, all things above, and the movement of the heavens in relation to the earth. We have seen their meticulous calendars and timepieces. This direction of above is often out of our minds in today's culture. Especially in many fast-paced Western cities, we spend most our time dwelling on earthly matters or forget that the Cosmos is alive and enveloping the earth.

The Cosmos is all the suns, moons, planets, stars, meteors, galaxies, dust, air, deep space, black holes, worm holes, and whatever consciousness exists in those sectors. Consider the Cosmos as the realm of cosmic consciousness. In connecting with this direction, remember you're part of the entirety of life—throughout the Universe in time and space. As you contemplate the heavens, imagine their mysteries and other worlds without being afraid of the unknown. Experience yourself as an inhabitant of our planet moving through space. Reflect on Indigenous American creation ideas and on stories of humans that have ventured forth into space from our planet.

We must do more than simply walk on the planet like an automaton. Consciousness is in the space above my head, above my roof, above my seat on an airplane. Though we might not agree with the concepts of extraterrestrial beings or their vehicles, we do have to acknowledge wisdom is in the Universe, if only because it maintains order.

March 27: Direction—Below

SACRED DANCE

Review the choreography given this week. After the marching pattern is completed, squat as low to the ground as you are comfortable while keeping the arms moving.

MEDITATION AND PRACTICE

Earth is our source of physical sustenance, and we walk upon it and navigate on its waters. The Indigenous Americans revere the earth and acknowledge it as a living entity, situated within the rest of the Universe. We are told that the earth's natural electromagnetic field has a frequency of 7.8 hertz, known as the Schumann resonance. When we meditate, dancing or otherwise, or live close to nature, the brain emits alpha frequencies like that of the earth, and our energy fields are in balance with the energy field of the earth. The result is an experience of more balance, alignment, stability, and health. As we learn from our Indigenous American ancestors and from our modern knowledge of science, earth's energy field interacts with the energy fields of the Cosmos. The energy field then interacts with the energy fields of living bodies here on earth, connecting all living beings.

Before electricity, the earth and people, who lived according to seasonal cycles, existed harmoniously. Microwaves, cell phones, computer monitors, and so forth add electromagnetic energy higher than the earth's. We live indoors, and, in modern Western culture, shoes prevent people from absorbing the balancing energy provided through the earth. Our modern conveniences disconnect us from earth's energy below us.

What kinds of activities, in addition to Sacred Dance Meditation, can you engage in that allow you to absorb the earth energies? Walking on the beach, hiking, going to the local park, and being outdoors in general can help reinvigorate this awareness of the sacred direction of below. When connecting to the earth, be mindful of it. If you're a technology user, can you consider reducing use of computers and other electromagnetic field–generating devices?

March 28: Spiritual Maps

SACRED DANCE

Practice the dance with the crouching and higher energy moves, and embody the eagle.

MEDITATION AND PRACTICE

A spiritual map illustrates your life journey—where you are, where you've been, and where you can head. Your spiritual journey began with your birth, and it leads to now. Spiritual maps include changes in spiritual identity and related practices as well as major events that push spiritual reevaluation and change. They may show beginning and ending friend-ships, helping a loved one transition, learning to be who you are, dealing with addiction and codependency, understanding or opening up to spir-itual reality, coming to terms with your physical components, and many more. You can associate moments along your spiritual map with each of the directions. Importantly, these points along the map are fluid and accessible to us regardless of our current physical age. These directional associations can be used to aid you in your spiritual mapping:

- North—Air, mental, elder-wisdom energy, movement, transformations
- South—Water, emotions, child energy, willpower
- East—Fire, spirituality, male energy, light
- West—Minerals, rocks, crystals, dirt, or soil, physical, inte-gration, female energy
- Above—All of the cosmos, Divine, ethers
- Below—Earth, stability, peace, electromagnetic energy

In your journal, or on a large sheet of paper, draft a spiritual jour-ney map. Start by placing a timeline across the page, which represents your life from birth to death. Next, add some significant moments perpendicular to the line, spacing them relative to their distance in time. The distance between them should be relative. Above these, add marks that represent peaks, valleys, and, importantly, plateaus where you coasted, or experienced deserts or wilderness. On your map, associate the four cardinal directions, and the above and below ener-gies, with main experiences. Now, look forward to chart a course, set a spiritual goal for your life, and consider how you will use the directional energies to move you toward your goal.

March 29: Setting Directional Intentions

SACRED DANCE

As you face eastward today, remember that you reside within a spiritual map. Become keenly aware of the directions that surround you. See if it's possible to be outdoors today.

With palms open to receive and arms outstretched, do the following:

1. Face south and say, "The warm winds of the south, Great Serpent Mother, show me how to let go and step away from ways of being that do not serve me. Allow me to walk toward beauty and attract beauty into my life and to those around me."

2. Face west and say, "Blessed winds of the west, Mother Jaguar, envelope me as I face my fears, anxieties, shortcomings, and uncertainty and teach me to transform these through loving kindness and compassion. Show me how to live impeccably. When needed, allow me to apologize immediately, without ego."

3. Face north and say, "Wise winds of the north, Royal Hummingbird and Ancient Elders, lead me through patient endurance so that I may experience peace and joy on this earth and in transitions. When time to shed my body, come to me during dreams as I travel the heavens."

4. Face east and say, "Winds of the Great Eagle with your visionary energy, remind me to lead from my pure heart, and guide me to soar to new places and not look back, to fly with my wings touching Spirit."

5. With one palm on the earth and another overhead, say, "Dearest Mother Earth, I pray for your healing. I melt into your wisdom, as I revere and nurture you as you do me. May I attune to your energies and leave positive and regenerative markers for generations to come."

6. Raise both arms to the sky and say, "Father Sun, Grandmother Moon, to the star gods and their nations, Great Spirit, the peoples know you by a thousand names, though you're not named or within my comprehension to name. Thank you for bringing me here and showing me the way to You."

MEDITATION AND PRACTICE

Indigenous Americans were known to set intentions using the energies of the cardinal directions and of the directions above and below.

Knowing where one was and what the directions represented were part of daily and cyclical life. Ceremonies were used to help the community align with the overarching intentions, and individuals used the energies to set their intentions. We can draw on this ancient ritual to aid us in journeying along the spiritual road ahead. Using the spiritual journey map you prepared or are preparing, and with the directional intention invocation previously described as your framework, set some intentions for each of the directions. Use them' as supports to propel you through your transitions.

March 30: Embodying the Spiritually Mapped Directions

SACRED DANCE

Review your directional intentions and spiritual map and the ideas you created for your life this week. Review the dance given this week. After gathering your instruments and your Sacred Dance Attire, connect your spiritually mapped directional intentions with the eagle dance.

MEDITATION AND PRACTICE

Our indigenous ancestors and many of those who have learned this sacred knowledge continue to enact these precepts. The eagle dance is connected to community and brings to the forefront a way of being that honors self, community, the earth, and beyond.

Say to yourself, *Spiritual energy is all around me in many forms, on many different levels and vibrations. The directions are the one form of support that can be drawn upon immediately, any time, and in any location.*

March 31: Incorporating and Integrating

SACRED DANCE

As we come to the close of March, gather your instruments for all the Mesoamerican and Indigenous American dances done. From the Olmecs to the Indigenous North American peoples, we have learned a great deal. We have leaped to life by finding our position, honoring the equinox, and meandering through transitions. Today when you assume the Sacred Dance Posture, speak to your Inner Mystic Dancer. Ask her to connect to these ancestors, giving thanks for them in the process, as you freely connect to the sacred dances for March.

MEDITATION AND PRACTICE

It's an amazing revelation to know that many who came before us already knew and practiced sacred dance and drew the power and energy contained in it. They paid close attention to the earth and its abundance, seasons of change, and the relation to the Cosmos. They devised systems to evaluate where they were in time and place and mapped these in addition to their spiritual maps. Their knowledge informs us today, which is important for unifying the planet at this juncture in our history. In this unity we can find strength.

Say to yourself, *Just when I think I am unable to learn more or do more, my Divine Self intervenes and leads me to new vistas. As I integrate all that I have learned and demonstrate in my body and consciousness, let me always remember that unlimited and boundless soaring and leaping is available to me any time I reach to the temple, the geomancy represented in my crystals, and my intentions that I set into motion.*

Multiplying Abundance

SACRED AUSTRONESIAN DANCE

In April, sacred dances of Indonesia, Polynesia, Tahiti, Hawai'i, and Australia guide us in learning to multiply abundance. Polynesian religion and mythology drew upon the people's relationship to the ocean. The Polynesians were master navigators and developed seafaring skills; furthermore, they valued interactions with nature. You see their affinity and reverence for these aspects of their lives in their mythology and religious works and Practices.

For the Polynesians, everything, including people, contained a sacred and supernatural power called mana. It is the foundation of the Polynesian worldview, linking the people to the ancestors, as you'll learn throughout the month. The way for humans to gain more mana was by *pono*, or good and balanced deeds that sustain the earth and its inhabitants in right ways. Sacred dance was imbued with mana and was considered a pono.

Tattooing is a sacred Practice of these ancient Polynesian islanders, which is discussed during Sacred Dance Meditations this month. Our word *tattoo* has connection with the Polynesian word *tatau*. Bodily markings served a variety of important functions. Because writing wasn't a part of Polynesian culture, tattoos were an important communication mechanism. They explained an individual's social status, rites of passages, lineage, and history. This will be discussed in greater depth later this month.

People from Southeast Asia arrived in Sumatra, Indonesia, around 500 BCE, and with them they brought sacred dance. From them came the Minangkabau peoples of West Sumatra who engaged in Tari Piriang. This sacred dance was based on daily movements, such as agricultural cultivation and meal preparation. It expressed joy, well-being, prosperity, and, most important, gratitude to the gods for abundance. Tari Piriang was danced after a plentiful harvest. Our ancient ancestors danced while they presented plates of food.

Differing from Tari Piriang, the ōte'a is characterized by rapid hip motions danced to percussion accompaniment of shells and drums. Such choreographies draw from sacred geometries—such as the symbol for infinity, or varu; a square, or otamu; a circle, or ami—while maintaining the hip movements. The ōte'a reenacts sacred daily life. The themes centered on spoils of warfare or sailing and depicted use of spears and paddles. The sacred dances tamure and paoti, which we practice this month, are from the ōte'a.

Ancient Hawai'ian hula, or ritual dance, is called hula kahiko. This dance was accompanied by certain types of chants, oli, such as those dedicated to the 'aumakua, or gods of hula. This sacred dance goes as far back as kumulipo, or how the world was made, first and foremost through the god of life and water, Kane. Hawai'ians believe that at the time Kane and the other gods, Lono, Ku, and Kanaloa, created the earth, they recited oli while they moved their bodies in reverence.

We end the month by practicing the dances of Indigenous Australians, but to see their wisdom, we must look some sixty-five thousand years ago. Although they likely migrated to Australia though the movement of the Austronesian New Guinea people, Aboriginal Australians aren't related to any known Asian or Polynesian population. They are now believed to be part of the migration out of Africa, a people that "split from the first modern human populations to leave Africa 64,000 to 75,000 years ago."* Today's Queensland would be where most of the population lived at the time, with some living in today's New South Wales.

---

* "DNA Confirms Aboriginal Culture One of Earth's Oldest," *Australia Geographic*, September 23, 2011, https://www.australiangeographic.com.au /news/2011/09/dna-confirms-aboriginal-culture-one-of-earths-oldest/.

PREPARATION

For each of the sacred dances presented this month, you'll have the opportunity to use instruments and sacred attire from several of the regions. If you aren't using those to embody the sacred from those regions, you needn't worry. Just use your usual Sacred Dance Attire, and use your imagination! Your incense and other supporting treasures are always welcome.

Please visit www.cswalter.org/sacreddancemeditations for video demonstrations. They are not intended to be step-by-step instructions but are meant to give you a view of the sacred dance.

APRIL 1–7

Landing on New Shores (Entry Point)

Directional Navigation

We have the internal compass to guide us, and we see clearly and follow wisely.

For the next seven days, we will embody the West Sumatra sacred dance of Tari Piriang. It is performed in small groups of three or five people, accompanied by people playing a *talempong* or a type of Minang kettle, and *saluang*, which is a Minang bamboo flute. Sacred dancers sometimes wear a bell attached to a ring. You may adorn yourself with these on your fingers if you're inclined. Invite others to join you if you'd like as well.

April 1: An Internal Navigation System

SACRED DANCE

Begin standing in a relaxed position with your gaze slightly downward. Slightly bend your knees. With your right foot on the floor, make a semicircle that crosses over the middle plane of your body, with your big toe leading. Then turn to the right a bit so that you're facing on an angle toward your right side. As you make the semicircle, engage your arms so they are bent at the elbows, resting at your sides, and then cross them over in front of you at the wrists, palms facing upward. Then spread them in front of you and to your sides as you turn your body toward the right. Place all your weight on your right foot, and then bring your left foot to slightly behind you. Hold this position for a beat.

MEDITATION AND PRACTICE

Ancient Austronesian peoples traveled great distances to realize the promise of a better life, to multiply their abundance. As they sailed, they likely experienced doubt, as they could see no horizons. Yet they continued anyway, knowing they were headed in the right direction.

Once they landed on the shores, they were likely encouraged and certain that their ancestors and the Universe guided them. We imagine the mental and emotional motivation needed to undertake such a voyage, such a manifestation. These are the same states of inner light that we need to travel the distances between ideas of lack and ideas of abundance, to realize what arriving on a new shore will bring.

What happens inside us individually and collectively to provoke travel to new, unchartered shores? Does change arise from circumstances outside ourselves, or does it come from realizing our own internal need to grow, change, or leave something behind? If we are going to a new place, what do we take with us?

New shore landings can include new ways of seeing and understanding and new appreciation for our experiences. What will you leave behind? What attitudes or ways of thinking are best suited for a new place? Does your change involve a physical move? Can people in your life come along with you? How will you inform them of your new direction? Can you chart a course? What are your expectations upon arrival? Multiply your abundance by being open to change, new challenges, and new opportunities while you make plans for new landings. Please, write down your thoughts in your journal.

April 2: No Limitations

SACRED DANCE

Repeat yesterday's dance, and after holding for a beat on the right, continue to do the moves on the left. That is, make a semicircle with your left foot that crosses the plane of your body, use your arms to cross in front of you at the wrists, and then spread your hands in front of you and open them outward to your sides. Step on the left foot, and bring your right foot to slightly behind you. Your gaze is slightly downward. The dance is slow moving and deliberate.

MEDITATION AND PRACTICE

The enormity of faith of the ancient Austronesian peoples had to do with their reliance upon their Divine Spirit to make the journey.

Crossing vast seas, calling on their gods, and using the stars and other guideposts, they went to new lands. Nothing held them back from getting to a better way of life as they cultivated and embodied a mindset that had no limits.

There is always a new course to chart and new areas of our mind to explore that lead to a better place. If nothing else, we can look for ways to come closer to our Higher Power or find new ways to give to others and thereby multiply our abundance. What habits of mind set us in limited roles and circumstances? If we are faced with change, either positive or negative, how do we react? It's said that our reaction to both should be the same because in life we have nothing but change. It's in how we view change that produces the internal position and propels or stymies our progress.

April 3: Wisdom

SACRED DANCE

Practice moving in each direction as you do this dance, and in between each direction add a knee-bend hold before you step to the next side. In other words, after you have moved to the right, do a knee bend. Your left foot will remain behind you for a moment, as you move your arms out in front of you and to your sides. Then begin the semicircle with the left foot crossing the plane of your body, and as you arrive on the left do a knee bend as you did on the right. Remember that you're facing slightly to the right, then slightly to the left. At each knee bend, twist your upper body a little further toward the foot you're standing on, and look over the same shoulder.

MEDITATION AND PRACTICE

Many Austronesians believed in animism. That means they thought that everything—tangible or not, sentient or not—had its own spiritual essence. In that light, everything is alive, whether it looks that way or not.

Animism is the oldest spiritual and supernatural perspective in world history. It dates to the Paleolithic Age, when humans communed with the Spirit of Nature. At this point was what we consider the origin of wisdom—the ability to evaluate, discern, and act upon life.

We develop such a faculty to let the Light of Spirit guide the way we live, and allow It to direct our thoughts, words, actions, and motivations. Sometimes it's a nudge, a hunch, or a follow-up on something heard or happened upon that stuck with us. Sometimes it's acting on a situation that has gotten us to our last straw or one that has driven us to look for new answers. Wisdom is that capacity to chart a course that leads to increased abundance even when on the face of it people may think we're misguided.

April 4: Contradictions

SACRED DANCE

Continue with this sacred dance as you did the last few days. Now move it in a circle, clockwise.

MEDITATION AND PRACTICE

It's no mistake that our Austronesian ancestors, as well as other peoples, were animistic before the onset of duality—perceiving by comparing and contrasting, making someone better than another, adding or reducing virtue. With the ancient perspective, everything had value and was valuable. The notion of separateness or distinction between mind and body didn't exist. Can you imagine a world with no feelings or thoughts of separateness and difference? It's a contradiction in many ways for Western societies to think as one people rather than separate humans. The time and energy spend on judgment—who is right and who is wrong—contradicts all that we are as Spirit Beings. Though we have come to rely on duality in the West, it isn't the best or only way of seeing existence or multiplying abundance. In fact, because of the feelings of, or beliefs in, lack, we often experience lack.

On our plane we're led to believe that if we give, what we have diminishes. But this isn't so. Genuine giving increases what we have, because we don't really live in a dualistic world—it only looks like we do. This kind of giving is healthy, not done out of obligation, pity, manipulation, or someone's conniving. Pure giving is done freely and with unconditional love. What are some healthy ways that you can give time, talent, or treasure? Are you giving in ways that aren't healthy, to people and organizations that are not serving you, the earth, or humanity well? Make or revise a giving plan outlining some ways you can give regularly. Watch your abundance multiply by keeping track in your journal of what you give, why, when, and what happens to your life.

April 5: Warfare Spoils

SACRED DANCE

Today you add on to what you've done this week. First, repeat the dance and add your personal style. When you're comfortable, bend your knees and pivot slightly so all your weight is on both feet, then lift your right foot and place the right heel or arch to your left knee. Then place it on the floor behind you. Pivot toward the right foot so that you're now facing in the opposite direction, with your weight equally distributed on both feet, with bent knees. Cross your wrists in front of you and then open your arms outwards, palms facing up, so that you reach a little over your head. Repeat these moves on the left side as well, then alternate four to six times.

MEDITATION AND PRACTICE

Through sacred dance, Ancient Indonesians expressed joy, well-being, prosperity, and, most important, gratitude to the Universe for abundance. Getting to a new location, like many migrations, often entails taking stances against resistance. Assuredly some people remained behind out of fear of the unknown, lack of courage, or inertia. Determination, faith, and preparation are needed to follow an internal nudge to move on, to meet circumstances that dictate we do so, to find new paths, and to create a better life.

In many of our travels to new locations, geographic or otherwise, we must fight for what we want or at least be uncompromising. The benefits of arriving at the new place, the new mindset, the new way of being are some of the spoils of that warfare. We get over the grief, the pain, the sadness; we learn how to let go. We use our ego appropriately to serve the good of all. We live in the present moment. Our past is behind us, and the future isn't here yet, so we savor today. We get new, better offers of material wealth to share with others. Our Divine Being becomes our central focus again, or for the first time, and pulls us forward. People may try to influence our decisions or beliefs to keep us in situations that no longer serve our Highest Good. But to manifest abundance often entails contradictions and moving forward in faith, with wisdom at our sails. They get us where we need to be. Untold rewards for making the trek multiply abundance.

What spoils of warfare have you received? In what ways did you step out on faith or fight for what you knew and needed? What do you need to fight for now?

April 6: Spiritual Markers

SACRED DANCE

Review the dance so far as you've learned it this week. Where you left off yesterday, you will swirl your left palm under, down, and around to arrive in front of you and step forward with the left foot. Then, swirl your right palm under, down, and around to arrive in front of you and step forward with the right foot. Pause between steps, and repeat these in a pattern, four to six times. Then return to the movement of making a semicircle with your foot that crosses over your body, as done throughout this week.

MEDITATION AND PRACTICE

Wanting to turn around in the middle of a new journey, as some of our West Sumatra ancestors undoubtedly did, can indicate that we're entering an unsupportive territory. Looking for positive, affirming signposts and Spirit markers gives a better course.

What are some signs that you may be engaging in a dangerous way of thinking or seeing the world? In some cases, we must distinguish between healthy imagining, wishful thinking, and dangerous acting. Wishful thinking is wanting a change that's impossible or something for which we don't want to put in the effort. When we enter dangerous territory, we may start doing destructive things, like not putting spiritual Practices first or breaking promises to ourselves. Do we stay in the past and ruminate on what we should have done or look too far ahead into the future, defeating our intentions? Do we lose sight of our motivations and destinations, either geographic or spiritual? Do we consider where we are on our spiritual map?

One way to check is to establish spiritual markers, or guideposts to see where you are and what is happening in the present moment. Ask yourself if your actions are in line with your intentions. Ask if you remember why you're doing what you're doing, going where you're going. Next, consider revisiting your spiritual plan, and dance again in the direction you have chosen. Give yourself some tangible actions to take when your doubt and fear arise, such as telling yourself you're okay and reminding yourself that being human has different mental states and that you can bathe in Light. Read something inspirational, listen to music, or do some activity that will get you out of yourself. What spiritual markers will let you know you're on the right path?

April 7: Perseverance

SACRED DANCE

Practice the Tari Piriang sacred dance in all its beauty.

MEDITATION AND PRACTICE

Along with animism, our Austronesian ancestors embraced dynamism and the monad. Dynamism concerns itself with matter, substance, and forces; it tells us that the first thing that came into existence is the monad, or Divine One, which gave rise to the notion of dyad (or two), which then set in place the numbers, which then led to geometry, the idea of finite and infinite lines, points, and so forth. Matter is in fact force, not divisible separate units of measure.

We can consider these beliefs a human universal, from which our sacred knowledge originates, stemming from before our Ancestors danced on this earth, and we have inherited it.

The monad was often represented as a circled dot, the Absolute, the Supreme Being, divinity, or the totality of all beings and things. Circled dots were drawn on caves and chiseled in stones. For the ancient Austronesians, the monad depicted the relationship between the Spirit and mundane worlds, showing the connections between dreams and rituals. In other words, life was intertwined with the Spirit, guided by the unseen, and no separation was between them. For indigenous Indonesians, dance let the people freely move between these two worlds.

How many spiritual Practices or other activities have you tried so that you can experience the Absolute? Make some notes in your journal. What kinds of support do you need to continue your sacred dance with oneness? What are you contributing to others by your way of being, to help them foster the awareness of oneness?

APRIL 8–14
Mana (Entry Point)

The power is within me.

All that is powerful lives right here and aligns with the energy fields.

For the next seven days, we will embody sacred Tahitian dances, the tamure for female energy and the paoti for male energy. For both energies, you may wish to wear a sarong, a large sash-like wrap that covers the hips, wristbands, headbands, or other adornments. Placing shells and other percussive instruments on your ankles and wrists would be great if you have these available. If you can arrange for a drumbeat, it would help set the trance state.

April 8: I Have It Inside

SACRED DANCE

For the tamure, stand with your feet together so they touch, and place fingertips on your hips. Your fingers should be close together, with the thumb in touch with all the fingers. Hold your elbows away from your body but relax your shoulders. Bend your knees as if you were going to sit in a chair. Keep your back straight and head held high. Then straighten one knee while keeping the other knee bent. Then repeat on the other side. Alternate straightening each knee while you lift your heel. Note that one knee is bent at all times, and the straightening of the alternate knee causes the hip sway.

MEDITATION AND PRACTICE

For the Austronesians, mana was an unexplainable supernatural power. Because Austronesians were animists and dynamists, aware of the monad, they understood mana to be attributable to peoples, governments, places, and inanimate objects. Any being or entity that embodied mana deserved reverence.

Mana was the possession of power but wasn't the source of it. Possession of mana was inextricably related to belief in the Divine. It was stronger in animated than in unanimated objects and was stronger in highly evolved beings than in simpler ones. People had more mana than animals, but its intensity was considered harmful for ordinary people. Because one's Shadow was an extension of oneself (see the sacred dances for January) and contained mana, people made sure that a shaman's Shadow didn't cast on ordinary citizens. Mana, like any other spiritual power, could be used for ill intentions. So whereas mana was vital for the interactive and interconnected Cosmos, in great concentrations or in the wrong hands it was dangerous.

There is so much expansive, giving, creative power available to you if you realize it and put it to right use. Power used rightly gives rise to personal and communal recovery from grief, alcoholism and addiction, depression, and sadness. It can snap people out of their sleepy dependencies on consumption, blame, and victimhood. It brings Light and love to all situations. It removes delusions, denial, and darkness. Power applied in the animistic and dynamic way transcends matter and is unstoppable. It gives you joy, abundance, healing, and love and allows you to live in reality, in the present moment. What are several ways you can expand your use of mana and provide new heart-expanding opportunities for those in your world? For yourself?

April 9: Sharing and Multiplying

SACRED DANCE

The paoti sacred dance for male energy begins with your feet together so that they are shoulder-width apart and your hands on your hips. Here, your fingers should be close together, resting on the front of the hip joint with the thumb resting at the back of the hip joint. Hold your elbows away from your body but relax your shoulders. Bend your knees as if you were going to sit in a chair, and place the weight on the balls of your feet. Keep your back straight and head held high as in the Sacred Dance Posture. Move your knees toward each other, then away in a rhythmic motion.

MEDITATION AND PRACTICE

Ancient Tahitians gave from their hearts to each other and to visitors, and they gave blessings through sacred dance. They revered the blessings from the goddesses and gods they worshipped. Most important, they realized that sharing inclusively created abundance and multiplied positive outcomes. Their relationships with the gods and goddesses and proper use of power, intention, and behavior ensured that. It's said that when this was not the case the gods and goddesses would need to be appeased with sacred dance so that it would go well for their people.

Giving is Source, Energy, and receiving; it is the antidote to any lack. Give appropriately, and give often. What can be given? Encouragement, understanding, a smile, a meal, a hug, or a sacred kiss blown across the room. A soft touch, an agreement, a nod. A visit, a phone call. An email. A card, a handwritten note sent by regular post. Participation at a service, rite of passage, or a child's endeavor. While referring to your giving plan, think of the ways you can give. Make some notes to augment your plan, and list things you can give every day. Consider those with whom you may be experiencing resistance. If you have no one in that category, give something anyway.

April 10: Fertility

SACRED DANCE

With each of the two sacred dances, practice getting rhythm for the lower-body movements. Then begin to rotate in place in a circle, in one direction and then turn the other. Keep your hands in place, knees bent, head held steady, back straight.

MEDITATION AND PRACTICE

Sacred dance in Ancient Tahiti put fertility in a revered position, and fertility was also used as a storytelling practice that documented ancestry. Each bloodline traced back to a specific *marae*, the ancient stone platforms imbued with immeasurable mana. These were places where people would offer sacrifices and pray, communicate with and worship their gods, and petition them for blessings in harvests or battles. At a marae, atua, or god, was summoned to earth by priests, called *tahu'a*, to supply people with mana, the Divine aspect responsible for fertility. Black pearls were sacred symbols in Tahiti, which Oro, the god of peace, war, and fertility, offered to Princess Bora Bora to express his undying and deep love for her.

Fertility shapes new ideas, new understandings, and new growth. April is an important month for fertility, with spring giving rise to new and renewed directions. Once planted in fertile ground, there is no limit to expanding spiritual relationships with ourselves and others, seen and unseen. However, anything planted must be shielded and nurtured until the nascent period concludes. Then, during a period of gestation, the idea develops, which involves contemplation and Sacred Dance Meditation. Only then can the idea find tangible expression. What will you plant today? Get excited about? What will you nurture? What will you detach from? How will you include your Higher Power in this?

April 11: Marking and Tattooing

SACRED DANCE

This sacred dance uses similar arm movements for both female and male energies. Standing in the Sacred Dance Posture, those identifying with the male energy first place the palms on the top of your head. After that, raise both arms to the sky, and then lower the right arm parallel to the earth and the palm facing down. Hold the left arm over your head so that it's straight toward the sky with the palm facing forward. Turn your head, and gaze toward the right arm. Now move to the right three steps while engaging the knees. Then, bring your right arm up over your head and place the left arm parallel to the earth, away from you. Now turn your head and gaze to the left, then move to the left three steps while engaging the knees.

MEDITATION AND PRACTICE

In Tahitian culture, people were believed to be children of heaven (Rangi) and earth (Papa), who were once united with each other somehow in a different time and place. The supreme goal of life on earth is to re-create and connect with that previous unification through one's lineage. The body is seen as a link between heaven and earth.

For Tahitians, the upper part of the body represents the spiritual realms, while the lower half of one's body is connected more closely to the sacred aspects of the physical earth. According to the ancient belief system, tattoos placed on these parts of the body are therefore symbolic representations of that sacredness.

Tattooing also indicated one's genealogy, history, and place in society. They were physical displays of a person's mana. For men, they were signs of wealth, strength, and ability to endure pain. For women, tattoos indicated maturity. As such, chiefs and warriors generally had the most elaborate tattoos, begun at adolescence and continuing for several years. All symbols in Tahitian tattoos were based on water, earth, wind, and fire. The tattoo was a communication device, with each telling a different story, and a traditional method of garnering spiritual power, protection, and strength. A sacred ceremony marked each tatau placement on the body, which was done with sharpened bone tools and ink made from the candlenut. Any sign of weakness while receiving the tatau meant one was unworthy. Sacred dancers were adorned with tattoos, which gave power to dance.

The body is a vessel for the Holy Spirit, and marking the body can demonstrate commitment to a sacred path. Monks, priests, and lay people all over the globe from time immemorial have worn distinctive clothing; tattooing and scarification is another method for showing one's place. Applying markings, tattoos, or other adornments helps you to remember that your dancing body contains the Spirit. What will you wear, or how will you signal that your body is a temple, a sacred vessel of the Divine?

April 12: Flowers Expressing Abundance

SACRED DANCE

Dances for those identifying with female energy use the same arm movements as for male. But instead of touching your head, bring your hands above your head, arms outstretched, palms facing the sky. After that, lower the right arm, holding the left arm over your head so that it's straight toward the sky, and hold the right arm away from you so that it's parallel to the earth. Turn your head toward the right arm. Now move to the right three steps while engaging the knees. Then, bring your right arm up over your head, and place the left arm parallel to the earth, away from you. Now turn your head and gaze to the left, then move to the left three steps while engaging the knees.

MEDITATION AND PRACTICE

Men and women both valued flowers in Tahiti; they were especially used to revere the *vahine*, the Tahitian woman. They were often worn around the head, neck, or wrists, or were woven through fabric.

Flower symbols also appeared in traditional tattoos. At gatherings, celebrations, rituals, and in everyday life, Tahitians made use of flowers to show their appreciation for life's transitions, joys, and sorrows.

The delicate white petals of the seven-petaled *tiare*, the sacred flower of Tahiti, stood for love. The scent was said to be hypnotic, spreading sweet and exotic aromas. Frangipani trees, also called tipaniers or plumerias, have been associated with life and fertility. Mure, myrtle, and indigenous *tamaru* orchids have also been used in Tahitian ritual.

In nature, patterns and structures govern particle formations and designs. This shows us how created things are interconnected and formed with an overall schema, and it really exposes our relationship to everything.

Perhaps we know this intuitively when we see flowers. They are beautiful forms of nature, giving healing and soothing to mind, body, and Soul. Their scents, form, colors, and energies touch our desires and needs without our knowing it. Flower gazing can lift our mood and bring our focus to beauty and wonder of nature's creative power. From that point flowers can help us shift our thoughts to awe and change emotional states from sadness to feeling loved and included and then to feeling joyful.

This is *floral power*. We can be drawn intuitively to a specific flower or flowers, guiding us to calmness and harmony. What flowers are you drawn to?

April 13: Choosing Responses

SACRED DANCE

Today we combine our energies to express the sacred dances of Tahiti. Female energies, after moving to the right and left, place both arms parallel to the earth, with your palms facing outward. Rotate in a circle to the left and to the right. Conclude the dance by bringing your palms together in front of you and holding the Sacred Dance Posture. Male energies, after moving to the right and to the left, stop, stand with knees slightly bent and feet about shoulder-width apart. Put your weight evenly on both feet, knees slightly bent. Bring your arms in front of you, holding them parallel to the earth, with palms facing downward. Rotate the right palm upward, and place it on the back of your head. Then rotate the left palm upward and place it on your head. Now, rotate the hips in a slow clockwise circle as you remove your right hand from your head and slowly point from left to right, then remove your left hand from your head and slowly point from right to left, each time looking where your hand points. Return your hands to the hips. Afterward, bring the arms parallel to the earth at the sides of your body, palms facing outward, and return the weight to the balls of your feet, knees slightly bent. Then repeat the knee clapping movements from earlier in the week as you turn in a circle in one direction, then the other. Conclude by bringing your palms to rest at your sides.

MEDITATION AND PRACTICE

The ancient Tahitians knew that the Divine energies of masculine and feminine were intertwined and that an affirmative response was always necessary in order to experience the love of life within the sacred environment in which they lived. When they felt like giving up, something in them kept them from doing so. Perhaps the realization that they were obligated to honor their Spiritual Being and the knowledge of being able to increase their power through mana and manifestation drove them to respond affirmatively. Knowing that they were the creators of their destiny and had the ability to fertilize ideas and places at will, along with wearing determination on their bodies through tatau, gave them the way of responding that allowed Tahitians to bring forth the flowering of Spirit.

April 14: Gender Multiplying Abundance

SACRED DANCE

Today, practice the sacred Tahitian dances that appeal to your energy gender identity. Honor both energies that swirl inside you. Acknowledge that Spirit is genderless.

—————————— MEDITATION AND PRACTICE ——————————

Tahitians and other ancient ancestors knew the interplay between gender energy and abundance. The Divine, they believed, used gender for creativity; both energies were required for the continuance of life and its enjoyment. The balance of gender energy was depicted in Sacred Dance Meditations.

The valorization of one gender over the other is a human intervention, part of the dualistic relationship created that causes separateness. We see the need for both energies in nearly every species. Healing principles stress the balance needed in our lives. Too much of one type of gender energy may block much-needed assistance, guidance, inspiration, love and acceptance, healing, or growth. We may see men a particular way and women another, which leads us to infer that men have particular habits, women others. Although past experiences may support these beliefs, they may not be completely true. Wear your gender energy as appropriate. Energies are fluid, so embodying one gender energy may be good for one situation but not another. What are your ideas and notions of male and female energies? When do you draw on them? Does one or the other hinder you from realization?

APRIL 15–21
New Horizons Setting Sail (Entry Point)

Altars of Perception

Bow before the altar each time you pass; acknowledge the forces that move and support you.

For the next seven days, you will focus on the sacred dance of hula. Ancient hula, unlike what is labeled as such in Hawai‘i nowadays, is called *kahiko*. Chants and percussive drumming generally accompany sacred hula, though you could perform the dance in silence.

April 15: Bowing, a Necessary Reverence

SACRED DANCE

Today we will focus on male energy in kahiko. Stand in the Sacred Dance Posture with your feet shoulder-width apart, knees slightly bent. Touch the heel of your right foot to the back of your left knee, return it to the standing position with a slight stomp, and do a deep squat. Repeat with the left heel to the back of the right knee. Now, hold your elbows out from your body, parallel to the floor with your fingertips touching, palms facing downward. Hands should be at the center of your chest. Practice these motions a few times, then add a turn between each squat before the next knee tap. That is, if you tap the right heel to the back of the left knee, stomp the right foot down, squat, then turn counterclockwise. After you tap the left heel to the back of the right knee, then stomp the left foot down, squat, and turn clockwise.

MEDITATION AND PRACTICE

Ancient Hawai'ian shrines and altars honored Spirit and ancestors; sacrifices occurred there, and more mana was manifested. Sacrifices sometimes conjure up discomfort for us. But they shouldn't. If the ancestors sacrificed an animal or part of a harvest, that was essentially the same as us giving to a worthy cause or tithing.

So often, we have no time for remembering. We increasingly need to reconnect to Spirit to return to our intentions. We need to recognize and remember miracles, or unseen assistance, and be in the present moment, mindful of our many blessings. Putting together an altar or shrine helps. The altar could be so simple that no would recognize it, or it can be ornate.

You can create altars in your home, at your workplace, and in your vehicle. You could simply set up a table in the corner of a room, where you place small crystals, a picture of a person or deity you respect, and a small vase of fresh or silk flowers. You might also include statues, jewels, beads, and incense. The sacredness of the area depends on the way you imbue it. You can also carry an altar in your pocket or purse—an altar could be a sacred stone or a wristband with reminders of your sacred symbols. And if you have an "internal altar," you could connect with Spirit through the day. Simply visualize your physical altars and your intentions, and realize you're never alone or disconnected.

April 16: Sacrifice

SACRED DANCE

Review the dance given yesterday. Now, you'll add some arm movements. After you touch your right foot to your left knee, stomp, and squat, your left arm is going to extend at shoulder length with fingers outstretched and palm still facing down. The right elbow remains parallel to the floor, with your palm facing downward and fingers touching. Look over your left middle finger. The position energy is that of a warrior, with a strong stance and firm arm movement. Keep your arms in this position as you turn counterclockwise. Repeat on the other side, making sure your gaze follows the right arm and turning clockwise.

MEDITATION AND PRACTICE

The ancient ancestors acknowledged that their abundance came from reliance on the Divine and the belief that life is sacred. They often performed sacrifices on their altars and set up monuments to remember. When they saw altars in their temple or in their homes, they were reminded of the Good of the Universe.

Some believe that we should feel jubilant all the time if we are connected to Spirit. This is not the case. Low spots, disappointments, sadness, and delusions still happen. Moreover, sacrifices are often needed to move forward. They can be involved or shallow, such as declining to engage in old behaviors, memories, or thought patterns. We could determine to deeply listen to someone without being distracted by media. If we intend to start a new business or career or to back away from working, we need to sacrifice spending or be mindful of our return on investment. In working through meditation, we may have to sacrifice watching television or online programming. What do you need to sacrifice to live your intentions? Whom will that affect? What would be the impact on them and you?

April 17: Great Crossings

SACRED DANCE

After you have completed several turns with the arms outstretched, to the left and to the right, stand with feet shoulder-width apart, knees slightly bent. Bring your hands together at your chest, palms facing outward, and raise them up over your head. Your gaze follows your palms. Bring them down briskly and clap both thighs loudly with your hands. Bring the palms back to your chest and focus your gaze outward, and then, making fists, circle them over one another as if you were rolling twine around a stick. Repeat the arm movement over your head, clap your thighs, and circle your fists one over the other.

MEDITATION AND PRACTICE

The ancestors who sailed to the Hawai'ian Islands really made the trip on faith. The belief that they would arrive whole and cared for propelled them forward. Likely, they had moments of doubt. Yet, they persevered and arrived. Great crossings required great sacrifices, and upon arrival shrines were erected to honor the gods and goddesses that facilitated the transition from one home to another.

Sometimes the distance between here and there seems too far. The journey is too difficult and the reward seemingly doesn't justify the effort. Changing our behaviors and interactions with others, accepting our unanswered questions, and facing our circumstances head-on can often be demoralizing. Without pretending everything will be better "over there," focusing on one small change each day can help us complete a metaphorical journey. Time is limited on earth; one day we will make the ultimate great crossing when we dance in Spirit with the Divine. Make some notes in your journal to help you focus on one thing you can do each day. Allow your Divine Self to chart the course, recognizing you aren't in control of outcomes but understanding that you have identified a direction.

April 18: Receiving Immigrants

SACRED DANCE

Today we introduce hula kahiko for the female energy. Stand in your Sacred Dance Posture, with feet shoulder-length apart and knees slightly bent. Start with tapping your feet in front of you, alternating left and right. Meanwhile, hold your arms close together and extended to the front of your body, at hip level. Point your palms toward the ground, and slowly scoop them upward and to the right and then over your head to reach for the sky, arms outstretched, palms flattened and facing outward. Gaze toward the sky over your fingertips. Keep your feet moving!

MEDITATION AND PRACTICE

There is no telling whether the ancient Polynesians thought they were going to find acceptance or rejection when they arrived on the shores of their destinations. The sacred dances tell of the voyages, the welcome they received, along with the challenges and obstacles they faced. As soon as they arrived, they built *hale*, or homes, and *heiau*, or temples. So they set up shrines and altars, in gratitude for the completed journey.

It's nice to have a welcome when we arrive at our destination, although we don't always. When people enter new cultural systems, even just neighborhoods or workspaces, we need to welcome them, with a genuine offer of time and attention. Immigrants have traveled long and difficult distances in many cases. Some have Hawai'ian certainty. But some arrive poor, scared, traumatized from being incarcerated, and alone. Things can be easier if friends or family can help, but the environment is still new.

Can you can aid an immigrant in reconnecting to the sacred? Can you learn from them new ways of connecting to the Divine?

With one heart and mind, all are from the same Source seeking the same peace and joy.

April 19: Settling In

SACRED DANCE

Review the dance sequence given yesterday, and get into a rhythm. With your arms reaching to the sky, place the right hand on the right chest area, palm facing downward and your arm parallel to the earth, while you move the left arm toward the earth, palm facing downward, stopping when it gets to shoulder level. Your gaze follows your outstretched arm movement. Now, bring your left arm to your left chest area, and move your right arm outstretched upward over your head and then toward your right, palm facing down, at shoulder height, and following your gaze. Keep your feet moving!

MEDITATION AND PRACTICE

Ancient Hawai'ians believed that *hana*, or work, was noble and respected, and laziness was shameful. The phrase "E ho'ohuli ka lima i lalo," which meant the palms should be turned down, communicated the idea that idleness, associated with upturned palms, was detrimental. Work was anything done to contribute to community and family prosperity, with a spiritual framing. This, along with relying on gods and goddess for support and increased mana, led to interdependency and abundance.

Navigating a new place can be fraught with wrong turns, frustrations, and false starts. Once-familiar routines suddenly require deep thought. In a new environment you must discover new places to provide for your needs. Settling in on new mental and spiritual shores is much the same. You are used to thinking or reacting a certain way, yet you know you can't go back to the place you've outgrown. Sometimes, out of fear, you may ignore Spirit calling you to dance forward to new horizons. Make some notes in your journal about your experiences and hesitations.

April 20: Expectations

SACRED DANCE

Review the dance given yesterday. Repeat the arm movements four times in each direction. Then touch your shoulders with your fingertips and raise both arms over your head slightly in front of you, making a sort of arc toward the right. Your gaze follows your hands, palms facing forward. Next, touch your shoulders with your fingertips, then raise both arms over your head again, this time with the arc toward the left, your gaze following your fingertips. Remember to keep your feet moving!

MEDITATION AND PRACTICE

Ancient Polynesians exploring the Hawai'ian Islands expected to learn and succeed when they relocated from their former home to the new shores. Failure was not considered. They traveled by outrigger or double-hulled canoes lashed side by side; in the space between the canoes, they stored food, hunting supplies, and nets. On these long journeys, the ancient Polynesians used natural navigation aids such as the stars, ocean currents, and wind patterns to arrive at their destination and, later, to gain awareness of flora and fauna behavior. These techniques required constant observation, memorization, and awareness of the surroundings. They would return to their original place to bring others who were willing to go forward. Locations were taught to other travelers by dance and song.

Expectations are a powerful driver. Some traditions teach that we should have none, so as not to get caught in future thinking at the expense of the present or in situations with unreliable people. We know people in our lives who let us down, yet we love them anyway. We learn to dance away from them. We also plan for many experiences, but other factors interfere with them. We have no control over those circumstances. Even so, we must have high expectations for ourselves—for the good, for Spirit to lead us to excellent health, peace, and joy. Still, like the ancient ancestors, we must navigate our mental and emotional oceans, to reach our new spiritual shores. We must balance action and expectation.

How do you navigate your next spiritual move?

April 21: Rejuvenation

SACRED DANCE

Today we will repeat the male-energy rendition of the hula kahiko dance from April 17. After rolling the fists one over the other, place the palms at chest level, fingertips touching, and elbows out. In rhythm, tap the back of the knee with the heel, on the right and left sides. Come to a standstill, and gaze toward the sky with knees slightly bent. In the feminine-energy version, bring the fingertips together at chest level, palms facing downward, elbows outward.

MEDITATION AND PRACTICE

A long voyage into the unknown requires energy. Then, after recovering from the demands such a journey placed on the body, mind, and Spirit, some celebration would be required. Ancient Polynesians rejuvenated themselves with sacred dance, songs, chants, and reverence to the gods and goddesses. They took time to celebrate in community and build new relationships with their environment and the people in them.

With much of the Western world's attention diverted to current events, sound bites, and a hurried pace of capitalism, many of us are exhausted, yet we don't realize it. To make a spiritual journey, we must rejuvenate ourselves. Retreats, workshops, and just being alone can aid us in reaching the promised land. Once we arrive at the destination, we will need to spend time away to celebrate and express gratitude. Rejuvenation also requires sacrifice—again, a contribution of our time, talent, and treasure to honor our Divine.

✳ ✳ ✳

Protecting Sacred Treasures (Entry Point)

Were you daydreaming?

Sleeping or awake, I am always meandering into sacred knowledge.

This week we embody the sacred through two Aboriginal Dances of Australia. There, dancers clap sticks, rattles, flat rocks, and wood for instrumental percussive sounds. Some people put shells on their ankles or tie leaves around their necks. Women more often than men use a drum in ceremonies, and the drums are made from emu, snake skins, or kangaroo hides. The drum beat accompanies singing when a didgeridoo, used mainly by men, isn't played.

The dance this week is high impact, though you can adjust the pace, according to comfort, for a low-impact form.

April 22: Happening Upon the Sacred

SACRED DANCE

Start out striking a medium- to fast-paced rhythm with your instruments if you chose to use them. Then bend slightly forward and step first right then left. Repeat that a few times before dragging your right foot on the floor and quickly lifting it as if you're going to touch the heel to the back of the right thigh. Place the foot down, and tap it. Then, repeat this movement on the left. Do this several times, getting a rhythm to match your music.

MEDITATION AND PRACTICE

The Dreaming or the Dreamtime referred to a time of primordial creation in Aboriginal understanding when supernatural deities, ancestors, or heroes created the world. These supernatural beings gave the earth form, substance, and context. During the Dreamtime, supernatural beings were said to have instilled consciousness and physical awareness in humans. Through Aboriginal sacred dance and rituals, Australian Aboriginals entered the Dreamtime for one reason: to experience primordial creativity.

Aboriginals mastered the protection of sacred treasures. The mechanisms for imparting sacred treasurers were only shared with the initiated—those who were emotionally, spiritually, and mentally ready to receive it. While all are beings of Light, some have yet to come close to the realization of their Divine capacity.

Which of your sacred treasures—Practices and places—benefit from being protected from overexposure? Just as we don't expect children to act in adult ways, we often must help companions by meeting them where they are.

April 23: The Value of Sacred Secrecy

SACRED DANCE

Review yesterday's choreography and get into a medium to fast-paced rhythm. As you're ready, hop on to the right foot with the left leg out in front of you, knee bent and the foot slightly crossing over the middle of your body. Hop three times on the right foot, then place the left foot down, and hop on the left foot, with the right leg bent and the right foot slightly crossing over the middle of your body. For low impact, bounce up and down, on tiptoes if you're able, rather than hopping from one foot to another.

MEDITATION AND PRACTICE

Manifesting the power needed to transcend to the Dreamtime was paramount, and sacred dance was the method. In the Dreamtime, one's aspirations and knowledge of creation was apparent. Returning from that sacred place, sacred dancers kept their visions held deep within.

We've all experienced the thrill of an idea or a direction. We're motivated. We know we can make our bed every day, start a new meditation Practice, or even decide to change our professional lives. Then we share it with someone, and he or she responds with the well-intended "that's great, but ..." followed by words of caution. And our excitement or motivation might falter.

Of course, not all ideas manifest our abundance, and talking things over with a trusted spiritual advisor or friend might be a good idea. But many ideas don't even see the light of day. So consider what you share and with whom. What ideas do you have that you should hold in secret to help them multiply your abundance? Make some notes.

April 24: Guarding Spiritual Sites

SACRED DANCE

Repeat the moves from yesterday a few times on the right and left, in the low-impact version if you desire. Then walk around in a circle, first to the right, then to the left, in rhythm to the music.

MEDITATION AND PRACTICE

To the indigenous people of Australia, land had spiritual value. Indigenous spiritual sites included trees, rocky outcrops, waterholes or clearings, and specific places that the ancestral spirits were associated with. Ancestral spirits sometimes left their human energy at these sites or would take the form of plants or animals. To enter a sacred spiritual site, or have knowledge of it, one had to be initiated. Because ancestral beings continued to live at the sites, Indigenous Australians believed their duty was to cherish the land and take only what was needed.

Male ceremonial sites used for initiation were often off limits for women. Men weren't allowed to enter female sites, such as those used for childbirth. Women had extensive spiritual and religious power and were the keepers of special knowledge transmitted through sacred dance.

We can make places where we dwell, work, and walk sacred, guarded spiritual sites, where we have epiphanies, conduct Practices, and express gratitude. Our spiritual sites need to be guarded, as do our sacred directions and commitments. We think carefully about how we can "initiate" our friends and loved ones before showing them our spiritual sites. We can bring them to the outermost circle, to the middle circle, or to our innermost circle if we feel comfortable. We can gauge their respect for our spiritual sites by noticing if they make small compliances, such as removing shoes, abstaining from substance consumptions, or speaking in loving tones.

What are some spiritual sites in your life? Who can be invited into them? Do you need to establish them? Which rituals and ceremonies can you use to remind you that you're entering upon sacred spiritual sites? Make some notes in your journal.

April 25: Stolen Identities

SACRED DANCE

Before today's dance, realize the land before you, without any pollution, and its relation to the Universe. Review and practice yesterday's moves. After you have hopped three times on the right, step on the left foot, scoop down to the ground with your right hand as if you're gathering spiritual sustenance, and bring it up to your chest. When you reach down to scoop, you'll turn your body in that general direction; when you finish the scoop, begin the hop on the left and repeat four times. Then step on the right foot as you scoop with your left side.

MEDITATION AND PRACTICE

Indigenous Australians knew that one couldn't limit the Divine. They acknowledged many sacred dance paths leading to Spirit. And this was part of the Dreaming.

Selfishness can only proliferate when we believe in separation. We are not separate; we have shown that over and over. Yet over time, empires and principalities have exploited or eradicated peoples and destroyed sacred places. No society in human history hasn't experienced this. But no one can take You from you. How do you cultivate your identity? How do you keep your whole authentic self from being plundered, stolen, or otherwise subsumed in something you disagree with? Are you loving in your delivery, or do you use anger to get your points across? How do you help keep the connectedness threaded through your identity when interacting with uninitiated others? Make some notes in your journal.

April 26: Commitment to Spiritual Practice

SACRED DANCE

Let's practice what you did yesterday until you're comfortable with the moves and you have a personal rhythm. Find a way to look up toward the sky as you scoop spiritual sustenance.

MEDITATION AND PRACTICE

Aboriginal ancestors used ceremonies to act out the Dreaming. Along with their other duties, men typically protected spiritual sites when carrying out ceremonial rituals. They would ritually care for the physical site in a way that would allow spirits to thrive there.

When first encountered by colonizers, sacred sites and rituals were misunderstood. The newcomers used their own perspective to interpret the behaviors of the Australian Aboriginals, and they judged Aboriginals as unacceptable. Even so, the ancient Aboriginals committed to their spiritual Practices, which are still performed today. We see such perseverance in many spiritual Practices considered unacceptable or misunderstood by colonizers. When we encounter an unknown, commitment and perseverance must be tempered with compassion and understanding. That is, live and let live. There are nearly as many spiritual Practices as there are human beings and cultures. All of them ultimately serve the same purpose.

April 27: Men's Business

SACRED DANCE

Review the dance from April 22, clapping, jumping so your heel almost touches the back of your thigh, and tapping your feet as you alternate sides. Do this several times, getting a rhythm to match your music. Now, hold your arms out in front of you as you then hop onto the right foot while you hold the left leg out in front of you, with the knee bent and the foot slightly crossing over the middle of your body. Hop three times on the right foot, then place the left foot down, quickly touch the floor with your right palm, and hop on the left foot, with the right leg bent at the knee and the right foot slightly crossing over the middle of your body. For low impact, bounce up and down, on tiptoes if you're able, rather than hopping from one foot to another.

──────── MEDITATION AND PRACTICE ────────

In Australian Aboriginal sacred dance, some ceremonies were for men only—called men's business—and others were for women only—called women's business. Both men and women had their own spiritual and sacred objects.

If we are to define ourselves, let's do so as we want to be spiritually. Let's talk about the ways we contribute to personal and communal spiritual growth and acknowledge our gratitude to ancestors, and the Divine. Sometimes particular work is needed to complete, influence, or transcend an outcome. Interdependence is required, and each of us has business to conduct.

April 28: Women's Business

──────── SACRED DANCE ────────

Review and repeat what you did yesterday. Now between the right and left hops, you will quickly bend forward and slap the floor with the palm opposite the leg you're hopping on. You can do a quick punching gesture if you can't reach the floor. When you have done this a few times, walk around in a circle, keeping your instrumental rhythm going.

──────── MEDITATION AND PRACTICE ────────

As guardians of special knowledge, Aboriginal Australian women used sacred dance to facilitate entering the Dreamtime and to bring back messages of change and encouragement into the created world.

Everyone can contribute to well-being and abundance. People can turn toward the Light at any time. What is particularly required, though, is the special knowledge that one way of interpreting the world isn't the only way.

Abundance requires that in times of both expansion and contraction we know, deep down, all is well. Nothing is permanent, except the energies that govern the Universe, and even that is vibrating with change all the time.

April 29: Balancing Energies

SACRED DANCE

Practice and embellish what you have done this week.

MEDITATION AND PRACTICE

Aboriginal Australians did not valorize men or women. They were considered equals who lived together doing their work to share the elements of the Dreaming.

Many cultural rules and regulations govern the way men and women behave or what they are supposed to do. They are ingrained in our societies. But do we have to accept them? We see a great movement shifting the expectation of men's and women's roles, yet this doesn't necessarily get Spirit moving.

Do you perform men's or women's business? Do you protect sacred sites, carry special spiritual knowledge, or both? Did you decide? Do you want to make a different decision? Being deliberate in spiritual commitment is required of you, as is knowing when to shift your business focus. Multiplying abundance involves doing the mundane as well as aligning your vision and using your energy for the good of you and the community, the earth, our ancestors and generations ahead.

April 30: Spirit Prevails

SACRED DANCE

You can embody this week's sacred dance to trance it out. Find your Sacred Dance Attire and your Inner Mystic Dancer that connect to the peoples of ancient Australia, who are connected to those of the present day. Imagine the Dreamtime and what you want to manifest in your Soul. Use your music, instruments, and awareness of the energy you hold and the business you're called to do.

MEDITATION AND PRACTICE

The ancient Aboriginals ensured that Spirit prevailed, through placing sacred sites secretly and connecting them to sacred inner places of the people and ancestors. They protected the Dreamtime so only the initiated could enter it, and they honored the lands. Dreamtime could never be eliminated or found by those who sought to harm it.

No one has the right to take one's Spirit, to dictate the way one's spiritual Practice evolves, unless the human permits it. Respect for other Practices, beliefs, and ways of worship are required for our great abundance. In addition, remaining free from judgment, duality, and sense of superiority multiplies compassion, connection, understanding, and wisdom. We are more the same than we are different.

Will you dance for truth? Will you take up the business you were called to do? Do you know that the business you do is always changing, much as the Dreamtime creates as time moves on? Although it changes, there is always business to do. You must be aware of that. What is your business?

Making Laughter Spiritual

IBERIAN SACRED DANCE

The Iberian Peninsula was a place of sophistication and creativity. By the eighth or ninth century BCE, it was known among the Greeks. The inhabitants had their own language, a literature, and a legal system more than six thousand years old. There is also a Phoenician influence, seen in eighth century BCE. Gades, at the tip of the Iberian Peninsula and what we know today as Cadiz, Spain, is traditionally considered to have been founded by Phoenicians in 1104 BCE.

Some believe that the Iberian people are descendants of Noah. Some believe that Gades was really founded by Hercules, who was Zeus's son, as one of his twelve labors to atone for killing his family. Others believe that the Iberians came from Atlantis and the northwest part of Africa and settled in southwest Europe before the Egyptians settled in northeast Africa. Some suggest a close relationship between the people of Iberia and the ancient inhabitants of North Africa. They believe a "connecting ridge" in the sea united Africa and Atlantis. Whichever story we believe about their origins, one thing is certain: dance was an important part of worship for ancient Iberians.

Ritual Iberian women's dances came out of the worship of Astarte, the Phoenician goddess of fertility. Men and women danced in a chorus and as couples. A chorus was a meeting point between the human and Divine realms, where they danced in sacred circles and lines. For these ancients, dance and music were intimately linked, providing wholeness and well-being, spiritual connection and community. The female goddess arose through female deities, who were associated with dance, including the muses, the nymphs, the maenads, Artemis, Aphrodite, the graces, Dimitra, Persephone, and Cybele. The ancient Iberians considered horses as sacred. They were included in worship, being directly tied to nature, particularly the health of fields. Horse figurines can be found at many sites throughout Iberia.

Iberians worshipped in natural sites and sanctuaries, where people sought blessings of health and protection. These sanctuaries are found in areas believed desirable to the goddesses. Iberians danced in outdoor open places as well as in hidden places like caves. Water was important to the rituals performed at these places too.

The Iberians, or people of ancient Hispania, evolved under the influence of the Tarssians, Phoenicians, Cretans, Greeks, and Romans. Because the history of Iberia draws from a melting pot of cultures, mythology, and lore, our sacred dances are drawn from Basque Country, Asturia, Galicia, Catalonia, and the Iberian Peninsula.

One immediately feels the way the people express sacred Soul laughter and happiness when watching Iberian sacred dances. They are high energy, done in a circles and lines, and include both men and women. The sacred dance attire is colorful and bright, and the entire function of the dance is to uplift the spirits. This month we realize the way laughter and sacred dance bring wholeness and healing to our thirsty Souls.

PREPARATION

Many of this month's dances could be done outdoors. If you have access to the shore, open spaces in parks, or a private outdoor space in your dwelling, you may consider one as your Sacred Dance Studio this week. As was the case in previous months, Sacred Dance Attire varies a bit by the different sacred dances of these peoples, but they are characterized by colorful, blossoming, flowing, airy types of clothing. Additionally, the musical accompaniment ranges from the accordion to the sound of the wind. As you work through the Sacred Dance Meditations this week, consider how sacred sounds support spiritual laughter.

Please visit www.cswalter.org/sacreddancemeditations for video demonstrations. They are not intended to be step-by-step instructions but are meant to give you a view of the sacred dance.

Making Laughter Spiritual (Entry Point)

Laughter is divine.

When you laugh, your whole being is healed.

For the next week our focus turns to Ancient Iberian Basque sacred dance. The music with this dance features an accordion, and the dance is best done in a group and outdoors. This month, we are working with higher-impact movements, so please make sure you're warmed up to prevent injury. You may always take the low-impact approach. Long, colorful, and loose garments may be placed over your Sacred Dance Attire if you're inspired, but they're not required.

May 1: Sacred Laughing

SACRED DANCE

Begin in your Sacred Dance Posture. Raise your hands over your head, so that your arms are slightly bent and elbows are in line with your ears. Once there, snap your fingers of both hands. Keep your arms in this position and continue snapping your fingers throughout the dance. Quickly turn in a clockwise circle, and then counterclockwise, in place.

MEDITATION AND PRACTICE

Basque peoples were one of many ancestors of Iberian descent. Since at least 1500 BCE they enjoyed the sacredness of dancing, merrymaking, celebrating, and laughing. Not everything has to be serious, stern, hard, or otherwise controlled in our Sacred Dance Meditation and Practice. We all can laugh and do it sacredly. Sacred laughter helps us to let go of assumptions, pushing for outcomes, and seeing the humor in the Divine's direction for our lives. Rather than holding tightly to the game of whack-a-mole that seems to be human life, we can realize how funny life is and, with that, how human we are.

Do you have a sense of humor? Do you know that laughing creates a sacred space? Have you laughed with the Divine lately?

May 2: Laugh at Self

SACRED DANCE

Review the instructions given on May 1 to refresh your memory. As you rotate clockwise, incorporate a rhythm into your movements by shifting your weight from right foot to left, in almost a hopping motion. Shift left to right four times. On the fifth shift, kick your right foot forward, and hold it out away from your body just a moment to accent the kick. Repeat on the left. Remember to keep your arms up over your head and snap your fingers!

MEDITATION AND PRACTICE

In Iberia during times of stability, many traders came from faraway lands to buy and sell goods. It was a wonderful luscious time of abundance, and people were content and aware of their Spirit and power. From Phoenicia, to Crete, to Greece, the landscape was ever shifting but thriving and alive. Given the way that the Iberians celebrated sacred dance in their lives and the ways it transmuted over time, it's safe to say that they took life seriously enough but also knew how to laugh at it, to enjoy it, no matter what shifting sands were beneath their feet.

One way to enhance a daily spiritual experience is to laugh at yourself when you're trying to be perfect, controlling, right, and planning outcomes, believing you know what someone will do or say. You may assume today will be like yesterday and tomorrow. Most times this is true on macro scales, but not always, and on the micro scale, variations always exist between the days. Change can come unexpectedly or gradually. Can you slow down enough to notice when you're being too serious, first noticing your thoughts and then your behaviors? Laugh at yourself whenever you're agitated, depressed, anxious, rushing, impatient, scared, procrastinating, anticipating catastrophe, blaming, regretting the past, or thinking in ways that make you crazy. Remember where you stand in the grand scheme of the Universe, and determine what changes you can make, what you can't control, and let go. Maybe carry your journal with you today to note the times you laugh at yourself.

May 3: Laughter Therapy

SACRED DANCE

Repeat what you've learned of this dance meditation. Now, as you kick, turn your body slightly in the direction of your kicking foot. Smile with happiness and contentment, if you're able.

MEDITATION AND PRACTICE

What did the Iberians do to keep such a pleasant perspective on life? They likely told jokes, understood their place in the Universe, and embraced being human. They celebrated on most days they lived. The results may have been unplanned or unintentional, but celebrations and laughter were deliberate parts of their way of being.

Seek out ways to laugh. Watch comedy, go to comedy clubs, or read funny stories or jokes. If you have dogs or cats, they can make you laugh hysterically if you play with them. The key is to get laughter therapy, to keep a healthy point of view. Of course, we shouldn't laugh at others' pain or make fun when it's inappropriate. What's your plan to incorporate laughter therapy into your schedule weekly, monthly, and daily? There are so many ways. Please make notes in your journal about your sacred laughter plan.

May 4: Jokes, Stories, and Truths

SACRED DANCE

Today, raise your arms above the head and snap the fingers. Step left, right, left, then shift back and forth—right, left, right, left—then cross the right foot over the left. Repeat in the opposite direction. Switching direction normally involves a small jump, but you can do this without jumping by bending the knees and keeping the feet close to the floor.

MEDITATION AND PRACTICE

Jokes tell stories of truths, pains, and desires—about us, our cultures, and our histories. Ancient Iberians probably knew that.

Things are often funny when they strike a chord of truth. We laugh with people because we can identify with them. Or satire is funny, when situations are truly insane or unbearable as they are. Someone has had your problem, felt your pain, joy, sorrow, excitement, hope, loss; someone has experienced what you feel because we are human. We need to tell our stories; sometimes we can do so in a way that makes others' loads lighter. Spiritual leaders, mystics, and many others know this too! Laughing helps ease the pain or inspire others.

You can search online for religious jokes and other kinds of humor. See if you can reframe a situation or retell your story with some humor, and make a few notes in your journal.

May 5: Lighten the Load—World Laughter Day

SACRED DANCE

With your arms, up, smiling happily, start standing on your right foot, then shift left to right four times; on the fifth shift, kick your right foot forward, with a bit of a hold away from your body for a moment to accent the kick. Repeat on the left. Remember to keep your arms up over your head, and your fingers snapping! Now, do these moves in a circle, clockwise and counterclockwise, where you're standing. Remember to keep your arms up, and fingers snapping. As you kick, you'll turn your body slightly in the direction of your kicking foot. Next, perform these moves in a large circle around the room, first clockwise and then counterclockwise.

MEDITATION AND PRACTICE

Iberia was a busy trading post rich with spiritual resources, and people from all over visited for rest, relaxation, and ways to lighten their loads. Stories of the Iberians living lives of happiness, conquering foes, and enjoying abundance dominated their mythology. Their culture looked forward to the crossing of the Great Sea of Life with confidence and happiness when one finished life on earth.

You can celebrate World Laughter Day each May, on the first Sunday. But every day can be celebrated with laughter. How do you see your load in life? Some loads are heavy because of the way you interpret them, others because you don't let go of them when the time has come. What can you lighten your load with today? Could you look at a past situation with people or institutions with a different perspective? Recall fond memories of people and situations? Or realize that in the scheme of time spent on earth, it's a waste of your precious energy to do anything other than revere and embrace the present moment? Try looking for the laughter. Make some notes of the happy times you shared with others who may be departed or here but haunting your memories and your Spirit with sadness.

May 6: *Planning Laughter*

SACRED DANCE

Review the Sacred Dance Meditation presented on May 5, and then add on stepping to the left, right, and left. Then do a small double shift with the feet, and cross the right foot over the left, as given on May 4. Then do the moves in the opposite direction. Switching direction involves a small jump, but you could instead bend the knees and keep the feet close to the floor. Now, move in a circle around the room, first counterclockwise, then clockwise.

MEDITATION AND PRACTICE

Glee—that word isn't used much nowadays. But why not? Maybe it's not cool or considered acceptable to be full of glee? Laughing hysterically is a Divine right. The next time you're invited to a celebration, go with glee. Show up everywhere with the result of planned laughter guiding your Spirit. Your attitude will be contagious, and those who don't share your glee will still feel it. Your planned laughter outcomes will encourage them too.

May 7: *Envision a World with Laughter*

SACRED DANCE

On the concluding day of the Sacred Dance Meditation for Basques dance, we engage with it fully, letting go of any concerns of doing it right. We hold our arms up, snap our fingers, and step to the left and right, shift from left and right, and feel glee and giddiness. Carry this into the dance meditation until you feel a deep sense of meditative calm, where your Spirit is free and you free others from their taking life too seriously.

MEDITATION AND PRACTICE

Some people hurt others by laughing at them. Even people who do that were embraced at one time, though. They were also given encouragement to laugh at themselves.

We have all had situations in which we were laughed at or imagined we were. And we have laughed at others, too. It hurts. It sometimes raises feelings of shame and embarrassment. If you have laughed at and hurt others, it may be beneficial to follow the apologetic process with them. If you have been laughed at, laugh at yourself for being so serious, and let it go. Now envision the world you live in with healthy laughter, healing and endearing, that lifts you and others to higher realms of awareness.

※ ※ ※

MAY 8–14
Laughter as Joy (Entry Point)

Laughter puts Spirit first.

Laughter is an expression of joy. Joy has been described as feeling of great pleasure and happiness, a byproduct of our approach to living.

Asturian and Galician Iberian sacred dance gets our attention this week. The sacred dance is upbeat, high energy, and lively, so you will want to warm up a bit as you prepare. You may want to have hand-held castanets or another percussive instrument. The background instruments used for this dance are bagpipes and drums.

May 8: Expressing Joy

SACRED DANCE

Raise your hands over your head so your elbows are in line with your ears and you can see your hands peripherally. Keep your neck and head held high in your Sacred Dance Posture. Set a medium-paced rhythm with your hand-held instruments. Keeping your arms up, kick the right foot in front of you, and then place it back as you kick the left foot. Bring this up to tempo by adding a bit of a hop as you alternate kicks.

MEDITATION AND PRACTICE

Joy was expressed in Galicia with swirling dances to music played on the *gaita galega*, the indigenous Galician bagpipe in boisterous village festivities.

Here are some ideas about joy: One idea, paraphrased from Gautama Buddha, is that when the mind is pure, joy follows like a shadow that never leaves. Joy is "the emotional dimension of the good life, of a life that is both going well and is being lived well," according to Miroslav Volf. According to George Bernard Shaw, joy arises from "being used for a purpose recognized by yourself as a mighty one ... being a force of Nature instead of a feverish selfish little clod of ailments and grievances complaining that the world will not devote itself to making you happy."

One element that leads to joy is engaging with spiritual laughter, the few moments that you can let go of ego-driven self, judgments, resentments, and all thoughts that drive you to separateness. Maybe you could think of a few times you have felt joy and write them down. Recall what you were doing, where you were, and how it arose. If you haven't experienced joy, please refer to your plan for engaging your Practice, and increase your activities associated with it. If you don't have a plan for your Practice, now is the time to develop it. Life is meant to be lived in a state of joy.

May 9: Laughter as Elation

────── SACRED DANCE ──────

Review the sacred dance given on May 8. Today you'll kick, hop, and slightly brush your foot on the floor rather than just placing it on the floor. The move is subtle but gives smoothness to the transition between left and right feet. At the end of the kick, you'll ever so slightly move the foot so that it's lifting behind your standing leg. Keep your arms up with the castanets going. Your gaze is straight ahead of you, head held high and face portraying a sense of peace.

────── MEDITATION AND PRACTICE ──────

Asturians emphasized enjoyment of life, people, the land, and food and drink. Elation was a way of life, perhaps due to the way their ancestors led them to engage with Spirit.

Elation is exhilarating joy, is expansive, and sometimes gives way to light-headedness. We cannot stay in a state of elation, but it would be great to experience it more regularly. Elation can't be anticipated, but it can be caused by several experiences, and rarely from laughter alone. It often is a byproduct of spiritual awakening or accumulation of experiences developed through practice. Have you ever felt elation? Make some notes.

May 10: Laughter Is Present-Moment Stuff

────── SACRED DANCE ──────

Today you will repeat what you've this week so far, doing the kick-hop-drag sequence eight times, four on each side. At the end of the sequence, turn to the left by placing the right foot in front of you, take three steps and swing your right arm in front of you, keeping the left arm held high. Then, turn to the right by placing the left foot in front of you, take three steps and swing your left arm in front of you, keeping the right arm held high.

Ancient Iberian peoples performed their rites in the open and maintained sanctuaries in groves, springs, and caves. Men, women, and children engaged in celebratory sacred dance. On the Iberian Peninsula, home of modern-day Spain and Portugal, the cultures of Africa, Europe, and the Mediterranean all mingled. Humor and laughter infused the culture and complemented their sacred dance.

As with sacred dance, all peoples naturally know how to laugh. When you're doubled over laughing, the present moment has taken over, and this is a wonderful feeling.

May 11: Laughter Is the Depression Antidote

SACRED DANCE

Stand in your Sacred Dance Posture, arms held high, holding your castanets. Today you will shift your weight left and right in a forward and backward hopping motion, tapping your foot in between your weight shifts. Shift to the left and right eight times, and turn your body slightly in the direction of your tapping. Keep your arms up while clicking your castanets. After you've done the sequence, return to center and swing your arms down, up, down, up, while shifting your weight from left to right.

MEDITATION AND PRACTICE

Ancient Iberians were unstoppable in their abilities to conquer territories, and they adopted Practices from the surrounding cultures. Though the Iberians faced many threats and many uncertainties, the record suggests they triumphed for centuries over external and internal foes. It was a result of dwelling in their present, not taking life too seriously, and believing in themselves. In those times of change, men danced much more than women, but both genders engaged in the sacred movements.

Perception informs everything. Can we triumph? Often, we can by just a change of perspective. Like the Indigenous Iberians, our thoughts should be *I'm unstoppable at being who I am in this present moment.* Laughter can help with this even in the face of old histories and memories and projecting into the future. We imagine the proverbial other shoe will drop at any moment or we'll get shortchanged. That could be true. However, engaging in laughter every day can help deflect such nagging thoughts and stop or blunt an unhealthy perspective. This is not to say we should live irreverently or ignore issues that render our lives unmanageable. No, it means that incorporating laughter and humor can help.

May 12: Laughter as Celebration

SACRED DANCE

Review the Sacred Dance Meditation from May 11. After familiarizing yourself with the dance sequence, move in a clockwise circle around the room while performing the choreography. When you return to your original position, move in the counterclockwise direction while performing the choreography. First, create a large circle in your space, then bring it back to a small circle. Repeat the pattern a few times in each direction, and return to center.

MEDITATION AND PRACTICE

It was common for the Ancient Iberians to celebrate transitions. They celebrated when their community had life-based events such as in weddings and births or harvests. But they also celebrated to acknowledge and fulfill their spiritual obligations. Sacred dances, always a part of these, were linked to religious sacred worshipping and ceremonies. The space was filled with laughter and music, feasts, and praise. Love connections were made with the community through and with Spirit as these Practices were enacted.

The thought of laughing in a sacred space may be foreign to your understanding of honoring Spirit. But do you think the Divine wants you to be so reverent that you don't celebrate with laughter? Some religious doctrines promote that life is just a burden to get through to the next passage. It's not! Celebrate your life, challenges, and evolving spirituality. Celebrate with laughter and sacred dance. If considering this causes anxiety, you may want to enter some thoughts in your journal.

May 13: Laughter and Letting Go of Control

SACRED DANCE

Today, combine what you learned on May 8–10. Remember to keep your elbows in line with your ears, keeping the rhythm with the castanets the whole time.

MEDITATION AND PRACTICE

Although Indigenous Iberians had much to celebrate, they weren't exempt from the human condition. Much was beyond their control.

So much is beyond our control. We do our best; we plan, envision, and intend. For the good of all, say, "Or something better" at the end of a prayer request. We can't know the outcomes; we can only request, affirm, and let go. Laughing can remind us that we aren't in control of outcomes, only inputs. And realize this is the situation for many of our companions on this spiritual path.

May 14: Spiritual Laughter as Practice

SACRED DANCE

Review this week's dance in its entirety. Feel the joyfulness of the movements as you tap your feet and move in circles.

MEDITATION AND PRACTICE

Indigenous Iberians, as with all the other peoples who sought union with the Divine, had wayward children, difficult spouses, enterprises to manage, and coworkers who gave them angst. Their communities were inhabited by the poor and wealthy in a stratified social structure. Tribes were challenging their territories all the time. The weather impacted their plans and altered their directions. But they laughed and celebrated anyway.

Look for the Divine in every situation. Try to see the events in your life from multiple perspectives.

※   ※   ※

MAY 15–21
Laughter, a Personal Dance Flow (Entry Point)

A smile carries us across. Smile from the Inner Spirit.

When we smile from within, others notice. The smile coming from personal contentment, deep joy, elation, celebrating all humanity is the one that gets people's attention and changes our world.

Meditative flowing and deliberation with the air characterize the sacred dance this week. Being outdoors would be ideal. Dark-colored Sacred Dance Attire would also help. You may wish to remain silent when doing this week's sacred dance and even to use prerecorded meditation music.

May 15: Enter into Your Personal Laughter

SACRED DANCE

Begin this dance facing east, slowly walking in a circle to your right. While you do so, lift your right arm upward and downward slowly, as if you're moving it through water. Then do the same for the left arm. Alternate them in this pattern as you step gingerly, as if you're stepping on footstones dotted across a flowing stream, while you move around the room in a large clockwise circle. The arm movement should be large but not fast. Your upper body should shift a bit as you alternate the arms. You have a very relaxed expression on your face. Repeat this part of the sacred dance for sixteen breaths.

MEDITATION AND PRACTICE

Our Iberian ancestors had no organized system of religious beliefs or tradition of discourse about ritual. There was no religious authority structure and no peer pressure to adhere to a set of beliefs. But they gathered often to celebrate and engage in sacred dance.

Pagan is a term applied out of ignorance and fear to a group of people. Instead of accepting misapplied or derogatory labeling, our terminology must involve knowledge, understanding, and compassion. As you internally absorb the correct historical spiritual record, you reflect that externally. Laugh as you dance into a different set of spiritual labels.

May 16: Have Fun

SACRED DANCE

Review and repeat the sacred dance piece given on May 15. As you complete the circle of sixteen breaths, raise the left arm up toward the sky, and let your elbow curve so that your palm is facing up over the center of your head. Turn to the opposite direction as you continue to gently move around the room in a circle. The right arm is gently outstretched to your right. You'll step in the counterclockwise circle for eight breaths and then alternate your arms so that the right arm is over your head and the left arm is outstretched as you step for eight breaths. After alternating the arm position, stand for a moment with both feet together. Bring both arms up over your head with the palms facing away from each other, the back of the wrists nearly touching, and the elbows pressing away from the front of the body. Your fingertips are relaxed, and your gaze is toward the floor.

MEDITATION AND PRACTICE

Seeing people as something other is often a result of fear, which transforms into domination and control. But these ancestors were open to encounters with different people, with fun and without shame and judgment. They handled challenges in such a way as to invite equanimity and communications.

In our general day-to-day world, we encounter difference all day long. People label; people judge. It's how we've been conditioned at this point of our evolution. But we can counter it by responding in a fun-loving way and creating opportunities for fun in our daily Practice. And Practice is not limited to any particular time.

How are you going to respond this way when you encounter difference, and how will you notice when you're labeling? Are you going to laugh about it while you adjust your perceptions? Your journal awaits your thoughts.

May 17: Be with People

SACRED DANCE

Today stand with your arms outstretched to the sides of your body, palms facing outward. Lead with your right foot to move in a clockwise direction. After four steps, place the right foot across the left one so that you may slightly turn with the left shoulder leading you around. Then step with the left foot behind the right foot, alternating this so that you move turn in a circle. Your arms gently move up and down along the sides of your body; your palms and wrists loosely glide through the air. After four breaths of alternating the stepping and turning, bring your arms again up to over your head with the palms facing outward, wrists touching. Gently step in a clockwise circle around the room.

MEDITATION AND PRACTICE

Sacred dancing with other humans provided increased feelings of connectedness and community. Descriptions of the ancient Iberians, and other sacred dance cultures, show this.

Sometimes we live as if we can be alone without consequence, that we don't need people to help us. Devices keep us company, or we have loving relationships with our pets and maybe relationships with humans that don't require commitment to them and their well-being. Committing to be with people is scary, especially people who may be different or who ask us for things we don't want to give, like changing our beliefs. Being with people can lead to new awareness or to disappointment, sadness, or other emotions we'd just as soon avoid. But being alone doesn't allow us to avoid these feelings either. Being with people who are appropriate for us, who can be reciprocal in the relationship, who are safe, is a required aspect of enjoying the beauty of life and celebrating existence with one another.

Have you been with any different people lately?

May 18: Gliding on Laughter

SACRED DANCE

Glidingly rotate your upper body in a clockwise direction, moving your arms out to the sides of your body in a wavelike motion, with your palms pressed outward. Your gaze follows your torso around the circular motion. Repeat for eight breaths, then alternate the motion in the counterclockwise direction for eight breaths. Next, bring the arms up over the head, with the palms facing outward and wrists touching; then sweep the right arm down as you turn in a clockwise direction 360 degrees. Repeat on the left side. Then bring both arms back to over the head with feet shoulder-width apart. Step with your right foot to move in a clockwise direction. After four steps, with the next step on the right, place the foot across the left one so that you may slightly turn with the left shoulder leading you around. Then step with the left foot behind the right foot, alternating this so that you turn in a circle. Continue gently waving your arms through the air, near your body. After four breaths, bring your arms again up to over your head with the palms facing outward, wrists touching.

MEDITATION AND PRACTICE

Ancient Iberians revered nature and fully expressed life. They realized complications and intricacies of day-to-day living made life unpredictable. These wise ones accepted the sacred, or Divine feminine as equal to or greater than the Divine masculine. At the same time, they realized that individuals were sacred, highly attuned manifestations of the Divine.

They say pagans don't follow a mainstream socially accepted religion. Perhaps lessons can be learned about shedding imposed forces—those that keep us in locked positions and mindsets—so that we can expand and laugh while acting when systems try to control us. Spirit isn't a controller; Spirit is a facilitator, moving us to acknowledge who we really are.

Can you imagine the notion of people being equally valuable? Can you laugh at the idea that a gender can be considered any other way? Can you write down other doctrines to have a good laugh about?

May 19: Uplift Others

SACRED DANCE

Today we practice bringing the sacred dance together from the first few days of this week. Review and practice the dance motions from May 15 to May 17 until you feel comfortable doing them all together.

MEDITATION AND PRACTICE

The root religion of humanity—the religion from which all other religions eventually evolved—is speculated to have begun around 22,000 BCE. The ancient Iberians were said to have used myths and rituals to increase their relationship with the land. Birth and death rites, gatherings and plantings, celebrations, and worship were aspects of the root religious Practice that these ancients engaged with. Giving thanks through song, dance, and feast was a part of life and community. Evidences of circles in reliefs on stones point to the solar as part of Iberian worship, dating around the third millennium BCE.

One fascinating depiction of the ancient worship and Practice is found on the Woman of Willendorf. She is said to represent a goddess and was carved into stone that has survived since 22,000 BCE or earlier and originated within or near the Iberian Peninsula. The body depicts a goddess of plenty.

We can take on the thinking of the ancient Iberians that comes to us through the millennia. They thought that every life form has a level of consciousness. Further, they believed consciousness transcends death and exists simultaneously on multiple levels of reality. Perhaps we can uplift others, understanding that everything has consciousness and therefore needs our affirmation and love.

May 20: Dance Spiritual Humor

SACRED DANCE

Today, review the sacred dance moves from May 17 and May 18. Practice them together until you can do them comfortably and in a flow.

Some Indigenous Iberians performed sacred dances to their "goddesses": to enhance their virtues and place in society or to humor or to delight in physical pleasure and share it. For others, sacred dances were associated with natural forces such as creation and growth or with social endeavors of running a community and producing loving citizens. They enjoyed sacredly dancing just to be in the presence of the goddesses together, having fun doing so. They knew that feeling free and having fun were something to treasure.

Nowadays, some still draw on rituals that come to us from ancient Iberia. Polytheists continue to honor their deities with sacred dance and spiritual humor. The purpose is to develop a deep relationship with their deities so that they live with more spiritual effect and visible affect.

May 21: Creating an Inviting Environment

SACRED DANCE

For today, combine the sacred dance sequences given this week and find yourself lost in them. Your swooping and circular moves can be free and full of laughter as you imbue the dance with your spiritual signature.

MEDITATION AND PRACTICE

Indigenous religious Practices with their renditions honoring their goddesses and gods lasted into the medieval period. These Practices included festivals used for healing and increasing the fertility in the ground and in humans. Magick was used in celebration and petitions to garner input from deities and beings from the Spirit world. Those celebrations set out to revere nature or the Divinity that creates and sustains a happy, laughing, loving, and free-flowing life. Magick was part of the people's effort to understand how one could shape the world.

In general, like our ancient Iberian ancestors, we celebrate nature and spirituality and encourage taking care of the environment.

Equality and social justice are truly important. Believe that Divinity is in the living world; in laughter and through sacred dance and laughing rituals we connect with the Divine.

❋ ❋ ❋

MAY 22–31

Sacred Play (Entry Point)

Play, and play some more—a spiritual assurance of winning the game of life.

The purpose of life is to enjoy living, to love, to be in conscious contact with your Higher Power or Higher Self, and to remind others to do this too. Playing is being engaged with Spirit in a Divine dance of pure pleasure, without purpose other than the dance itself. In play, earthly problems suddenly become left behind and released to the past. In play we accept the unimagined and incredible.

Wear flowing red and black Sacred Dance Attire, with a sash around the torso. Sacred music this week comes from bagpipes. You may wish to dance outdoors this week, with people, if possible. The sacred dance is of medium impact this week, but you can also work in a low-impact method if you choose to.

May 22: Playing Is Sacred

SACRED DANCE

Stand in the Sacred Dance Posture, and start out skipping in place like perhaps you did as a child, for eight breaths. If your Sacred Dance Attire is flowing, gently hold it away from your body with your fingertips so you can imitate the wind. Spin in place to your right and then repeat the skipping in place for another eight breaths. Spin in place to your left. Your face is full of joy, and you smile widely. Repeat this sequence until you feel like you're floating on clouds. Skip and spin, skip and spin. The sacred dance moves are light. If you're inclined, march in place and then spin.

In the fifth century BCE, ancient Iberia was what is now Catalan. Over time, the Catalans developed *seny*, or common-sense planning, mindful action, and reason, and *rauxa*, which was unplanned activity inspired by impulse and instinct. Rauxa was considered play—activity driven by creative and spontaneous energy. It embodied risk-taking, passion, and expression.

During rauxa, children played at being water-women, who symbolized fertility and life-giving virtues of water. Exceptionally beautiful, they had high self-esteem and tried to bring wealth and well-being to the areas they inhabited. Water-women came out at night, with shimmering long gold or red hair and emerald or deep blue eyes; they wore fine, lavish clothes and, when the moon was full, enjoyed viewing their reflections in lakes. Some were said to have beautiful, colorful wings. Many carried magic wands carved from hazel, a wood used in casting spells. Some said they were witches who could take down a whole community at will, especially if it'd been bad!

Taking on aspects of good and evil characters helps playing children cope with the real world. But they know the difference between the real world and an imaginary one. In fact, play wouldn't be play if children did not recognize that distinction.

For us adults, play helps to balance our energies and recognize the part of us that wants to be free from the human condition. Even for those who haven't had joyful childhoods, play helps to re-create childlike moments. Imagine you're a child again and that you live in circumstances that support your being a child.

May 23: *Learning Optimism and Imagination*

Repeat what you did on May 22. After the second set of skipping and spinning, lift your arms up above your head. Step to your left, lift the right knee high, and place the right foot down in front of the left foot. Repeat this four times, then step to the right, lift the left knee high, and place the left foot in front of the right foot. There is a bit of a skip and brush on the floor with the stepping foot. Keep your arms held up high and wide and away from your head, and smile. At the end of the Sacred Dance sequence, bring your arms down to your sides, lean forward a bit and with your fingertips grasping your Sacred Dance Attire if it's loose, and hold it away from your body. If you aren't wearing loose-fitting attire, simply keep your arms down and away from your body, with your fingertips touching.

MEDITATION AND PRACTICE

People used ritual and play and all things in between to make sense of life. The stories and beliefs were myths, but they served the sacred as both fictions and functions, supporting real life and community. With sacred stories and games, ancient Iberians understood that a Great Reality inside each person loves to play.

Sometimes our Great Reality gets obscured or forgotten by concentrating solely on obligation or tasks. Imagination doesn't get exercised. Some of us must learn optimism to let that Inner Beauty come out, to guide our lives and give it freshness. Playfulness shapes our Souls and helps us be optimistic, especially if it includes other people.

Imagine you're a child again. If you had a great childhood, recall times when you were most playful. Write them down in your journal. If you didn't enjoy childhood, imagine that you lived in circumstances supporting your childhood. You had a support system, good food, and nurturing by loving family and friends. Write the real or imagined experiences in your journal.

May 24: Play as a Spiritual Practice

SACRED DANCE

Review and repeat the dance from May 23. When you hold your Sacred Dance Attire away from your body, tap the right foot in front of you, then transfer your weight and tap the left foot in front of you. Turn your torso and shoulders in the opposite direction of your tapping foot, which will occur naturally as you swing your body. Move forward for four breaths and backward for four breaths as you do this. When you have completed the last tap, transition to the skipping movements for sixteen breaths. Keep holding your arms away from your body, holding your Sacred Dance Attire if it is loose. Keep smiling.

MEDITATION AND PRACTICE

Catalans were used to playing with the numerous deities of their times, consulting with them regarding all sorts of matters and including them in celebrations. Sacred play seems to have been initiated through unseen forces. Cycles of change and the flow were integrated with playful sacred dance ceremonies, as well as with imaginative stories of how goddesses helped people achieve their imaginative dreams by interacting with other worlds such as Atlantis. Rauxa was the energy given to this effort by the goddesses.

As people shifted from interacting with a pantheon to participating in monotheism, spiritual Practices became less playful for many. At a certain point, fear replaced play, especially under a hierarchical spiritual structure. Gods and goddesses weren't playmates anymore, but "He" evolved into a punishing god that made people afraid. Would it be possible to return to the notion of freedom through spiritual aid without punishment? Would we be able to let go of the idea that we must be serious all the time? Trace your beliefs around seriousness and spirituality. What do you find? Are you able to play with your Higher Power?

May 25: Playfulness Is Divine

SACRED DANCE

Repeat the dance from May 24. After you have completed the skipping, add spinning in place to your right and then repeat the skipping in place for another eight breaths. Spin in place to your left. Your face is full of joy as you smile widely.

MEDITATION AND PRACTICE

Life is full of negative happenings, and people always have experiences and responses to them. Ancient Iberians were no different. Politics and change happened, people died, people were born, the sun rose and set. Through it all, there was time to play, to imagine, and to create. The goddesses and gods were there for them, encouraging, helping, guiding—through play. So people were freed from being so attached to day-to-day foibles. Freedom was inherent to play, and the gods were thought to live with freedom. Playing freely was an end in itself.

Most spend time working rather than playing. Some teachings seem to make play a behavior to be avoided. What would you do with your days if you didn't have to "work" at making a living? Or work to please others or take care of others? Could you be free to play? Would you be able to adapt? How would your interaction with your Divine Being change? Use your imagination to visualize the way life would be if you played and play was the norm rather than the exception.

May 26: *Playing in Spiritual Community*

SACRED DANCE

Review the sacred dance from previous days this week. Today we bring the dance all together. When you practice it, focus on your shoulders and torso as you do the steps and the skips. Feel the air move around you as you spin. Feel the way the fabric moves, and how lightly and gently you can hold it between your fingers without dropping it.

MEDITATION AND PRACTICE

Imagine your life as a perfect creation: Everyone lives in perfect alignment, authenticity, and harmony with the environment and community. You're okay and can be who you truly are, without judgment. You are self-realized and live from a place of wholeness. You rely on your intuition to navigate your direction with direct guidance from the goddesses and gods. This is how many Indigenous Iberians lived.

To keep our Inner Mystic Dancer in communication with the Divine, we must keep playing sacredly. It brings out the best of us and contributes to our well-being. And the more opportunities we create in which we are playing, the closer we get to experiencing sacred play. The gods themselves join us in play. Playing freely, playfully together, we realize, remember, and reconnect to the Sacred Being we have always been.

May 27: Healing Through Spiritual Play

SACRED DANCE

Today you embellish the dance with your combination of skips, spins, steps, taps, knee lifts, and grasp of the Sacred Dance Attire as you move around the room. Open yourself up to freely letting go and do the Sacred Dance as you remember it.

MEDITATION AND PRACTICE

We can't go back in time and talk to the Indigenous Iberians; we can only see what they left us through sacred dance, their stories, and their relationships with the goddesses and gods. Their Practices reveal that sacred dance plus sacred play equals spiritual enlightenment.

Play embraced as a spiritual Practice enables us to reclaim our bodies as temples of the Spirit and develop a sense of abundant creativity, to reclaim the spiritual gifts of hearing a waterfall, feeling the air in our nostrils, or disappearing into games for intervals of time. We don't focus on tomorrow or yesterday. We don't have regrets or aspirations; we're in the present. Like sounds of nature or placement of flowers in a room, play is a simple statement about all that is wonderful. It's the realization of wholeness.

May 28: Develop a Play Plan

SACRED DANCE

Perform the sacred dance given this week while letting go of trying to do it right. Feel every part of your body, and be aware of this moment. Remember to hold a pleasant look on your face.

The Iberian legend of the Home dels Nassos, or the Man of Noses, tells of a man who had as many noses as the year had days. He lost a nose every day, and his actual person could only be seen on December 31. Children played and searched for him on the last day of the year. Some people on the streets told the children they'd just seen him passing by through a nearby street so they'd run to see if they could find him. On the last day of the year, the Man of Noses had one nose left, and it could be anyone.

All sorts of things can be morphed into play and are easy to do if you focus on life in the moment, laughing at problems, and making them a game. Like prayer, laughter and play can be healing to the body, mind, and Soul. When we play, and when we pray, we abandon our stress and allow our Spirit to breathe and re-create.

Make a play plan. Schedule time for a hobby, but find joy in the process, not in the outcome. The cool thing is doing something with other people for social interactions. Try classes, workshops, leagues, and groups that cover what you like. Don't know what you like? Try a bunch of stuff! Your gaming can be spontaneous, like racing people on the escalator, visiting a park or playground, swinging on the swings, or hanging by the jungle-gym bars. Practice mindfulness as you notice the changing leaves, feel or smell the seasons, or allow yourself to jump in a rain puddle. Your play plan may include regular or occasional activities, and it should include other people and be sometimes outside.

May 29: Playful Thoughts

Repeat yesterday's instructions. When you hold a pleasant look on your face, imagine a world you'd create if you were a god or goddess.

According to myth, people in ancient Iberia were from Atlantis, reached via a natural bridge from Northern Africa into Iberia. Those people spread from the Mediterranean to the Pyrenees; a powerful people, they attempted to conquer the then-known world. Ancient Iberians were characterized as impetuous, merry, and hospitable. They were remarkable for their vivacity and grace and easily traversed the complexities of spirituality and humanity. By creating a place that was utopic, the balance between spirituality and humanity was accomplished by playing between those spheres and having the goddesses and gods help.

A spirituality of play helps us live with the mystery, paradox, and spontaneous nature of life! It helps us come to know ourselves, as spiritual beings having a human experience.

May 30: Play as an Act of Pleasure

SACRED DANCE

Perform the dance as you did yesterday.

MEDITATION AND PRACTICE

Seriousness is not godliness. Play and creativity, framed within the confines of responsible action and observance of natural and spiritual laws, was like the Divine. Seny and rauxa coexisted in the Indigenous Iberian ancestors' Spirits and ways of being.

What types of play and spontaneity are on your list? Make changes to your list if you like.

May 31–Play to Surrender

SACRED DANCE

Revisit the sacred dances given during May. You may like to choose your favorite one to do or select them all. Or you might improvise and bring the dances together in a new way. Wearing your Sacred Dance Attire, recall sacred laughter, joy, and play.

MEDITATION AND PRACTICE

Our Iberian ancestors expressed their connection with the Divine in many ways. Although numerous deities informed their lives, they seemed to basically have been connected to inner wisdom.

As you practice playing and laughing, pause to notice what's happening in your inner world. What are you feeling as you play? What sense of your Higher Self do you have when playing? How does the Universe meet you during play?

Honoring the Triad of Higher Self

TIBETAN SACRED DANCE

Transformation is our theme this month, and we honor that through Tibetan dance traditions. Tibet is between India and China. Mountain ranges near it form a border between Tibet and China, while the Himalayas divide Tibet and India. Indigenous people appear to have inhabited this area about twenty-one thousand years ago. The area has had tremendous change and upheaval over the centuries with India and China and then with the West.

Indigenous Tibetans practiced Bon in ancient days. It arose in the Zhang Zhung kingdom around 500 BCE; the inhabitants had migrated from the Amdo region of Tibet. Modern Bon is a conglomeration of Buddhist and indigenous Practices—an attempt to return to a time before Buddhism. Tibetan spiritual Practices have been touched by all sorts of politics, as has been the case in many indigenous sacred dance regions.

Before the arrival of Buddhism and the codification of Bon, the main religion among Tibetans was shamanic and animistic. For the indigenous Tibetans, like other ancient sacred dance cultures, every part of the natural environment was considered alive with sentient energy. Whether in mountains or trees, wetlands and streams, organic or inorganic substances, the heavens or earth, there was Spirit energy. Every region identified its own native supernatural beings, and people living in these areas worshipped and honored them. To ensure their favor, Tibetans made offerings, performed rituals appeasing them, and sometimes refrained from going to particular places.

They believed the earth was fraught with dark beings and demons, energy flows that must be channeled or neutralized, and these are taken seriously even if one is a practicing Tibetan Buddhist. But because trouble is everywhere and can pop up in an instant, our ancient Tibetan ancestors enlisted the help of the Spirit world all the time. Tibetan sacred dances were celebrated and practiced as part of the way of life in this region. They reach backward to the beginnings of time.

Monks traditionally danced at monasteries in two main forms: *cham* and the five elements dance. The cham dance was performed by both monks and nuns, in addition to lay people. Monks played music on traditional Tibetan instruments as an accompaniment. The sacred dance embodied moral instruction on compassion and was a type of prayer to invoke blessings. This Sacred Dance Meditation had the power to transform evil for the benefit of the entire world.

Tibetans usually engaged with the cham dance during the Monlam, or Great Prayer Festival. The reason for the festival was to pray for the gurus so they lived a long life, to bring a rapid spread of dharma to people, and to engender peace around the globe. Several stages make up a cham; in its full form, it lasted for several days. Dancers wore colorful but oversized masks and brightly colored robes.

The five elements dance was a complex sacred dance that involved creating a sacred mandala within a fire, where powerful spiritual forces, the purified or "enlightened" form of the five elements of water, earth, air, fire, and space, dwelt. Then various symbolic offerings were placed in the fire, as a method of purification of the sacred dancer's elemental body and mind. The dancers were often dressed as the Five Wisdom Dakinis, or embodiments of the feminine aspect of fully transformed psyche and soma.

PREPARATION

For sacred mystical Tibetan dances, you might want to avail your-self of colorful outfits, masks, and headdresses. The masked faces and dancers represent the enlightened deities, and their move-ments are different forms of enlightened activities.

Prepare a fragrance of your choice, such as Tibetan incense, which can contain thirty or more ingredients. Available through healers and monasteries, authentic Tibetan incense was originally used for medicinal and spiritual purposes, following a lineage of monks. Tibetan incense produces a rich, earthy, and pure scent, which can help soothe and calm a restless mind. It's widely used to purify the environment, cleanse a home, and aid meditation and relaxation. You can now find authentic incense products online or in temples with stores. Use them so the smell will linger with you in memory and in the place where you dance. State your intentions as you prepare your Sacred Dance Studio space.

Please visit www.cswalter.org/sacreddancemeditations for video illustrations.

JUNE 1–7
Transformation (Entry Point)

Look at yourself today; remember yourself tomorrow.

Transformation is dynamic and occurs with or without our consent. Be awake to it so you'll find the secret meanings of all the Unseen.

June 1: Three Prongs of Spirituality

You may wish to use a mask for this week's sacred dance to help you assume the role of a deity. Masks can be very elaborate or very simple, and you can find them with a general online search for them. You may wish to add bells or other Tibetan music to your Practice. Your Sacred Dance Attire can include colorful loose-fitting garments and beads worn around your wrists and neck. Face east as you open your awareness and move into the Sacred Dance Meditation.

SACRED DANCE

Stand with your left hand in front of your heart chakra, with your palm open to your right side to attract and generate energy. Your right foot is behind your left, and knees are slightly bent. Lift the right knee as you shift your weight to your left and bring the knee up high. Then bring it around to the right and place it on the floor behind you. Your right palm comes to your heart chakra as your left palm drops behind you. Shift your weight to both feet as your right foot arrives on the floor behind the left foot, keeping your knees bent. Hold here for four breaths. These movements are very meditative and slow. Repeat on the other side, lifting the left knee, and placing it behind you, moving your palms through the heart chakra and down to the right side of your body. Hold the stance with your right foot behind you for four breaths. Bring the left knee up again to the hip height, and place the foot on the floor so that the feet are parallel. Bring your palms together in front of your heart chakra.

MEDITATION AND PRACTICE

Tibetan Bon ancestors applied magical sacred dance Practices by focusing on a specific spiritual goal. For example, perhaps they wanted to counter negative energy, give testament to a need, and foster wellness, long life, wealth, or inner transformation. The sacred dance contained drum sounds that vibrated the spiritual and earthly realms to make deep transformations. All forms of Tibetan sacred dance could spark instantaneous enlightenment, since any person in the ritual might happen to understand the heretofore and otherwise secret meaning of the sacred. They all had the goal of achieving three-pronged spiritual desires: the need for connecting Unseen with the Higher Self to bring about transformation, for honoring all Beings and setting aside differences, and for thinking and acting from the Divine in decisions affecting the community.

Transformation is based on what's revealed, on action, and on knowing from experience. Yet, sometimes we must set seeing the revealed as the goal. How do you honor your three-pronged spiritual desires?

June 2: The Element of Surprise

SACRED DANCE

Review the Sacred Dance entry from June 1. You begin today with your palms together in front of your heart chakra, standing in your eastward position. Open your palms as you reach forward, keeping them in front of your heart chakra. Flip them in a slow circular motion twice in front of you, then place them in a mudra, or hand pose, with the index fingers and the thumbs touching. Circle the wrists with your fingers in the mudra pose for several breaths, then open the palms to face the floor and press them around from the wrists in circular motions for four breaths. Then return the fingers to the mudra position and circle the wrists with your fingers in the mudra pose for another four breaths.

In the Tibetan dance, the motions, mantras, songs, and devotional thoughts that accompanied sacred dances were offerings to a deity to attend the dance and bless all present. From these sacred dances arose *terma*, hidden teaching that was key to transformations of people from one level of awareness to the next. Tibetan tradition held that terma could also be dance or hidden physical objects, like rocks or crystals, plants, trees, water, or the sky.

When have you had a memorable transformation come from an unexpected direction? What is your reaction to the notion of the Divine Feminine? How do you handle spiritual surprises? Is your mind open? Your heart? Do you have all the methods to achieve your three-pronged spiritual desires?

June 3: Subtle or Grand Transmissions

SACRED DANCE

Today's dance continues from where you ended on June 2. Facing east, stand with your feet shoulder-width apart, knees slightly bent. Change the position of the mudra for each hand so that you have your thumb touching your ring finger. Using your wrists, alternating left and right, point the mudra upward and then forward, while hands are in front of your heart chakra. Imagine making a semicircle away from your body with the fingertips, and then pointing them back toward you. After eight breaths, return to the thumb-to-forefinger mudra, rotate the wrists again so that the palms face the ceiling, then cross the wrists and bring the arms to your chest with the wrists crossed, hands closed in a loose fist.

MEDITATION AND PRACTICE

Termas were of two main kinds: earth-intentioned treasures or mind-intentioned treasures. Earth terma was physical. The mind terma was constituted by space and transmitted from one enlightened human to another. Mind terma could be realized through Sacred Dance Meditation, removing evil forces. Sacred dancers were representatives of humans, animals, creatures, and the Divine. They were considered a sort of Tibetan medicine.

Setting intentions for earth or mind termas could simply be a way of remembering who you really are and setting your course to follow that. Some realizations occur in Sacred Dance Meditation and some while sleeping, taking care of your body, or engaging in other activities of everyday life. Even if you have a "negative" experience, it gives food for thought, a way to synthesize the event and set yourself on a course or in a direction. You see many instances of people taking up lineages in rites of passage, such as taking vows, getting baptized, and so on, so they can be in the receptive state of earth and mind termas. Some have chosen to follow a guru with teachings and scriptures. Others have chosen a path that has very loose directives found in contemporary books. What are your termas generators? Who are your gurus? Read one of their texts again today and see if there is new information for your transformation.

June 4: Mandalic Transformation

SACRED DANCE

As you begin today, think of the space of your Sacred Dance Studio as a sacred geometric form, in which you're encircling to create transformative energies. Imagine your Sacred Dance Studio as a location on earth in relation to the solar system.

Review the Sacred Dance Meditation given on June 3, and begin with your hands in the closed fist position, knees slightly bent. Now place your palms facing each other at your heart chakra. Move your right palm away from your body as you lift your right knee up and behind you to place it down on the floor behind the left foot. After you pause in this position for a few breaths, move the left palm behind you and bring your right palm to your heart chakra. Lift the left knee up and around to place the foot on the floor behind your right foot. Pause here again for a few breaths. Shift the weight onto the left leg, and lift your right knee so that the thigh is parallel to the floor and your right palm moves in a circular pattern just above the right knee. The knee and the palm move simultaneously in this circular pattern four breaths as the left palm rests on the left hip. On the fourth breath place the right foot down on the floor and the right hand to the right hip. Swing the left arm outstretched and around to the front of your body, and, placing the weight on the right foot, bring the left knee up and around to the front of your body. You will naturally rotate your body as you do this. Keeping the left knee up, engage in the circular movement with the left knee and palm facing the floor for four breaths. Place the left foot down next to the right, slightly bend your knees in a bowing motion, and bring the left hand to your heart chakra, palm facing right. Hold here, and breathe for four breaths.

MEDITATION AND PRACTICE

Ancient Tibetan sacred dance was mandalic—in other words, it employed a sacred geometrical form that represented the Universe. Mandalas assist with healing and transformation. Dancers whirled around the mandala, encircling a representative deity stationed in a central location in the sacred temple until they merged with the Divine. Their movements were clockwise and formed a ring around the space to protect it and develop a safe space for transformation. By revolving around the center counterclockwise, they danced as they thought the planets did, around the sun. The mandala space was sanctified and empowered by the circling of the dancers.

Your transformations necessarily, though maybe not intentionally, include the transformations of others. What are your thoughts on a transformative process being extended to or systematically applied to others as you engage in Sacred Dance Meditation? Can you transform yourself and the Universe and its interaction with humanity? What thoughts need your transformation? Actions? Behaviors? Who or what do you consider when thinking of transforming? Please write some things down in your journal, without judging them.

June 5: Countering Negativity

SACRED DANCE

Revisit the sacred dance given on June 4. At the end of that last breath, jump slightly upward on the right foot, bringing the left knee upward and both arms reaching to the sky. Place the left foot over to the right so that it's in front of it with both knees bent. Bend over as you swing the arms around to the right side of your body, as if you're going to reach for the floor. Then swing around, and bring the right knee up with a small jump and arms reaching to the sky. Place the right foot down in front of the left, and swing the arms to the left in a big sweeping motion to complete a full 360-degree rotation. Bring the left knee up as you complete the turn, and bring your arms up to the sky with a little hop upward on the right foot. Then place the left foot on the floor in front of the right. Repeat on the left side, and place the right foot on the floor parallel to the left foot. Bring the arms down in front of your body as you open your palms toward the floor. Hold this pose for four breaths to close the dance meditation.

MEDITATION AND PRACTICE

Ancient Tibetan mythology proposed that from the nothingness came Light and darkness. Male and female darkness lay down together and produced a poisonous egg. When it hatched, planetary disturbances were created. That made earth full of illnesses and physical handicaps, and from it emerged a monster, black life. It had awful eyes, gnashing teeth, and hair with blood reaching to the heavens. It wielded a black cross of power and a lasso from which to spread disease.

In all cultures, stories explain bad actors and how they came to be abound. Now, some people want us to believe that all we need to do is think positively or imagine only attracting what we want, and this will transform us. To a point that is true. But really, it's a matter of encasing your entire self to prevent negativity and negative energy from limiting your transformation. We need to repair the earth, and help people who are suffering, but to do that we have to take action. And given the alarming increases in the exploitation of the environment, we need harmony to heal the planet.

What are you doing or what will you do as part of your Practice to counter negativity on the physical, spiritual, and mental planes? Is it not repeating or sharing something? Is it consuming or producing certain services or products? Do you increase your time in prayer and meditation? Pick something difficult to place on your list as you make notes in your journal.

June 6: Go Off Script

SACRED DANCE

Practice what you've learned this week by reviewing the sacred dance given the last five days. Commit the movements to your memory. Take as much time as you need.

MEDITATION AND PRACTICE

Sacred Dance Meditations in ancient Himalaya used the efforts from the shaman to help people recover from illnesses and to aid the community in recovery from the effects of illnesses. Sacred dancers were often themselves considered as shamans. This required not only a knowledge base of wisdom and sacred dance but also a willingness to engage with the visions as they were shown to them in the Sacred Dance Meditation. There was no list of prohibitions or precepts, but rather a shaman had to see the Spirit in humans to facilitate their healing.

Transformation comes about in the present, often unexpectedly. Our bodies influence and carry what we think and feel. Oftentimes, we don't focus on what is happening but on what we imagine, which limits our forward movement. Engaging the body in sacred dance reveals fears that accompany apocalyptic beliefs. As you continue your journey, let go of any expectation of how it should unfold, and stand in the Light of the Truth in the transformative process as you embrace the idea of knowing both nothing and everything at the same time.

June 7: Being Alone

SACRED DANCE

Today, try to do the week's sacred dance from memory. Repeat the sacred dance movements until you have focused only on it, the power it holds, and the knowledge that the dance sets your mandala in motion and gives you a powerful force to apply to your transformation of yourself, your community, and the solar system. Feel the energy flowing in and out of your feet and hands, feel the mandala, and imagine it in your mind.

MEDITATION AND PRACTICE

Ancient Tibetan sacred dance was transformative for both groups and individuals: the group Practice was energizing to the community. The individual would need to be alone, though, to sense what was being conveyed, even as they practiced together. The individual's own inner compass would move the person forward.

We all come to the earth alone, and we leave alone. While we are here, we crave knowledge and deep spiritual connection, but these desired outcomes are often redirected as we are forced to associate with unappealing conversations or images, misinterpretations, persecution, and vilifications. Negative labels and suggestions can obscure knowledge and redirect our thoughts and behaviors. We may know that many of the peoples, if not all of them studied so far, have had their Sacred Dance Meditations revised or in some cases obliterated. We know that the Ancient Tibetans believed in their sacred Practices, and they lived in impossible conditions, on steep plateaus with harsh weather. Harmony is one of the beacons to transformation. That means acceptance of people with unconditional love while not condoning poor behavior and honoring belief systems of others while also helping to bring Light in contexts of where people are. How will you be in community with people who hold beliefs that don't resonate with yours and speak to them and yourself through loving kindness?

※　※　※

JUNE 8–14
Tantric Transformations (Entry Point)

Chart the path, and stay the course.

Tantras pave the way to peace and contentment, to leave the crazies behind, to laugh and play, and to share these qualities with others.

This week, it may be good to envision a mandala of the Universe and hold it in your consciousness. If you have a revered spiritual guide, you can bring that person into your awareness as well. Your Sacred Dance Attire can include colorful loose-fitting garments and beads worn around the wrists and neck.

June 8: The Lower Tantra

SACRED DANCE

Begin with the right palm facing toward the left side of your body at your heart chakra, with the right foot placed behind the left in the manner of a walking stride held in place. Jump up on the left foot, raise the right knee up, and bring both arms up into the air over your head and away from your ears. Place the right foot down in front of your left one, bring your arms down toward the floor, and jump up on the right foot, as you raise the left knee and arms. Repeat this six times alternating sides.

MEDITATION AND PRACTICE

Some of the ancient Tibetans pursued *siddhis*, magical powers such as extrasensory perception and liberation, which included sacred dance, along a tantric path of transformation. Ancient Tibetan tradition has two main types of tantra: lower tantra and a higher one. On the tantric path, the afflictive emotions seen as unwanted and problematic in revealing one's true nature aid in achieving transformation. In lower tantras, sacred dancers completely transformed themselves into a certain deity by embodying its characteristics. The sacred dancer visualized the entire Universe as safe and full of perfection and wisdom. In practice, the dancer worked with the knowledge being, the symbolic being, and the action being. Bringing in consciousness or awareness was done through the symbolic being, which could be a chosen deity, a deity's mantra, the mandala that was the focus of visualizing, or any form of subtle energies. The knowledge being represented the positive qualities of the chosen deity, felt in the mantra or invoked in the deity. The knowledge and symbolic beings unified as an action being, a transformed state free of guilt, anger, fear, or any of their forms.

Because we are Spirit by nature, we can see ourselves as deities. Therefore, we ignite the potential to be who we truly are: compassionate, loving, caring, and always kind, thinking of others first. When we visualize being a deity, we invoke a quality to fulfill our needs and bring it into our daily lives, and that allows reconnection with the unchanging, pure, innate Self.

When we are distracted by everyday life, bombarded with messages and directives, it's hard for us to recognize our innate Good. Through deity visualization we can utilize the concepts of tantra. If we focus on the word's meaning—*tan*, to elaborate on and understand profound matters in reality and within sacred mantras, and *tra*, to provide liberation—we can incorporate tantra into our Practice.

When you hear *tantra* what do you think? Many of us in the West have been given a false definition of the word. Make some notes in your journal as you ponder.

June 9: The Higher Tantra

SACRED DANCE

Review the sacred dance from June 8. After repeating it six times, alternate sides to wind up on the left side. As you put the right foot on the floor, take two steps, and then swing around with the left foot on the floor. Jump up, put the right foot down on the floor, bring the left knee up, and extend the leg in front of you as you jump around in a clockwise circle on the right leg for eight rotations. Hold your arms up away from your body, elbows at shoulder height, palms facing forward. On the last rotation, place the left foot down behind you. Walk forward on the right, then the left, and turn to change directions.

MEDITATION AND PRACTICE

The goal of higher tantra Practice was unification of bliss and emptiness. Its two stages included the generation stage, during which visualization provided an encompassing nurturing cocoon, and the completion stage, when the essence of Practice was manifest and transformation emerged. In the generation stage, feeling or sensation was unified with emptiness. Feeling led to bliss, but feelings of any kind, blissful or otherwise, weren't allowed to become attachments. The unification of blissful feeling and emptiness yielded wisdom. Perception had to be free from afflicted thoughts and full of emptiness to help reach the process of transformation. Clearly, ancient Tibetans honored the higher tantra Practices so that people could be loosed from desire, attachment, craving, or even vacillation, liking, and disliking.

In Sacred Dance Meditation, we endeavor to evoke our own completion stage, manifesting transformational change. Like the ancient Tibetans, we know that it's human nature to be attached to what we want and what feels good. Doing only what feels good often separates us from achieving enlightenment through a transformational Practice. This is fine if we *consciously* choose that. Usually, this behavior chooses us, though. Fear of intimacy and fear of not getting what we want or losing what we have puts us in a constant state of flux and imbalance. Emptying these drivers of emotions and replacing them with what is truly good is the key.

What are some of your addictive behaviors? We all have them, regardless of our stage of transformation. Do you desire to be liked? Feel it difficult to face a truth about one or more of your relationships? Do you spend more money than you should? Allow ambition to drive you? Are you addicted to spirituality? There are millions of addictions that are subtle. Jot down some of yours. What are some ways you can unify a blissful feeling with emptiness to yield wisdom?

June 10: Tantric Mantras

SACRED DANCE

Review the sacred dance given yesterday to the point where you're familiar with it and can add on to it today. Jump on the left foot, and raise the right knee again bringing your arms up, then place the right foot down on the floor in front of the left. Step forward with the left two steps, then jump on the right foot and raise the left knee, arms up, and jump in place for eleven rotations. On the last rotation, step forward on the right, then left, foot. Next, jump up on the left, raise the right knee, lift the arms, step forward—right, left, right—then jump up on the right foot, and raise the left knee.

MEDITATION AND PRACTICE

Tantric mantras produced almost instantaneous results. The mantras' power came from awakening primal energy, which in turn spurred spiritual growth. Mantras had four successively progressive and powerful layers. A word was chosen based on the meaning it was given, how it felt, and the awareness achieved through repeating it or vibrating it. When done repetitively over time, it became a part of the practitioner's inner wisdom and provided a location for understanding and generation of compassion. In using it with higher and lower tantras, the mantra expressed a higher level of reality than the mind itself could fully grasp.

We strive for simple peace inside and around us, in addition to some joy and happiness. Using a mantra has untold and nearly unlimited benefits. Rather than letting the mind race everywhere it wants all day and night, which can make us feel depressed, anxious, sad, or disconnected, we can use the tantric mantra to tune into the vibration deep within. Emotions come from thoughts, and thoughts can be guided.

Write down a few mantras that you may use as we continue this Practice. Names of your deities, ancestors, sacred songs or prayers, or syllables that can be hummed—any will work. Select one to use today and for the next several days. You will begin using one of them tomorrow, so please prepare.

June 11: Tantric Dance Mandalas

SACRED DANCE

Please select a mantra from your list. As you engage in the sacred dance today, practice vibrating the mantra as you move. You might hum the words or syllables as you jump or exhale and inhale. You can slow the word down to match your movements, or you can verbalize one syllable on the exhale and one with a movement. Review the dance from June 10. Repeat jumping and raising the knee, alternating the jumping foot, taking two steps in between, and raising the arms. Walk in a clockwise circle on the last jump, and bring the palms together in front of your heart chakra to conclude. Vibrate your mantra.

MEDITATION AND PRACTICE

Mandala is Sanskrit for "circle," but it also was a symbol representing the Universe. Tibetan ancestors and sacred dancers realized the tantric mandala within the human body. Divine mandalas had the energy of the Universe contained in them and were represented as deities. The goal was to have their forms brought within the body. Advanced internalized tantric mandala Practice was very obscure and secretive, only shared with the few. People visualized the mandalas as inner sacred and spiritual bodies.

Where the mind goes, the body follows. Thought is visualization with the power to transform. What we focus on dominates our being and can shut out the Light if we're not careful. Ancient Tibetans knew this too, and so we can be assured that it's human nature to be this way. However, the goal is to figure this out, get over limitations, and awaken. Where you focus your vision creates what shows up in your life. Understanding that is how you live with energetic awareness. When we visualize a mandala while vibrating or repeating a mantra, we are working with a syllable on a lotus petal at our heart. Tantric body mandala is an inner Sacred Dance Meditation. The focus is on the divine enlightened presence of meditational deities, bringing the transformative energy within. Write some notes about how you feel about this.

June 12: Creating a Personal Mandala

SACRED DANCE

As you tune into your chosen mantra, begin with the right palm facing toward the left side of your body at your heart chakra, with the right foot placed behind the left in the manner of a walking stride held in place. Jump up on the left foot, raise the right knee up, and bring both arms up into the air over your head and away from your ears. Place the right foot down, in front of your left one, bring your arms down toward the floor, and jump up on the right foot as you raise the left knee and arms. Repeat this six times, alternating sides.

MEDITATION AND PRACTICE

Mandalas have been used in many ancient cultures to symbolize the Universe, its relation to human beings, and comprehending wholeness. They were found on ceramics, glyphs, monuments, and sacred sites. This meant that they had to be first conceived in the mind-body to be drawn by people. Creating a mandala strengthens your connection to your mantra, which you're attuning to with the Sacred Dance Meditation. In turn, your mandala is a geometrical form, a vivid image of objects or beings. It's a cosmic diagram that reminds all of us that we are part of the infinite Cosmos.

Our personal mandala triggers something within us, a sacred geometry in which we see ourself and our place in the Cosmos. Today, create a mandala in your journal. You can also generate a mandala from software, if you can access it easily. Keep it simple; gather a pencil, ruler, and eraser. If you feel inclined, you can also get some colored markers or crayons. First construct a square and then mark a dot in the center of it. Then from there you can draw lines and additional circles. Many resources for mandala drawing are available, and you can download a mandala from the web. Or if you have already created mandalas, feel free to use one or more of them. The idea is to have one readily available.

June 13: Sound Connected Mandala

SACRED DANCE

Please have your mantra memorized and your created or chosen universal mandala available to see for today's dance meditation. You will bring the sacred dance into your body memory today. Repeat what you learned on June 12 six times. Next, put the right foot on the floor and take two steps forward. Then swing around with the left foot on the floor, and jump up. Put the right foot down on the floor, bring the left knee up, and extend the leg in front of you as you jump around in a clockwise circle on the right leg for eight rotations. Hold your arms up away from your body, elbows bent at shoulder height, palms facing forward. On the last rotation, place the left foot down behind you. Walk forward on the right, then the left, and turn to change directions. Jump on the left and raise the right knee, bringing your arms up, then place the right foot down on the floor in front of the left. Step forward two steps starting with the left foot, then jump on the right foot and raise the left knee, arms up, and jump in place for eleven rotations. On the last rotation, step forward on the right then left foot. Next, jump up on the left, raise the right knee, lift the arms, step forward—right, left, right—then jump up on the right foot, raise the left knee. Repeat jumping and raising the knee, alternating the jumping foot, taking two steps in between, and raising the arms. Walk in a clockwise circle after the last jump, and bring the palms together in front of your heart chakra to conclude.

MEDITATION AND PRACTICE

Sound was involved in sacred dance, and the inner mandala was a given in ancient Tibetan spiritual Practices. Our ancestors helped people hear directions from the deities through embodying them and experiencing their knowledge.

The general human condition is always alive and well among all peoples, past, present, and surely in the future. We aren't unique. Addictions, wants, sufferings, and living in the past or future are a part of being human. The key is to use those energies to move forward, placing the human condition behind the spiritual realm and elevating the body mandala and vibrated mantra.

June 14: Internalizing the Tantric Mandala Mantra

SACRED DANCE

Review the two videos of the Sacred Dance Meditation if you need to. Repeat the sacred dance as you create a trance moment, while vibrating your mantra and visualizing your mandala.

MEDITATION AND PRACTICE

Whether Tibetan ancestors originated tantras, mandalas, and mantras remains a mystery. However, the wisdom of understanding how humans internalized awareness of Spirit was key in the way they conceived sacred dance.

Womanists advise us from their experiences that it behooves one to connect their tantras, personal mantras, universal mandalas, and sacred dance to form a multidimensional transformative process to both know one's actual deepest desires and dance sacredly toward them. Note in your journal your energy levels today and your outlook on your day-to-day life. After incorporating Tibetan methods into your Practice for a while, write in your journal to see if you're more energetic, more intuitive, and more faithful to your Higher Self. Are any of your intended directions being manifested? How do you feel?

※ ※ ※

JUNE 15–21
Six Aspects of Transformation (Entry Point)

When we are enlightened, we can handle anything.

The great reality is recognizable when we encounter it. The people of ancient Tibet practiced immediate transformation.

June 15: Dharma

SACRED DANCE

Stand with feet shoulder-width apart, knees slightly bent, your palms facing each other at your heart chakra, elbows held away from your body, with bells on your wrists and ankles. Swing your arms as you twist your torso to the right and left, turning your head as you swing each arm, allowing them to wrap around your body freely. Do this on each side once. Then raise your right hand as in an offering as you raise your right knee and then step forward on it and bow, holding your left palm close to your chin. Stand up, and step backward with the right foot as you again swing your arms while turning your torso to the right and left. Repeat three times.

MEDITATION AND PRACTICE

Each ancient Tibetan village had a temple in which Tibetans engaged with cham dance, which differed from temple to temple. The sameness was that the sacred dance served the people's spiritual needs and honored the local deities.

Masks were used to help the sacred dance meditator transform the forces of wrathful deities within them. Although masks were meant to evoke terror and fear in evil spirits, they also provided tranquility, protection, and calm to the practitioner seeking enlightenment. Masks were extensions of expressions of the spontaneous flow of enlightened energy. Such energy is provided to us through transmitted truths. Some call this dharma.

Dharma is three-fold: a spiritual teaching, a spiritual path, and an existence. In this work, dharma connotes the intrinsic nature of something or someone. Just like the dharma of sugar is sweetness and the dharma of water is wetness, the dharma of a sacred dancer is simply the way it is for *you* at a point within these three aspects. It consists of your experience, strength, and hope over time. Dharma includes the progressive spiritual teachings you follow, your spiritual path, and how these evolve to aid your enlightened existence. The question "Who are you?" is asked in this context. How do you answer it? Do you consider any of your answers to this question to be a "mask" that you can wear to transform unwanted or unwelcome feelings and thoughts? Your dharma may be, for example, impatience. A mask could be gentleness, and three aspects you practice may have come from studying the teachings of the Christ, or the Buddha, and how that personage responded to challenges of impatience. Did these teachings inform or change your spiritual path? How did they lead you to an enlightened moment? Ponder this, and write some notes.

June 16: Living in the Body

SACRED DANCE

Review and repeat the June 15 dance. When you have completed the sequence three times, jump up twice on the left leg (not too high off the ground), as you keep the right leg up with the knee at hip height. With the jumping motions, your arms are bent at the elbows with hands just opposite your ears and reaching for the ceiling; your gaze is toward the sky. Your wrists engage in circular motion away from you. Now step down on the right foot, bow forward, and continue the circular wrist motions, keeping the arms and hands held in the same position. Repeat this sequence twice.

MEDITATION AND PRACTICE

Physical gestures and postures in cham were powerful. Doing them could trigger healing through spiritual experiences that allowed people to overcome negative feelings and thoughts.

The sacred dance gave rise to the experience of nondual awareness of the true nature of a human's Being. Nondualism was a mature state of consciousness, in which the illusion of "I" versus "you" was eliminated and awareness was described as centerless and without dichotomies. Ancient Tibetan cham had a seriously liberating role in helping people progress on their path to enlightenment and diminished suffering. It was often a Sacred Dance Meditation that freed Souls just upon seeing it.

Often, mind and Spirit must follow the body. After practicing for a while, we begin to have awareness from the body that lets us know we are fundamentally safe, whole, and free. The idea of the body knowing that there is no duality and that we live in this container is really body dharma. It existed long before we came to be. We just happen to be looking out on the world from within it. We have space to step aside and let "deities" show us the way if we will but trust.

June 17: Identify Distractions

SACRED DANCE

Stand with feet shoulder-width apart, knees slightly bent, your palms facing each other at your heart chakra, elbows held away from your body, with bells on your wrists and ankles. Begin by swinging your arms as you twist your torso to the left and right, allowing them to wrap around your body freely. Allow your head to turn with each swing of your arms. Do this on each side once. Then raise your right hand as if making an offering as you raise the right knee, and then step forward on it and bow, bringing your right palm forward as you do so, and holding your left palm close to your chin. Stand up, and step backward with the right foot as you again swing your arms as you turn your torso to the right and left. Repeat three times. Then jump up twice on the left leg (not too high off the ground), as you keep the right leg up with the knee at hip height. With the jumping motions, your arms are bent at the elbows, hands just opposite your ears and reaching for the ceiling. Your gaze is toward the sky. Your wrists engage in circular motion away from you. Now step down on the right foot, bow forward, and continue the circular wrist motions, keeping the arms and hands in the same position. Repeat this sequence twice.

MEDITATION AND PRACTICE

Just watching a sacred cham dance communicated powerful messages on the same level as enacting them by generating new awareness of enlightenment, knowledge of the presence of divinities nearby the onlooker, or repetitive engagement through visual connection to the dance. For instance, while watching the variations of the Sacred Dance Meditations, people might be reminded of the cycle of life and death, karma, rebirth, and the process of liberation. Observers understood the dance's significance and power displayed. Cham wasn't an entertainment, pastime, or distraction, but an entertaining path to enlightenment.

Distractions and boredom come and go. Thinking we have an eternity to focus our attention on the Supreme Being is one. Ruminating on the past and fearing the future are distractions. Many of us are familiar with focusing on lack rather than abundance. Comparing ourselves to others can cause us to act like scavenging squirrels! But the issue is that we search outside ourselves to relieve our ills rather than remembering the Higher Self is where our focus and comfort lies. Take a small journal or other device with you today so you can note the number of times you feel distracted by your thinking, what that does to your feelings, and how these relate to your body dharma. Try to replace those thoughts with your mantra.

June 18: Dzogchen Remembering

SACRED DANCE

Review the dance given on June 15, and then repeat it but on the opposite side. So twist to the left: Stand with feet shoulder-width apart, knees slightly bent, your palms facing each other at your heart chakra, elbows held away from your body, with bells on your wrists and ankles. Begin by swinging your arms as you twist your torso to the left and right, allowing them to wrap around your body freely. Allow your head to turn with each swing of your arms. Do this on each side once. Then raise your left hand as if making an offering as you raise your left knee, and then step forward on it and bow, bringing your left palm forward as you do so and holding your right palm close to your chin. Stand up, and step backward with the left foot as you again swing your arms as you turn your torso to the left and right. Repeat three times.

MEDITATION AND PRACTICE

According to an ancient terma, Dzogchen originated eighteen thousand years ago, when Tonpa Shenrab ruled Tazik, west of Tibet. Dzogchen classified outer, inner, and secret teachings. Dzogchen was couched in the ideas of ground (*gzhi*), sometimes called basis, and gnosis, or knowledge (*rig pa*). Ground represented the nature of being, and gnosis the limits of the knowledge of nirvana. Dzogchen described nirvana as the true expanse of the Higher Self.

Basis was humanity's original state before realization produced Buddha, and nonrealization produced sentience. The state of basis or ground was nontemporal and unchanging. According to the Dzogchen, ground had three qualities in humans: First was an essence, oneness, or emptiness and purity of being. Second was one's nature, which consisted of luminosity, lucidity, or clarity (as in the luminous mind of the five pure lights). And last was the power to utilize and call upon universal compassionate energy.

Gnosis described the state wherein people were reflexively self-aware of primordial wisdom and unbounded wholeness. Dzogchen masters suggested that humanity's true nature is like a mirror, which reflects complete openness but isn't affected by the reflections. It is like a crystal ball that takes on the color of the material on which it's placed without itself being changed. Sacred knowledge ensued from recognizing this mirror.

Knowledge has three aspects. People began with a sense of purity, being unaware of the self as separate and lacking any concept of separation from others. With that, people came with knowledge that could influence others. At the same time, people were by nature innately compassionate in responding to situations and people in them.

Dzogchen teaches us how to remain balanced with ten thousand things distracting us from remembering our true Selves. We are tossed from good to bad to indifferent experiences, with wants and desires shifting us all the time. Our conditioned human nature is to be attracted to pleasure, comforts, and the familiar. If something makes us feel uneasy, we try to avoid it or get out of it. Dzogchen Practice prepares us to live with the moment so we aren't beholden to the changing tides of human existence. The idea is not to be elated with good news or depressed with bad news, not to see yourself as separate from others or detached from G-d.

Say to yourself, *I have compassion for myself and others; I keep this awareness when confronted with likes and dislikes and crazy unending distractions.*

June 19: Watch the Stream Flow By

SACRED DANCE

Repeat the dance as given on June 17.

MEDITATION AND PRACTICE

Dzogchen was beyond conception and above grasping and having to let go—that is, it was an unchanging state with awareness and no clinging to wants and desires. Sacred dances helped people to enter this balanced conception.

Dzogchen drives individuals to be open and present, to realize self-liberation. They can liberate themselves in every second, in every situation, by responding from their true nature rather than from conditioning.

The practice allows us to leave things alone and simultaneously to exert influence over them without judgment. In leaving them untouched and unjudged, we allow space for them to change and manifest. From a point of equanimity, we can draw on our compassion to be connected and understand other persons in a situation, to feel what they feel and know what they need. We may not be able to fulfill a given need, but we can do our best to remain compassionate, loving, accepting, and forgiving.

Think, *The stream of life will flow by like a newsfeed on social media, no matter what I do.*

June 20: Stay in Reality

SACRED DANCE

Repeat the dance as presented on June 18, followed by the dance as presented on June 19. Perform this sequence twice on each side.

MEDITATION AND PRACTICE

The ancient Tibetans were very aware of the duality of openness and presence. In their quest for enlightenment, they also faced each moment as it came, without fear and judgment. The consciousness of space being comprised of both emptiness and awareness was reflected in their interactions with people and the environment. And the ancient Tibetans embraced living life on earth as an important function while also living in eternity. The two existences happened simultaneously.

Sometimes because we're impatient, we interrupt progress before we can show our compassionate heart. That obscures our wisdom. Such interruptions prevent us from gaining clarity and acting appropriately. But in Dzogchen Practice, we get clarity through wisdom and being aware of a situation without the distraction of impatience. We learn to be stable and respond with equanimity. That way, when wisdom and compassion both exist in the present, clear decisions come forth that work best for the situation without being based on fear.

June 21: Know What Is (Summer Solstice Today)

SACRED DANCE

Repeat the sacred dance movements from this week until you're able to get into a flow.

MEDITATION AND PRACTICE

Dzogchen was the understanding that embodied human consciousness manifested in the first place because beings failed to recognize that all phenomena arose as the creativity of the nature of mind. Beings missed their own luminescence or didn't recognize the qualities of ground and knowledge. In other words, they didn't "recognize their own face." That led to sentient beings arising, and people forgot they were enlightened, nirvanic beings. Sacred dance was a way to help people who were driven by an inner leading to restore that memory.

The clarity gained from Dzogchen Practice helps us recognize that whatever emotion we experience is not separate from the true nature of the Soul and Spirit. It's our body dharma in action. This recognition is wisdom. Wisdom gives us the strength to accept things as they are while taking appropriate action in a very Spirit-connected way. We accept our feelings but don't allow them to rule our life even for a split second. We do not allow them to obstruct our path to nirvana.

Disappointment may make you angry. Anger may flow right into hatred (outward expression) or depression (inward expression). Either is hurtful. You can trace the impact of excitement in this way too. If you're excited about something, you form an expectation of it. Then when expectations aren't meant, or the excitement subsides, you might desire more of it. When it isn't forthcoming, you can get angry. Thus, you begin that cycle over and over. By the very nature of living on this plane, everything arises, abides, and then departs. It doesn't stay forever.

❋ ❋ ❋

JUNE 22–30
Transformation Through Healing (Entry Point)

Constantly tap into yourself.

We never see how many times a sculptor taps a stone; we only see what emerges after innumerable faithful taps.

June 22: Transformative Healing

SACRED DANCE

For this week's Sacred Dance Meditation, you may want to avail yourself of Tibetan flowing clothing to wear over or as your Sacred Dance Attire, to connect to the Divine feminine. Begin with a pose:

your right foot held up with the knee at hip height in front of you, and the left hand held at your heart chakra, palm open and facing right, with the right arm gently placed at your right side. Make a quarter turn, swinging the right foot behind you and then to the floor as you pivot on the left foot, keeping your palm at your heart chakra and allowing your right arm to swing slightly behind you. Once the right foot touches the floor, lift your arms wide and away from your ears, elbows bent at shoulder height, and lift your left knee to hip height. Make a quarter turn back toward where you started, placing the left foot on the floor behind you. Keep the arms up, and now lift the right knee to hip height and swivel around and place the right foot on the floor behind the left. You should be facing in the opposite direction now. Keep the arms up, lift the right foot, with the leg straight this time, and swivel in a counterclockwise direction, holding the right leg out in front of you as you keep the standing leg slightly bent. Step forward on the right foot, and now swing the left foot out to turn in a clockwise motion, swiveling on the right foot, and place the left foot down on the floor in front of you. Practice the movements until you get the hang of them, and remember to have fun as you swing from one direction to the other.

MEDITATION AND PRACTICE

Ancient Tibetan religion, which incorporated both Bon and Buddhist thought, championed the idea of evolving into a dakini, or a female embodiment of enlightenment, the greatest enlightened being. Dakinis were energetic beings in female form who evoked movement energy along with the elements. The role was considered more attainable for women due to what was considered their innate connection to Spirit. Dakinis were associated with Bon healing principles and were linked to spirituality, health, and well-being through acknowledging the connection between mind, body, and Spirit.

Ancient Tibetans believed that human civilization originated with them. Their medicine, which emerged within the shamanic Bon era, incorporated the five elements (earth, water, fire, air, and space), which were considered the underlying mechanisms for human life. Ancient Tibetans employed the five elements dance to balance themselves and their humors. They believed that illness came from three mental poisons, or humors as they were called: ignorance, attachment, and aversion. Each person was born with a unique mental, emotional, and physical constitution and into particular lifestyles and circumstances. These formed the person's inbred health and wellness affinities and spiritual vitality. Of course, Sacred Dance Meditation played an integral role in directing wellness and wholeness, regardless of one's makeup at birth. Ancient Tibetans employed the five elements dance to balance themselves and their humors. The sacred dance could bring together and awaken "natural healing energies in the mind and body. The techniques [were] designed to deepen the practitioner's connection with the five elements … which are the energetic undercurrent that form and affect the physical world, including [human] bodies."[*] The sacred dance was therefore a sacred dance of manifestation, purity, and enlightenment, a calling to transform oneself into a dakini.

As we know, integration of mind, body, and Spirit is required for transformative healing. This means that our lifestyles must be congruent in what we eat, what we watch, what we say, what we think, how we act, and what we do. Ignorance, negative attitudes, and attachments to desires keep us from evolving into dakinis. The spiritual path is said to be the hardest path anyone can follow because of the constant evolution and awareness that happens to you and the seemingly miniscule and slow changes that manifest, all while still in human form.

What are your thoughts on mind, body, and Spirit congruity? Sometimes it seems like there's more to give up than to gain. Do you think you have to abstain from certain practices that the popular world follows? Does this abstaining incite your deepest longing for transformation?

---

[*] "Bon Healing," Bon Shen Ling: Tibetan Bon Education Fund, accessed July 2, 2020, http://www.bonshenling.org/bon-healing.

June 23: Lifestyle Transformation

SACRED DANCE

Review the sequence given on June 22 until you feel comfortable with it. When you reach the end, shift your weight to your right foot, and swivel as you lift the left leg out in front of your body, arms remaining up. Place the left foot down behind the right. Shift the weight onto the left foot, lift the right leg, and swing it around clockwise to bring the right foot down behind the left. You will alternate the shifting and swinging the legs several times. Practice until you're laughing hysterically and you forget you're trying. Try to coordinate your breath with the movements.

MEDITATION AND PRACTICE

The ancient Tibetans thought the five elements manifested themselves in the body as energy and matter. All illnesses were considered a result of imbalanced humors. The five elements Sacred Dance Meditation was used to return to balance and to bring forth the much-needed connection to the elements.

The mind has its movements, and we need to make sure it moves where we want it to, and not the other way around. That's one of the points of Sacred Dance Meditation: to direct the mind to act only for our Highest Good. Tibetan medicine explains that everything in the world derives from the mind and the five elements; all things depend on the mind's movements. It's the source and creator of every external and internal thing we see and feel. The mind then is responsible for good health. It's also the location of the three mental poisons of attachment, anger, and closed-mindedness, which are produced by not knowing or forgetting the power we hold. When sacred dance is connected to the mind, through mantras and intentions for the good of all, and as a result the elements are in balance, then the humors act on our behalf. As has been written, we transform ourselves by renewing our minds. Lifestyle transformations occur over time and can range from big sweeping changes such as finding a new career that supports our innermost Self, to better sleep practices so that we achieve better rest.

June 24: Consumption Transformation

SACRED DANCE

Notice how you feel today and if you feel out of balance from any recent thoughts, words, or deeds. Center yourself, and embody your Inner Mystic Dancer. When you're ready, review and repeat the sacred dance given on June 23. As you end the alternating swings with the legs straight, keeping your arms up, then with feet together turn four or five times clockwise by taking small stepping movements in place. Then pause, and repeat this moving counterclockwise. Be careful not to get dizzy!

MEDITATION AND PRACTICE

In ancient Tibetan language, *loong* was the subtle flow of energy circulating throughout the body and supported all movements and activities connected with mind, speech and body. Sacred Dance Meditation had the most powerful impact on the body because of that. *Mkhrispa* was heat energy, which circulated throughout the body and balanced bodily temperature, digestion, and vitality. *Bad-kan* was a fluid energy, which was associated with flexibility, bodily stability, and healing systems. Ancient Tibetans had knowledge of the interconnectedness of all the body's systems. They knew that these systems were intimately connected, and when they were unbalanced, the result was illness. Illness prevented people from reaching a dakini level of enlightenment.

These days, when we encounter someone with a unique daily spiritual Practice, we may judge that person or ourselves in our thoughts: *I wish I were as disciplined with my food intake*, or, *I think their clothing behaviors are strange and exclusionary*. Even those enlightened beyond belief still can be affected by consumerism in everyday life. We still need to make choices. Do we choose the sugar cereal, make our own, or stop eating cereal altogether because of what we learn about the origins of grains? Do we choose to avoid articles made of leather or other animal parts? The answers depend upon each person's understanding of what consumption means to their spirituality. Each person must decide what is needed and what to consume.

Recently, someone said that a person doesn't have to pay attention to any of these aspects of sacred awareness because they are not as important as focusing on responses given in human interactions. If you're inclined, write about your consumption and how it has aided your transformation, or how you think it can.

June 25: Being in the Elements for Transformation

SACRED DANCE

Review the sacred dance choreography given this week. Perform the dance presented on June 22, followed by the dance of June 23, and finally the June 24 dance. Just remember to have fun and let go with it, keeping in mind that you're dancing sacredly with the elements.

MEDITATION AND PRACTICE

The main healing methods in ancient Tibetan medicine were based on the proper intake of foods for nutrition, engaging in a proper livelihood to assist others in their spiritual development, and the use of Sacred Dance Meditations to balance the humors. Within the application of the five elements Sacred Dance Meditation, wind elements supported breathing and gave sacred dancers strength to move and to manage movements of physical powers inside them. Bile elements provided courage and the use of the intellect to apply to meditation and prayer. Phlegm elements strengthened the body and mind to continue to balance the sacred dancer in achieving the mystical aspiration of emerging as a dakini.

The body is active physically all the time. Some of the action is automatic, such as the beating of the heart and breathing of the lungs, and some is directed by what you tell your body to do, such as to lift your knee.

But nowadays, we understand from the work of Herbert Benson, MD, and others who practice transformative healing, that we can control many aspects of the body's physical activities by how we think, the kind of livelihood or work we do, how much we meditate and pray, and, of course, what we consume. An integral aspect of our transformation relies on these conscious decisions and routinely being physically in touch with the elements: water, earth, air, fire, and Spirit. Have you lay down on the earth lately? Bathed yourself in a natural water source? Pondered in front of a flame (controlled, mind you!), or been in the open air of a breathtaking, awe-inspiring countryside? Have you done any Sacred Dance Meditations outdoors? What plans do you have to regularly engage with the elements?

June 26: You Have to Rebalance

SACRED DANCE

Review what was done for the Sacred Dance Meditation on June 25. After the clockwise and counterclockwise turns and at the end of the sequence where you have your right foot out in front of your body, shift the weight to your right foot, and now swivel as you lift the left leg out in front of your body, arms remaining up. Place the left foot down behind the right. Shift the weight onto the left foot, lift the right leg, and swing it around clockwise to bring the right foot down behind the left. You will alternate the shifting and swinging the legs for several breaths. Try to coordinate your breath with the leg swings. You conclude with your arms up, feet together, knees slightly bent.

MEDITATION AND PRACTICE

The three poisons were desire, aggression, and ignorance. They came from imbalanced humors, what people did and consumed, and how they thought. But importantly, the ancient Tibetans thought that the three poisons were exacerbated by the influence of spirits. According to their beliefs, there were 360 female spirits connected with desire, 360 male spirits connected with aggression, and 360 water-dwelling and earth spirits connected with ignorance. The three poisons could be eliminated through Sacred Dance Meditation and other purification rites.

Desire in and of itself is perfectly fine. We desire nourishment and sustenance, a warm bed to sleep in, love from appropriate people, and so forth. But when it gets out of hand, we can't be satisfied; we beat ourselves up psychologically and cause internal stress. We wind up with headaches, back pains, indigestion. Then we find ourselves getting angry because life is not what we wanted. The multitude of spirits connected to the ancient Tibetans' three poisons means countless tiny but significant ways can get us off balance when we allow our desires, anger, and lack of knowledge to direct our path. The key is remaining in balance, but that first means we notice immediately when we begin the spiral down and choose not to go there.

Here is a perfect place where the point of Sacred Dance Meditation is useful. Use your body to change the desire, the aggression, and the ignorance. Remember the truth deep in your body's cells.

June 27: Spiritual Stress Transformation

SACRED DANCE

Let's put it all together today. Please practice the sacred dance given this week so that you're familiar with it without needing to review the video.

MEDITATION AND PRACTICE

In addition to the three poisons (attachment, anger, closed-mindedness) and the three humors (wind, bile, phlegm) that affected the body, the Ancient Tibetans believed in the five winds. They were associated with movement of energy down the body through the chakras: The creative wind resided in the crown chakra, ruling over bodily functions and sustaining life. The breath contained Spirit and animated human beings and allowed them to make choices, pray, meditate, and engage with Spirit. The ascending wind resided in the throat chakra, enabling speech, keeping people well-colored, and helping memory. The pervasive wind resided at the heart chakra, pervaded the whole body, and allowed for all movements. The wind of the sacral chakra was considered fiery and allowed transformation.

Lastly, the descending Wind, located at the root chakra, expelled waste and eliminated unwanted thoughts and emotions.

Appropriate use of desire is needed to transform and eliminate spiritual stress. Spiritual Stress causes the imbalances in the first place; that is, you're out of alignment with what you are here on earth to do. Each desire that arises in you should be subjected to the five winds, so that you can really discern their underlying nature. Everything needs to be examined with this lens, from when you arise in the morning to when, where, and why you take vacations. This kind of evaluation can happen at lightning speed with the human mind on its own. Yet your thoughts need to be placed in this energy-movement filter first to determine what you'll keep in mind, what you do and say, and what you'll expel as waste. It all starts in the head, and with Spirit leading. Otherwise you have the thousands of spirits taking hold and jerking you every which way.

June 28: Using Prayer Flags for Transformation

SACRED DANCE

Practice the sacred dance today, and find ways to improvise and own the choreography and sequences. Try holding the idea that you're moving the five elements in your body while you balance the three humors as you dance.

MEDITATION AND PRACTICE

In addition to the five winds, the ancient Tibetans valued the five biles and the five phlegms. The five biles impacted aggression; they resided in the intestines, liver, heart, eye, and skin. The bile that resided in the heart and in the eye caused desire, aggression and ignorance, which in turn impacted the other two. The five phlegms were to be used for consternation, to contemplate ideas, actions, or subjects. From these phlegms, one's likes and dislikes were created to produce feelings of wholeness or separateness.

Through using the five elements, Sacred Dance Meditation seekers endeavored to rebalance their desires and appreciate knowledge, warding off the negative spirits. To do so, sacred dancers often utilized prayer flags, which represented the elements, to enlist Spirit in aiding them to rightly place and realign their desires, to detach, and to reduce aggression and delusion. Prayer flags were handmade of natural fabric and hung outdoors in the elements so the gods and goddesses could see them and make themselves available to the sacred dancer, getting rid of hundreds of spirits that interfered with opening the way for clarity.

It may be difficult to believe in or validate the different biles, but it's not difficult to use prayer flags to remind us of our deepest desires, which we align with G-d's desires for us and which can reduce our spiritual stress. Prayer flags are hung where the wind can touch them. Their movement creates emanating vibrations, which in turn create natural positive energy. On a spiritual level, this energy protects you and others from harm and brings harmony to everything the wind touches. Before hanging a prayer flag, you vibrate intentions and prayers on each segment of the flag. Make a prayer flag for yourself and your community today. Buy swatches of colored fabrics that represent the five elements, and as you sew them together with cords or thick yarn, imbue them with your intentions and prayers. You can hang the prayer flag somewhere outside your dwelling where the wind will carry your intentions. No one will know what the flag stands for unless you explain. But recall secrecy is a key practice in this work.

June 29: Five Pure Lights

SACRED DANCE

Practice and improvise today as you hold the idea that you're moving the five elements in your body, in your Sacred Dance Studio, and out in the Universe while you balance the three humors as you engage in Sacred Dance Meditation.

MEDITATION AND PRACTICE

The Five Pure Lights was an essential teaching in the ancient Tibetan Dzogchen tradition. Knowledge was the absence of delusion. Seeing the Five Pure Lights produced the rainbow body, a nonmaterial body of light manifested through the transformative Practices of Sacred Dance Meditation and other rituals. Everything the sacred dancer sought and felt as the body mandala was purified and realized by the Five Pure Lights. A kind of sanctification returned them to their awareness of singularity and union with the Divine. The perceiver and the perception were continuous.

Reaching the state of the five wisdom dakinis is our aim when merging the body-mind with Spirit. It's a level where we are not bothered by anything, choices about right acts and decisions aren't debated, resentments and anger don't enter, we aren't deluded, and we know to our core that we are here on earth doing G-d's work for the good of every being, seen or unseen, that was here or will be here. And through our way of being, we influence the people in our lives to want what we have because they see our peace, fruits, and Higher Power.

June 30: Great Perfection in Transformation

SACRED DANCE

Dance until you reach a trance, as you have brought the dance into your body, mind, and Spirit.

MEDITATION AND PRACTICE

As taught in the ancient Tibetan traditions, each of the Five Lights in the Five Elements Sacred Dance had meaning.

The luminous white light of wisdom, associated with the element of water, was the manifestation of knowledge's immaculate, pure, and completely pacified nature. If meditated upon, white cut the delusion of ignorance and turned it into the wisdom of the ultimate reality.

Blue, associated with the element of Spirit, was associated with purity and healing. It was believed that when meditating on this color, anger could be transformed into wisdom. The blue light symbolized the unchanging nature of knowledge, a state beyond all confusion.

Red light, linked to the element of fire, was related to the Life Force and preservation. Meditating on red transformed the delusion of attachment into the wisdom of discernment. The red light was the manifestation of the quality of knowledge that included, attracted, and magnetized.

Green, linked with the element of wind, was the color of balance and harmony. Meditation on this color transformed jealousy into the wisdom of accomplishment. The green light meant that knowledge manifested as compassion, love, and wisdom in all interactions.

Yellow, associated with the element of earth, symbolized rootedness and renunciation. Yellow transformed pride into the wisdom of sameness when visualized in meditation. Yellow symbolized a fully manifested knowledge, meaning the enlightened wisdoms necessary to overcome emotions, ignorance, and delusions that were present.

In perceiving our Light correctly in line with the elements, we experience perfected transformation into the rainbow body.

JULY

Celebrating Epiphanies

GRECIAN SACRED DANCE

Ancient Greek Sacred Dance Meditation aids us in understanding and interpreting our freedoms this month. We have many freedoms, and no freedom is separate from Spirit. Even in situations with untreated codependency, grief, and recovery, there exists a level of spiritual opportunity. We take lessons from the indigenous Greek peoples to propel us forward in our spiritual journey to freedom. The Minoans, the Pelasgians, the Mycenaeans, and ancient Greeks give us insights into how we can celebrate and own our freedoms.

THE MINOANS

Crete was home to the Minoan people, who lived from around 3000 to 1400 BCE. A significant Minoan ritual was epiphany, or when the goddess appeared in the community. Getting an appearance was individually driven and involved Sacred Dance Meditations. In this epiphany scene, the deity descends from the sky, her hair waving in the air. Or sometimes she is rendered as receiving the supplications of the faithful in a sacred enclosure close to a pedestal or a sacred tree.

Almost all the community celebrations had a sacred character and used Sacred Dance Meditation and supporting accouterments. Sacred dance brought enchantment and connection and contributed to epiphanic visions. Sacred dance was relied upon as a communication vehicle. Ritual celebrations were part of Sacred Dance Meditation and worship of nature goddesses. People used music, dance, and prayer to achieve a state of ecstasy, putting them in touch with the sacred feminine. The worshippers came to the sanctuary or near to the vision of a goddess with their torsos inclined backward and one hand on their head. Other gestures included raised hands, outstretched arms, and crouching, for supplications, prayers, and devotion. They may represent the successive phases of sacred dance movements when, for example, the hands were extended forward and then drawn back close to the body.

THE PELASGIANS

The Pelasgians were the ancestors of the Greeks and Minoans and indigenous peoples near the Aegean Sea. These ancients survived in several locations of mainland Greece, Crete, and other regions of the Aegean. They were inhabitants until around 1700 BCE, when some natural disasters and wars began to minimize the kingdoms.

According to the Pelasgians, creation is attributed to the goddess Eurynome. She manifested from chaos, the great nothingness, and the void before time and space, and her first act separated water from the sky. Next, she danced across the water. As she meditated on existence, she danced in the four cardinal directions and eventually to the south, swirling so that wind came up behind her. Eurynome turned and grabbed the wind between her hands and formed it into a stream, which resembled a serpent. She called this stream of wind Ophion and gave it energy and masculinity. He watched as the goddess danced and felt drawn to the love and power contained in her sacred dance.

She created the seven planetary powers, appointing a titaness and a titan to rule over each; this will be discussed in greater length later this month. Eurynome was the goddess, mother, creator, and ruler over every person, place, and thing. And she partnered with Ophion to create living beings on earth, and they moved into Mount Olympus, dwelling there until the time came when Ophion and Eurynome had to part ways, due to his desire to take credit for creating the Universe. This began the change of the way that Sacred Dance Meditation went forth with the Mycenaeans.

THE MYCENAEANS

The Mycenaean civilization rose to prominence after the Minoan heyday and flourished until 1100 BCE. Lore tells us that the Mycenaeans were originally from Crete, their ancestors were Minoan, and aspects of the sacred feminine prevailed. Some suggest that the Mycenaean spiritual Practices provided the foundation for the Greek religion. Since the Mycenaeans came from Minoa, they were sacred dance meditators who inherited the Practice. The priestess and the attendants prayed and meditated through sweeping circular and processional dances, supplementing them with offerings and sacrifices in gratitude. They danced in the countryside, in rocky landscapes, under sacred trees, and around altars, with men playing the lute and harp. The dances were aimed at provoking the visual appearance of the goddess to her worshippers, the so-called epiphany.

ANCIENT GREEKS

For the ancient Greeks, sacred dance was the spiritual sustenance for people. They followed the traditions instituted in Crete, which they conquered around 1500 BCE. The ancient Greeks considered dance an essential part of both spiritual development and education, so it became widespread. Ancient Greek leaders differentiated Apollonian and Dionysian dance. Apollonian dance incorporated thoughtful and slow movements, carried out during religious festivals and sacred ceremonies, like funerals and weddings. Conversely, wild and feverish dancing was associated with Dionysus, who represented passion, pursuit of ecstasy, and desire.

Ancient Greek dance evolved to include both men and women. Dancers circled around an altar, with a votive offering of personal objects left as gifts to the gods. The people believed that anything dedicated to the god being revered was retained within the god's *temenos*, which was a sacred wall encircling a sanctuary. This type of offering was both a private devotion and a pious act with public recognition, which came at times during sacred dances accompanying processions. In general, men and women danced separately. Greek sacred dancers covered themselves completely with sacred clothing when dancing.

PREPARATION

You may want to add some very flowing garments, decorative or charged beads, and scarves to your Sacred Dance Attire for this month. Draped scarves and headbands with gold or silver colors may be part of it. In addition, you may want to use music that includes slow melodies using lyres, lutes, and kitharas. You can continue the practice of setting up incense, but for this month you may want to establish a fragrance bowl, using fresh citrus, rose, gardenia, and eucalyptus oils infused in water. Use a large glass bowl from your kitchen, and deem it sacred by stating an intention over it and removing it out of circulation for eating and cooking. Or buy a bowl for this sacred purpose. Alternatively, you may want to use an infuser for fragrance.

Please visit www.cswalter.org/sacreddancemeditations for video demonstrations. They are not intended to be step-by-step instructions but are meant to give you a view of the sacred dance.

Freedoms (Entry Point)

The crucible exists in our minds. What we think can alter our reality.

Epiphanies come through our choices and actions. This is the root of mindfulness.

This week, a long silk scarf or other lightweight fabric would be good to complement your Sacred Dance Attire and may set a particular feeling and state of mind.

July 1: Thought Freedoms

SACRED DANCE

Begin facing east, bending forward from the hips with knees bent. Imagine you're an idea being generated and simultaneously generating new thoughts that you've never had before. Unfurl your body, but keep the knees bent as you float your arms up over your head, then bring them to shoulder height and twist your torso slowly as your bring the right arm slowly to the front and the left arm to the back. Your palms face each other and are lightly cupped. Then swing the left arm across your body and the right arm behind you. Step forward on the left foot with the left arm leading and your head tilted to the right. Sweep the right arm in front of you as you walk counterclockwise to face the opposite direction. Keep moving but then change your energy to walk clockwise, with the right arm leading and the head tilted to the left. Repeat these meditations twice on each side.

MEDITATION AND PRACTICE

The Minoan society was based on a matriarchal and goddess-based spirituality. Ancient Cretans danced in circles, around trees, around altars, or among mystical creations to free themselves from the mundane, enter divine discourse, and experience change. Through these dances, often accompanied by music, it was normal to experience an epiphany, an experience of intimacy with a goddess descended from on high to greet the seeker.

Though Crete would yield to the Greeks later and influence their philosophies greatly, before then the people freely thought about their interactions with the Divine with little interference. From them we know that we have freedom of thought, conscience, and ideas. We have abilities to consider and revise our points of view, practices, beliefs, and knowledge apart from what others think or believe or what others want us to believe. This is the key to all our freedoms and the basis for the international human-rights laws. An epiphany happens when a new thought or experience revises us. Some people have them when they realize they have moved to another spiritual plateau without trying. Have you ever had an epiphany? Do you have freedom of thought? What do you spend your time thinking about?

July 2: Thinking and Seeing the Divine

SACRED DANCE

Prepare your Sacred Dance Attire as you did on July 1. Imagine that you can live outside of any preconceived set of beliefs and that what you see with your eyes is only a limited glimpse into a tiny portion of the Universe. Repeat the sacred dance given on July 1 until you're roughly back to the starting position. Then swing the left arm across your body and the right arm behind you. Step forward on the left foot with the left arm leading and your head tilted to the right. Sweep the right arm in front of you as you walk counterclockwise to complete the circle, then sweep the left arm in front of you as you walk clockwise to complete the circle. Repeat this twice on each side. Reach into the sweeps and tilt your head; breathe.

MEDITATION AND PRACTICE

For ancient Cretans, an epiphany was experienced by seeing the feminine deity physically in a person who interacted with the practitioners during a Sacred Dance Meditation, and, as a result, the Cretans revised their beliefs.

The ancient Cretans expected to interact with the Divine regularly and without any fear of ridicule. They apparently thought freely and weren't restrained. Of course, we don't know for sure that they weren't coerced into saying they saw something when they didn't or into toeing the line when they secretly rejected a belief system. Assuming their reports were authentic, the interaction with the Divine occurred daily. Perhaps, though, the interactions weren't on a grand scale but were subtler, such as when disagreement with systems of thought could be expressed and supported. In other words, the Cretans likely allowed themselves to see clearly and to align their thinking with their most desired Highest Good.

Do you allow new information to revise your spiritual knowledge? Are you thinking freely enough to interact with the Divine?

July 3: Divinely Inspired Free Will

SACRED DANCE

Today, imagine that you have unlimited wonderful paths to follow and that you have just been made aware that you have been locked in an illusion, trapped in time and space, but that now you're free. Revisit the sacred dance movements given on July 2. Picking up where you left off, take two forward steps starting with the right foot. As you sweep the arms up away from your body to the left, step backward two steps, lower the arms, and then reach upward and arch your back to the right as far as is comfortable. Take three steps forward, and sweep the right arm in front of you. Take three steps to the right, lift the arms up, and take three steps backward. Sweep the arms down, and bend your torso forward; sweep the arms to the right, and step around in a clockwise circle.

MEDITATION AND PRACTICE

Sacred dances in ancient Crete were created and taught by Zeus's mother, Rhea, and presented in her temple, built at the palatial and matriarchal city of Phaistos, Crete, where she was from. Through her, Cretans thought about their relationship with each sacred dance experience, and it was part of daily life. Yet, according to legend, she finally saw during her sacred dance one day that her husband Kronos devoured her ideas that had come through her in the form of babies. In an epiphanic moment, she decided to hand him a rock dressed up like a baby instead of her baby Zeus, who was her last-born. The Divine had given her a vision; it was idiosyncratic, a specific personal epiphany only for her.

If you consider that it takes a year for a human child to be born, ten years may have gone by before Rhea could trust an intimate connection with the Divine to exercise her free will. If we take the birth of a child to be a metaphor for an idea or change to manifest and the devouring her husband relates to ideas squashed, we can find some compassion for ourselves. What actions or nonactions are eating us alive? Do we have a free will in it? Yes, we do. Time is eating us alive. We must wake up! So much of what we want to create is lost to a poor use of time. The thing about free will and free thought is that it's up to us. No one can see what we're thinking until we act.

July 4: Choices Made

SACRED DANCE

Today, think about the courage Rhea embodied when she gave Kronos a rock dressed in blankets instead of her child. Picking up where you left off on July 3, lean forward, and sweep the arms down toward the earth. Then sweep them backward clockwise, and lean backward to your level of comfort, all the way around. Then, bend your knees, and bring the arms down in front of you. Turn counterclockwise, and walk in a circle as you sweep the arms to the left. Then lean forward, and sweep the arms down toward the earth. Next, lean backward, and sweep them counterclockwise. Repeat on both sides. Facing the opposite direction that you started in, roll down through your spine, bend your waist and your knees, and rest your elbows on your thighs; bow your head. Hold for a few breaths to conclude.

In Crete when the Minoans were influential, priestesses led worshippers, and women engaged with sacred dance to honor the snake goddess. The serpent was associated with the renewal of life because it shed it skin, was considered the protector of the house, and signified wisdom and fertility. The snake goddesses in Crete wore a sacral knot as a part of their Sacred Dance Attire. It represented the sacred feminine and, by association, eternal enlightenment. The snake goddess held the snakes in a proffering stance, to convey great revelatory authority and power from deities dwelling both above and below the earth. The sacral knot was the symbol of holiness, a gift from goddesses who only showed themselves during an epiphany to those who could see.

The sacral knot can be considered a symbol of an enlightened choice made by the people of ancient Crete. The sacred dance enabled them to experience epiphanies, which in turn opened their eyes to an array of choices perhaps they'd never imagined. It's been said that we are the sum of our choices. What we think shows up in every aspect of our lives—whom we marry, how we feel, where we live and work, how we worship, what our beliefs are—and in this way people see what we think of ourselves and our abilities. Write some notes in your journal about what people see about you and your choices. Do you think it's too late to explore all your choices? Have you had ideas about choices and just dismissed them because you thought they were impossible, too late, too hard, too expensive? Or do you just disallow them?

July 5: Imagining Impact and Welfare Through Thought

SACRED DANCE

As you prepare today, imagine that you can sense positive change coming to you from all directions and there is no limit of the good available to your mind, body, and Spirit. In our work today, we combine the pieces of the sacred dance from July 1, 2, and 3. Practice putting all the moves together in a fluid sequence.

In Ancient Crete, the labrys, an icon for the mother goddess, was an important sacred symbol of spiritual Practice associated with female goddesses. For the Minoans, the symbol represented the sacred feminine and earthly priestesses and was the image of matriarchy. Any Minoan woman with a labrys held a powerful position within Minoan society. When combined with the labrys, the sacral knot represented welfare in an ongoing eternal life. These sacred supports were used in dance meditations, which were held in Rhea's temple and other places.

The labrys represented transformation; when it was placed with a sacral knot, sacred manifestation was unstoppable. Like the sacred feminine goddesses of ancient Crete, we can imagine our impact if we open to our power. Sometimes the limits we put on ourselves or the expectation of good coming from a particular direction can squelch the impact on our own being. Can you imagine a situation in your life comparable to that of the ancient Cretans? That is, do you engage in Sacred Dance Meditations, avail yourself of, and interact with, powerful emblems, and seek epiphanies to continue to think freely? Do you have an open mind? Do you think only one method can lead to self-realization? Do you feel the flow of the Divine from all directions?

July 6: Palatial Freedom

In our work today, we combine the pieces of the sacred dance from the first four days of this week. You may review them if you like. Combine all the motions you've learned from July 1, 2, 3, and 4. Practice putting all the moves together in a fluid sequence.

The people who lived in ancient Cretan civilizations manifested their freedom by thinking palatially. It wasn't that they had to practice visioning excellence and good; they were just that way. The area was considered palatial, with abundance being the norm. At the time, no fortifications or controlling devices signaled a power structure intent on holding people in subservience. Rather, the Minoans were elegant, with fine clothing; their sensitive ways guided their interactions. They had refined tastes, loved luxury, and honored politeness and formal manners, while interacting in compassionate ways with their trading partners and neighbors. These were people gifted with spiritual intelligence who relied on deities and epiphanies to move them forward through their Sacred Dance Meditation.

We can learn a great deal about thought freedom from studying our Cretan ancestors and their Sacred Dance Meditations. So much of what we do and say is conditioned. In the Western world, where competitiveness and control have been the norm, we see the results of the lack of freedom to think positively and considerately of others. The orientation affects us on many levels and often puts us in the mindset of being victims or martyrs. Can you imagine being in a world of abundance, where you can think spiritual thoughts all the time? Although no one reads your mind, we see your mind in your life's manifestations. What do you spend most of your time thinking about? When you listen to your thoughts, who is speaking to you? Do any of your thoughts come from your heart, your Spirit? List three things in your journal you want to change in your thinking and what you expect to gain from that change.

July 7: Congruence in Thinking

SACRED DANCE

Please review the first day of this week to get a sense of the Sacred Dance Attire. We practice the dance meditation fully today, which was described fully on July 6. Review it if you're inclined. As the week concludes, free yourself to the sacred, and as you do embody the freedom of thought you enjoy and the decisions you have made to expand your epiphanies.

MEDITATION AND PRACTICE

The people of Crete inscribed a disc with signs drawn in a single spiraling line reminiscent of fractals, which they grouped together to form words separated by vertical lines. It was a sacred text used in dance meditations to honor the sacred feminine. These signs were also inscribed on the labrys. With this Phaistos disc, the sacral knot, and the labrys, the Sacred Dance Meditations, were ignited with praise. Each sacred dancer freely connected with the Divine to open his or her mind to receive repeated enlightenments.

Enlightenments, like epiphanies, occur all the time if we are progressing spiritually. Ancient Minoans believed that aligning one's personal epiphanies with outward reminders of manifestations aided one in harmonizing spiritual practice and life. Therefore, thoughts and prayers to the Divine, along with dance meditation and the knowledge of freedom and change, was completely personal. At the same time, one was free to not change, and this was also a harmonization between spiritual practice and life. So often we think and believe what we've been told to think and believe. Sometimes it's easier to do that, but ultimately we need to exercise the Divine right of freedom of thought.

JULY 8–14
I Do What I Do Like I Do Because I Do (Entry Point)

Out of chaos comes creativity.

The ancient Greeks knew that creation comes from chaos or nothingness. We embrace chaos for the good it has to offer, for the new creations awaiting our consciousness.

For this week's sacred dances, again supplement your Sacred Dance Attire with soft, flowy, loose garments and a long silk scarf or one made from another soft fabric. Soft and soothing music featuring primarily string instruments is ideal. You're completely free to use scented waters, low-light-emitting candles, and incense to create an atmosphere of tranquility.

July 8: Chaos

SACRED DANCE

Stand facing east, and think of the ancient Greek gods and goddesses and the freedoms they enjoyed, which were guided by ethos and principles. With scarves draped over your hands, slowly reach them upward toward the sky, and follow their reach with your eyes. Imagine the universe expanding around you as you look. Keeping your hands held high, slowly and deliberately turn clockwise 360 degrees and then counterclockwise 360 degrees, leaning slightly toward the direction you're turning. Repeat four times in each direction. Inhale when you begin to turn, and exhale when you complete a turn. Return to the eastward-facing position, and let your arms rest by your sides, keeping your scarves from falling to the floor.

MEDITATION AND PRACTICE

Chaos was the state of the Universe from which everything else came. At that point, chaos was all there was and was creation in potential. The ancients of Crete worshipped goddesses and sky gods and engaged in dance meditation to their benefit. Sacred Dance Meditation was the norm, and it was from within the matriarchal Divine sacred feminine aspect that we see chaos being handled.

We enjoy our freedom to be as we are, especially in the Western world. Some people are guided by commandments, and others are guided by precepts. Most of us have an internal set of principles that guides how we act and induces us to think in certain ways. But sometimes the beliefs we've adopted need revision, especially when life seems out of control. Sometimes we think freedom happens in isolation. But we are all connected, so what we do and think every day impacts everyone. And unbeknownst to us, we can create frenetic environments—otherwise known as drama!

One of the principles of chaos is called the butterfly effect. It supposes that power to cause a hurricane in Asia can come from a butterfly flapping its wings in North America. Though it may take a while for the effect to show up, the idea is that by flapping its wings at just the right time and place, the butterfly can start a hurricane. The point is that small changes consistently applied lead to drastic changes.

July 9: Choice Reactions

SACRED DANCE

Begin where you left off yesterday. Stand facing east and, with your scarves draped over your hands, extend them in front of your body. With your arms extended and moving from your shoulders, slowly make a clockwise circle with the hands, and then move your arms in the counterclockwise direction. Keep your gaze toward the horizon, tilting your head naturally as you repeat the movements eight times, alternating directions. Your face is relaxed, and you have a pleasant affect. As you do these moves, gently step side to side in the direction of the arm movements. Just let it flow, nice and easy, and feel comfortable with improvising.

MEDITATION AND PRACTICE

The goddess Eurynome came from chaos and separated the water from the sky. Next, she began to dance with a soft flowing movement, with Light coming from her Inner Mystic Dancer. With twirls and turns, she created sacred wind and other elements. She also danced in the cardinal directions, expressing the deep gratitude for the ability to influence the Cosmos. As she danced, she created her new Sacred Dance Studio between the earth and sky. Soon she imagined a partner and created him too. After she finished creating the sky, earth, and sea, and her Soul mate, Ophion, the two brought creatures forward to populate the world. It's said that Ophion and Eurynome ruled from Mount Olympus, which is in ancient Crete. Over time, it seems, her partner gave in to fear and was jealous of her creations, which led her to exile him.

We have all heard creation stories of something being created out of nothing and a relationship gone wrong. A god then reacts, or deities come in conflict. Power shifts to the male, and the female deity is silenced. The Sacred Dance Meditations we do with our human Soul mates is dependent upon balance and how we perceive the other and what we want from that person. If we can get into a position where we don't want anything but unconditional love and we want to give ours, we come from a spiritual place, rather than reacting to create more constraints.

How do you react to situations? Are you creating destructive winds behind you, or are you creating joyful breezes? Do you take people hostage, or do you hold them loosely? Do you realize that we have limited time on earth and that you leave your legacy with every reaction and thought? Can you accept a deep commitment to freedom?

July 10: Fluid Boundaries

SACRED DANCE

Stand facing east. With scarves in your right hand and the left hand reaching behind you, step forward with your right foot, inhaling, as you bring the scarves upward toward the sky and you look upward. Exhaling, you step backward on the left foot and bring the scarves toward the earth. Repeat this four times; come to center, change hands with the scarves, and repeat on the left.

MEDITATION AND PRACTICE

Eurynome was known among Pelasgians as the goddess of unity, peace, and balance. She was the icon of Sacred Dance Meditation and the creation of spiritual forces. This ancient Greek goddess embraced the chaos at the beginning of time and made order in the world. Through her sacred dance, the winds were born; from her imagination came the land and the stars. Then She created feminine and masculine rulers for each of the poles of the earth so that balance would be maintained. Pelasgian spiritual Practice was chthonic—that is, earth-focused, feminine in Spirit, matriarchal in structure, but embracing and valuing masculine energies as equal.

The people of Crete followed the goddess Eurynome as well as the snake goddesses and lived a prosperous life. Because of the power the Pelasgians wielded, the stories of these gods and goddesses were subsumed into the spiritual stories, Practices, and beliefs of the peoples that would follow them, including the Titans, Romans, and Egyptians.

In the Western world, sometimes understanding practices of others is difficult because many of us are taught to fear and compete. Getting to the core of this matter sometimes requires setting fluid boundaries. Before we rush to judge a group or an individual, it would behoove us to clearly understand some of the backstory. Most of the creation myths we hear nowadays leave out important parts, thereby giving an unbalanced understanding of spiritual Practices and their purposes. "Snake" and "serpent," for example, turn people off before they comprehend what the animals symbolize.

Do you have fluid or static boundaries about your Practice? Is it possible that a spiritual Practice can contain multiple directions, people, and stories?

July 11: Enough Is Enough!

SACRED DANCE

Facing east, with your scarves and flowing costumes serving as your Sacred Dance Attire, get into your Sacred Dance Posture and connect with your Inner Mystic Dancer. Think of the ancient gods and goddesses and their people and what they may have been feeling when they were secure in their knowledge of the Universe. Imagine the safety and security they felt, the freedom to travel between the earth and sky, and the knowledge of every mystery. Repeat the dance as described on July 8.

MEDITATION AND PRACTICE

Ancient Pelasgians, like many other cultures, sought the power of the serpent for answers to deep questions, growth in their spiritual journeys, and inspiration. A serpent named Ophion was Eurynome's partner, and he loved the earth from Mount Olympus on the holy island of Crete. It was Ophion who had enlightened Man. Over time he became known as the king and Eurynome the queen of the Pelasgians in Crete. Lore tells us that Eurynome and Ophion also ruled Greece and Egypt and the entire Mediterranean Sea. The sacred dances were manifested to celebrate transitions through stages of life, celebrations, and epiphanies. Sacred Dance Meditations were inscribed on seals and ringlets, on pottery and frescoes. Swirling and flowing, sacred dance movements created intentional directions to honor human and godly beings.

In the West, sometimes serpents are considered unpleasant, and people refer to them as demons. But this isn't the whole story. The word *demon* comes from *dæmon*, which is derived from the original Greek ΔΑΙΜΩΝ, meaning knowing, wise, or intelligent, or, as we see the word used today, a supernatural being whose nature is somewhere between that of a god and goddess and that of a human being. Eurynome got tired of fighting with Ophion, who increasingly wanted to dictate her life and take credit for her creations. She got fed up and, with love, cast him out of Mount Olympus, realizing she couldn't change him and that the only person that can be changed is one's self. Through changing our individual behaviors, we change the world and the course of history. What situations have caused you to say, "Enough is enough" and make a change in your behavior? Are you gentle? Kind? Soft-spoken? Slow to anger? Is there something or someone or some entity you need to cast out? Are you facing any of these decisions now? Make some notes in your journal.

July 12: Actions and Words Are the Language of the Heart

SACRED DANCE

With scarves in your right hand and left hand reaching behind you, step forward with your right foot, inhaling, as you bring the scarves upward toward the sky and you look in that direction. Exhaling, step backward on the left foot, and bring the scarves toward the earth. Create a semicircle with the scarves and a line on the floor with your feet. Repeat this four times. Come to center, change hands with the scarves, and repeat on the left. Stand with knees slightly bent. Drape the scarves loosely over your wrists so they will remain intact. Inhale, step forward with the right foot, bringing your feet together, and, beginning on the right side of your body, make four infinity signs with the scarves; exhale. Step backward with the left foot as your hands create a backward circle and come together in front of you. Inhale and repeat with stepping forward on the left foot.

MEDITATION AND PRACTICE

After Eurynome sent Ophion away from Mount Olympus, another period of chaos began. Eurynome engaged Sacred Dance Meditation to embrace it. She created the Seven Planetary Powers with which the gods and goddesses were set to rule. To Theia and Hyperion, she gave the sun and the power of illumination; to Phoebe and Atlas, she granted control of the moon and the power of enchantment. Dione and Crius received Mars and the power of growth, while Metis and Coeus had Mercury and the power of wisdom. Themis and Eurymedon ruled Jupiter and the power of law. Tethys and Oceanus oversaw Venus and the power of love, while Rhea and Cronus had Saturn with the power of peace. Eurynome steadied the balance of energies as she danced forth her words and actions through the language of her heart, and from her work we have these Seven Powers:

- Illumination—to see with Divine light
- Enchantment—to fill ourselves and others with great delight
- Growth—to change and grow closer to the sacred
- Wisdom—to discern what serves us and the rest of the cosmos
- Law—to understand the butterfly effect
- Love—to hold everyone in that space, including ourselves
- Peace—to design a world of unity, balance, and wholeness

It's time for freedom, or to put your loving and appropriate words and action into alignment. From that alignment, fullness, exuberance, and rapture prevail in your life. Reflect on what these seven powers mean to you and how you find them showing up in your freedom to be, freedom to behave, freedom to act. Make a note for each of them, and see if you understand what each of their meanings holds for you.

July 13: Freedom to Receive Feedback

SACRED DANCE

Repeat the motions of the dance you learned on July 8 and 9. Relax your face, and take on a pleasant affect. Remember you're free to move as you'd like, to behave in a manner beneficial to you and to others on earth. Think of your spiritual guides, the way they lead you, and where. As you do these moves, gently step side to side in the direction of the arm movements. Come to rest facing east.

MEDITATION AND PRACTICE

Eurynome was originally the Great Mother Goddess and Creator of All Things. Before that, everything was total chaos. As she danced and meditated, ideas began to come to her, including the notion that she could be with others and experience more than she could in her aloneness. She acted upon that feedback and created a whole new experience, a way to see the Cosmos, and a way to interact with it, for herself and many other beings.

Eurynome may have been pained by her realization because of not wanting to venture away from stillness and darkness. But deep within her the intuition came, giving her feedback about her life and the lives around her. Often our feedback comes from pain or seemingly unrelated events such as multiple betrayals or disillusions. We see that Eurynome had those too, even if she was a goddess. This is an indication that nothing stays the same and everything is always moving and changing. Being grateful for the feedback allows us to do better each day.

Even so-called negative feedback has something for you to see. Are you free to receive the gift of feedback?

July 14: Freedom to Yield

SACRED DANCE

Today, put the whole sacred dance together for this week, from July 8. Each time you lift your arms with the scarves draped over your hands, imagine the universe expanding around you as you look up with the light reaching through your hands and scarves. Repeat from the beginning for as many times as you feel comfortable.

MEDITATION AND PRACTICE

Not long after Eurynome split up with Ophion, Rhea and Cronus took this couple's place as the leaders of Sacred Dance Meditation in ancient Crete. Eurynome yielded to the new thinking and the turn of events that progressed. As a result, the snake goddesses were as all-powerful, loving, and knowing and received the ability to transmit epiphanies, to meet the sacred dance meditators in midair. The power of sacred feminine prevailed, though through the chaos, a new iteration of it was created.

The breakup of Eurynome and Ophion allowed them the opportunity for progress. Though their story is obscured within other stories, it gives the sense that every human being is free to create, to make choices, to behave in ways that benefit. The story also shows that the human condition has not changed, really, since the being of creation. We all must work at overcoming our deepest fears and letting go when holding on doesn't serve us well. Thankfully we have the freedom to yield, surrender, turn the other cheek, or otherwise allow the flow to continue. We are here but for an instant. Our behaviors should be uplifting but appropriate to the situation.

❄   ❄   ❄

JULY 15–21
It's My Spiritual Responsibility?
(Entry Point)

Standing at the Lion Gate: Sphinxes

"This is my doing," is what we have to say, always.

Stand facing east and think of the ancient Greek gods and goddesses and the responsibility that came with their freedom. Add music, lute, and the harp, if you're inclined to do so, along with sacred and charged beads to complement your Sacred Dance Attire. You may also want to have a large, clear, inflated plastic ball to represent the Universe as you do this week's Sacred Dance Meditations.

July 15: One Hundred Percent You

––––––––––––––––––––––––––– SACRED DANCE –––––––––––––––––––––––––––

Gently lift and expand your arms, with wrists loose and palms facing inward. Keep your fingertips from touching, and then make a wide space with them extending away from your body. Imagine you're holding the Universe in your upstretched arms. You have a variety of loving elements, such as stars or nearby worlds or the lighted heavens, surrounding you. The Universe feels heavy, but you can't drop it or let it go. Breathe in and out deeply through your nose if you're able; if not, breathe deeply as you're able. With your feet parallel and together, slightly bend your knees. Sway from your waist as you float the Universe from left to right, six or eight times in each direction, above your head. Slowly move the Universe from above your head to waist level, and continue to sway, equal times on each side, and then bend forward with the same swaying. Return to standing with the Universe held over your head.

Mycenae priestesses were associated with royalty in the palatial citics of Mycenae, Tiryns, Pylos, Athens, and Thebes from about 1600 to 1100 BCE and were usually wealthy. Women with authority over the sacred treasury of a deity were known as key bearers. In times of need, they could dispense funds and had the power to assess a situation and respond accordingly. Sacred Dance Meditations brought forth the certainty of sacred treasury for those who witnessed and engaged with them. They just needed to first claim their role in creating the situation.

What is a sacred treasury today? It could be money, but it could also be support, love, and consideration for beings. It's the unveiling of barriers that prevent forward movement and replacing them with solutions so the Light can shine. So, whatever anyone—parents or other family members, teachers, bosses, or anyone else, alive or transcendent—did to you that you perceive is wrong, you have to work in the present to overcome it and heal. Sadly, healing necessitates walking through the pain and coming to terms with it through intense scrutiny. If you blame anyone for that pain, you're betraying your spiritual promises to yourself. On the flip side of this treasury coin is taking full responsibility of how your actions—regardless of intent—impacted other beings, alive or transcended. Realize that you must never take responsibility for the thoughts and behaviors of others. These points are vital to enjoying freedoms and the vast wealth that comes with using the keys we have.

July 16: Owning Your Amazing Self

Begin with a review of what you learned July 15. Step forward with your arms outstretched in front of you slightly above your throat chakra. Starting with your left foot, take four or five steps on the balls of your feet, then turn toward your left, and take another four or five steps. Realize the energy coming into you as you embrace the Universe and the energy you give it from your Divine position. Stop, slightly bend your knees, and bring your Universe down your left hip, toward your back, then expand and contract your arms as if the Universe were alternating in contraction and expansion. Repeat four times each side. Breathe in with each expansion, exhale with each contraction. You're making fluid movements, gentle yet strong. Now, "toss" the Universe over your head to your right side, and step sideways to quickly "catch it." Keep your arms loose and in a circular frame. Repeat the alternating shrinking and growing, while breathing as described, four times. Step with the right foot, walking on the balls of your feet four or five steps, then turn to your right, back to the place you started. Gently set the Universe down on the floor in front of you. Return to a standing position.

MEDITATION AND PRACTICE

At the city gate in Mycenae, people were greeted with two grand lionesses on both sides of the entry archway. In this palatial society, the lioness, representing divine and mortal power, was associated with the goddesses known for Sacred Dance Meditation prowess and with the relationship between human mortality and Spirit immortality. They stood sentry and reminded the people that there was sacred love and compassion from the heavens and that they had power to overcome any barrier to sustaining plenty, never doubting for a second the greatness of one's life and abilities. These were sacred givens understood to be manifest for any person. These beliefs formed the basis of the Sacred Dance Meditations and allowed for creation of a reality that was fulfilling and focused on knowing the truth of being.

The biggest responsibility is to own our power and not be afraid of it. Realizing this deep power is freeing. Once we admit just how beautiful and amazing we are deep in our core, we freely live that truth. We don't hide by telling ourselves we aren't good enough or blame others for our own actions or worry we don't know what our truth is. We are beautiful, Light-filled beings, and we are freely responsible for that. We use that freedom to influence the Universe, to create worlds and circumstances, rather than let things "happen to us." How do you feel about your freedom, and your responsibility, to harness this power, and what will you do with that responsibility? How can you ignite or extend your responsibility? Please make some notes in your journal.

July 17: Keeping Spiritual Power

SACRED DANCE

Stand where you left off on June 16, with the "Universe" on the floor in front of you. Focus your gaze on that Universe, rise on your balls of your feet, and gently walk counterclockwise, to the other side of the Universe in front of you. Deeply inhale as you begin to walk, arms gently held outward at your sides but moving gently as well, with the rhythm of the music or with a flowing pattern, palms soft, arms curved. Exhale when you arrive on the other side. Bend your knees, inhale, rise onto the balls of your feet with your gaze on the Universe, and, again with arms gently held outward at your sides and flowing, walk counterclockwise to the starting position. Stand, bend your knees slightly, exhale, and glide the palms of both hands over the Universe in front of you. Place them at your sides, and inhale. Repeat the choreography, starting with the clockwise direction.

MEDITATION AND PRACTICE

Priestesses, carefully selected and nurtured as an elite group, served the goddesses and humanity by leading Sacred Dance Meditations, rituals, and ceremonies during the times of the Mycenae empire. They were responsible and accountable for their actions. A priestess was a vessel of eternity, a servant of the goddess, awake in her femininity and the power of the goddess as her Inner Mystic Dancer. The priestesses were lightworkers. They danced with the elements, practiced self-love, and worshipped in devotion to the goddess. They channeled wisdom and healing energies and harnessed and directed the Divine forces serving the greatest good. These characteristics were seen in sacred dances that were the primary communication vessels.

So many of you can do things no one else can because you're spiritually or psychically extraordinary. You must bring these gifts to the world—that's why you're here. Certainly, some people fear lightworkers, for example. However, there's need for healing. But if you deny your gift to heal, speak, provide foresight, teach, lead, speak with spirits, or what have you, you will cut yourself off from your own true nature. Yet because of negativity you may have difficulty staying in line with your spiritual power. It's so easy to slip back into defeatist thinking. Write some ideas in your journal that will help you remember your fantastic spiritual power, keeping it in the forefront of your mind and feeling it in your bones.

July 18: Truth in the Soul

SACRED DANCE

With feet at shoulder width, bend your knees deeply enough to reach over and gently embrace and then lift your Universe up over your head as you return to a standing position. Hold your arms widely away from your body but over your head. Inhale, step to the left, tap the right foot behind the left, and step on the right foot. Repeat this with the right foot. Exhale. A little bit of a hop when shifting between the two sides will naturally occur. Continue alternating the pattern of left, right, inhale, and exhale as you turn in a clockwise circle. After one complete turn, contract your torso with the Universe overhead, then repeat. Starting on the right foot, contract your torso. Slowly bend your knees, and place the Universe on the floor without letting it drop or bounce. Repeat the pattern of turn and contract three times on each side, alternating as you go. Return to standing, facing east. Hold the Universe in front of you for a moment before placing it on the floor, and take two slow steps backward. Arms rest at your sides.

MEDITATION AND PRACTICE

The goddesses, priestesses, and key bearers had attendants, women who were privileged to provide support for the women leaders of the spiritual community. Each of these women were also considered to be lightworkers and participated in the Sacred Dance Meditations for celebrations, feasts, funerals, and other rituals. The lightworkers were at times asked to support an action or direction that may have been questionable, such as when, perhaps, Ophion began entertaining self-serving thoughts that went against the Highest Good. In these instances, the Matriarchs were in the position to use their Light for Good, suppressing the action.

Everyone has one basic responsibility: to be true to his or her Spirit, to be what one was created to be. It's doing what is naturally done by trees, plants, and everything else in the created Universe. Beings express the essence of their own Inner Mystic Dancer. Anyone who is persistently true to his or her own Spirit will also always be in the rightful place in the Divine hierarchy, which provides sacred alignment within creation. However, sometimes one must say no when it's appropriate to stay true to oneself. A loving "no" given in response to inappropriate use of spiritual power can change the direction of entire social structures. But often, there is fear in saying no, mainly because of codependency, ego, and self-doubt. Or sometimes one is talked out of a "no" into a "maybe" or even a "yes."

To be who you truly are, are you ready to say no when appropriate? Something reverberates through all decisions and choices.

July 19: Innermost Desires

SACRED DANCE

Imagine now that you're deep within the Universe and unseen forces are holding it up. Standing with your knees shoulder-width apart, gently lift your arms upward in front of you, and then wipe them toward your head and shoulders, making large circles, moving from your shoulders as if you're sweeping and creating a vortex of energy just above you. Keep this going as you step toward your left side, sweep your arms four times, return to center, sweep your arms twice, then step toward your right, and sweep your arms four times. Return to center, sweep your arms twice, and then bring them to your sides, contract your torso, and come to rest.

MEDITATION AND PRACTICE

The ancient Mycenae people, along with their ancestors, considered Sacred Dance Meditations to be vehicles to manifest their innermost desires because of their beliefs about creation. In a sacred dance, the goddess followed her desires without having a preconceived outcome in mind. She knew it was her nature to enact the Divine dance, and so she did. The people of Mycenae followed this example, and so did the attendants, key bearers, and priestesses.

Trust your innermost leadings. They always point you to the right source of love.

The flow of the Life Force through pure self-knowledge generates sacred connections and loving desire. Remember that beauty, truth, and Spirit are one. In seeking one, all of them are received. This gives you a profound sense of freedom. Trusting the innermost desires and following them in truth and Divine respect is a spiritual right you have. In your lifetime, have you ever experienced an undirected result of following your innermost desires? When, what was it, and how long did you feel that way? Do you believe you have a right to live this way every day?

July 20: Know Thyself

SACRED DANCE

For today's Sacred Dance Meditation, review and practice the choreography given for this week. Today, if you can do your best to memorize the sacred dance, that would be great. Feel free to improvise and make the dance moves yours.

MEDITATION AND PRACTICE

By the time the ancient Mycenaeans were living in Greece, many changes had taken place. People from other lands and their gods were interested in shifting the conversation. Wars and unrest were common, other forces were trying to control how people knew lightworkers, the goddess, and epiphanies. This is exemplified in the story of the Sphinx, who was part goddess, lioness, eagle, and serpent. She stood at the city gate and asked people to answer a riddle: "Which creature has one

voice and yet becomes four-footed and two-footed and three-footed?"
She would eat whomever couldn't answer correctly. Oedipus solved the
riddle by answering, "Man—who crawls on all fours as a baby, then
walks on two feet as an adult, and then uses a walking stick in old age."
The Sphinx extinguished herself at his answer. From there, some people's inner knowing of the great goddess began to decline. Nevertheless, Sacred Dance Meditations continued, in caves, secret temples, and
secluded places, by those who recognized their truth within. Oedipus
exemplified change and transition though awareness of truth, represented by the death of the Sphinx.

Everybody's realization of truth comes through a form of love,
which is always underpinned by creative energy. None can avoid this
mystical law, which can lead to fulfillment of one's deepest desires.
Suffering results from not knowing or accepting this law. Acknowledging this law at any time can help every situation. However, the consequences of forgetting that mystical law are sometimes unchangeable.

Can you imagine the separation from self that led to Oedipus's
desire to answer the Sphinx's question correctly?

July 21: True Responsibilities

SACRED DANCE

Envision the situation with the Sphinx described in the entry for
July 20: that of having the answer to a riddle that was meant to keep
people safe from manipulative and dangerous visitors who would extin-
guish the Light. Imagine you're the sacred goddess now seeing this situation. Review the Sacred Dance Meditation choreography given this
week, which you made your own on July 20. Prepare your Sacred Dance
Studio, and get into your Sacred Dance Attire. Today you trance the
dance meditation and commit it to the body-mind to carry it with you
in a library form, connecting to your ancestors who knew of the power
of Sacred Dance Meditations long before that power was obscured.

MEDITATION AND PRACTICE

The Mycenaeans were perhaps the last of the ancient Greeks to
know the great goddess but they weren't the last to know their true

responsibilities. Although much of the actual history is lost, it is known that they knew that the greatest responsibility was to understand what was theirs and what wasn't. Everything came from chaos, and chaos always returned, because nothing was static in the Universe. From chaos order is sought. There was change from following the sacred feminine to following the sacred masculine. And yet, the ancient Greeks continued to engage in sacred dances, seeking to connect with the Divine and embracing their true responsibilities to live in love and harmony, even when these seemed to be foiled. The goddess knew she couldn't help Ophion, just as the Sphinx knew she couldn't keep controlling people's awareness that they were responsible for themselves.

As author and Akashic researcher Linda Rowe suggests, if a situation gives you energy, peace of mind, or satisfaction most of the time, it's a spiritual responsibility in line with your reason for being. Pay attention, however, if the "responsibility" is draining, causes sadness or anger, puts you in danger, or gives a sense of defeat. Such a situation is reminiscent of the saying heard on airplanes: put on your oxygen mask before you try to help another. To keep from feeling a sense of defeat or depletion, you must allow people to refuse your help and to live as they please. Doing so, you'd get out of the way of their natural consequences. These are the principles of detaching with love.

JULY 22–31
With Freedom, Responsibility Comes (Entry Point)

Make an offering, and be ready for the blessing.

When you ask, expect to receive but also expect to honor the responsibility that comes with the gift.

For this week, keep your scarves nearby if you have them. You can also use a bell or other handheld instrument if you're inclined.

July 22: Right Use of Spiritual Power

SACRED DANCE

Begin the dance facing east. Direct your gaze to the earth, place your left arm across your chest, and gently rest the palm of your hand on your right shoulder. Step to the left, place your right foot slightly behind the left foot, and rise on the ball of the right foot. Then move toward the left foot again. Keep the knees slightly bent. Curve your right arm so your palm is softly facing you or holding the scarf, and gently move your arm toward and away from your body as you move. Inhale and exhale six times as you move backward and to the left, diagonally. Then pause, bring your arms overhead, switch the scarf to the other hand, and place the right hand on the left shoulder. Repeat the choreography, moving forward and to the right, as you inhale and exhale six times. You will have created a *V* shape on the floor. Bring the arms overhead, and gently place them by your sides.

MEDITATION AND PRACTICE

Apollo was the god of Light and the god of Truth in ancient Greece, serving as an intermediary between gods and humans. In that capacity, he used his gifts of reason, harmony, balance, and prophesy. Form and structure, containers, and rational thought were his forte. Because of his truthfulness and integrity, he was granted the gift of prophecy and oracles. Apollo's sacred dances were reverent and thoughtful, deliberate and purposeful. Apollo's lineage traced back to Chaos, Eurynome and Ophion, to the Titans on Mount Olympus, from Rhea and Cronus, to Zeus. With this lineage, sacred dance expanded to allow men the opportunity to benefit from it, helping them deal with their realities and take responsibility.

The Greek deities epitomized dysfunctional families. We are all part of dysfunction as a result because we live with people, usually. Apollo had all kinds of issues, and drama was always going on in the lands. Boundaries were constantly violated, and power shifts were prevalent. People were controlled and forced into submission, in private and public situations. And while it's true that some of the sacred dances we enjoy today are from this lineage, so much was done to prohibit dance to obscure the power it holds. Or some placed the power into vessels for which it was never intended, so that what was presented to people in need of Spirit was sometimes deadly. This was a result of misuse of spiritual powers, and we see the fallout from it. Right use of spiritual power is critical to gaining access to a sense of peace.

You have freedom to use your spiritual power because of your sacredness. With this freedom, however, comes an enormous responsibility. Not only must you take responsibility for yourself and your life's circumstances, but also you must use your knowledge and wisdom to help bring the truth forward, without looking for gain. Are you in a dysfunctional family, tribe, or kin group? Maybe you're in multiple such groups, at home, work, place of worship, etc. Will you take responsibility that comes with your freedom even if it means you must go against the grain?

July 23: Open, Speak, Act to Remember Yourself

SACRED DANCE

Begin facing east again. Extend the right arm out in front of you toward the right side, on a slight diagonal upward, with your left arm extending behind you. Inhale, and take eight steps forward on the balls of your feet. Stop. Bring the feet together, exhale, then inhale, and then crisscross your hands in front of you four times. Exhale, hold your arms out from your body to your sides, and walk around counterclockwise 180 degrees in a small circle. Now, extend your left arm in front of you, placing your right arm behind. Inhale, take eight steps forward on the balls of your feet. Stop. Bring the feet together, exhale, then inhale, and then crisscross your hands in front of you four times. Exhale, hold arms out from your body to your sides, and walk around counterclockwise 180 degrees in a small circle. Bring your arms to your sides.

MEDITATION AND PRACTICE

Dionysus, the son of Zeus and Semele, was the god of wine, agriculture, fertility, revelry, ecstatic emotion, and drama in ancient Greece and was associated with spiritual intoxication. The poster child of a god unable to or unwilling to tame his passions, Dionysus led by instinct and displayed behaviors opposite to those of his brother Apollo. Sometimes called Bacchus, Dionysus was the last of the Twelve Olympians. His followers were satyrs and maenads; the maenads danced wildly at festivals mostly. These women devoted themselves to his care and eventually were called Dionysus's worshippers. The maenads practiced ecstatic sacred dances and led frenzied religious rites during which Dionysus possessed them. While in trance, they were supposed to have superhuman strength.

Characterizing sacred dance as frenzied or out of control became associated with women, whereas men who engaged in sacred dance accepted Apollonian thinking. These two manifestations of sacred dance might have brought forth their power depending on influence from the left or right sides of the brain or on the masculine or feminine duality.

Even out of the chaos of godly dysfunction and deceit, sacred dance prevailed. When have you been of two minds? When have you been spiritually intoxicated, willing to believe anything just to change how you feel or deflect responsibility? How have you felt when you're in these kinds of mindsets? Although spiritually intoxicated, you still have the responsibility and freedom to speak, act, and choose. You can choose to be self-seeking, to be cowards even for a time, and to be authentic, acting as we were meant to, doing what we were called to do while on earth.

July 24: Sacrifices

SACRED DANCE

Like you did yesterday, prepare with music and your Sacred Dance Attire, facing east. If you have them, please hold your scarves loosely in your hands. Slightly bend your knees, and inhale, moving your arms from the shoulder in opposing circles in front of you, then in sweeping circles toward you. Sway gently toward the left and the right, exhaling when you bring the circles toward you. Repeat this vortex-generating movement slowly for twelve breaths, swaying and moving your feet on the floor so that you move away from a fixed position. Come back to center and sweep the arms to the sides and in front of your body, and contract the torso after each, for another twelve breaths.

MEDITATION AND PRACTICE

Maenads were possessed by Dionysus's Spirit. They were his companions as he went from Thrace to Greece trying to have his Divinity validated. Dionysus danced on Mount Parnassos with Delphic virgins, and soon other women followed the maenads and danced, holding a thyrsus and wearing animal skins. They also put snakes in their hair to mark the ceremony as sacred. Snakes symbolized religious festivities during periods when reverence for the sacred feminine was the norm.

The sacrifices that the maenads made to continue to practice sacred dance and worship Dionysus couldn't have been easy. They were perhaps trying to hold on to their recollections of a spiritual past and sacrificing some aspects of themselves to do so.

Holding on to old spiritual behaviors when we've outgrown them can limit the progression forward. Instead of changing and taking responsibility, sometimes we want to remain as we are, where things are familiar. Or we want to have someone tell us what to do, whom to worship, when to pray, etc., without a true connection to Spirit. It doesn't work, so we must take new knowledge like a savior to help us move on to higher planes. That responsibility comes with sacred freedom.

Have you ever been "a maenad?" That is, have you ever been following a guru or leader who was a bit questionable? Make some notes.

July 25: *Making Offerings for Balance*

SACRED DANCE

Begin today's dance facing east. Review the choreography from July 22 and 23 until it becomes familiar to you.

In Ancient Greece during the time of Dionysus, satyrs were the counterparts to maenads. These creatures worshipped him and were his companions. He loved them, and they loved him, as they danced and played music in the forests. They led a life of pleasure and self-indulgence. But some of their dances were sacred meditations, calling forth the spiritual power to aid sustenance and growth and to appease the gods.

The satyrs offered themselves as the prototype for human indulgence. A balance is needed in recognizing those drives and offering them to Spirit so that they can be manifested in a way that helps everyone. As free beings, we're responsible for integrating every aspect of ourselves as we dance along this road. Excesses of any kind, including being too serious all the time or playing all the time, get us off balance. Denying our humanity is also counter to balance and to living in equanimity. Make some notes in your journal. What will you offer to the Divine (even when it takes a human form) today to respect your freedom and take responsibility to keep your balance between your humanness and your Spirit? Offer your time, your ear, your interest, your smile, your suffering, and your songs. Give it all away with gladness. It's not about what you get in life; it's about what you give away.

July 26: *Spiritual Loneliness*

Repeat the dance as described on July 24. Then bring stillness to the dance by closing your eyes and crossing your hands with the scarves across your chest.

Ancient Greek gods were lonely even though they had every opportunity to simply be, to use their powers in ways that were uplifting and edifying. Due to this loneliness, they enacted ways to use Sacred Dance Meditations. In some cases, the loneliness led to desperate behaviors, indulging in excesses, and being irresponsible.

Spiritual loneliness sometimes results when we have realized the truth. It's a deeply moving feeling in our Inner Mystic Dancer. We can enjoy the beauty, the fruits, the offerings found here if we remember that our sacred dance is short and our impact great. As we evolve to the highest planes, a few companions are with us. We are responsible for paving the way for any onlookers who remain behind.

Engage in your ceremony and rituals and include sacred dance. By doing so, you inform the mind that it has passed through the desert and found its way into the arms of Spirit. Writing in your spiritual journal what you'll want to say at your death and engaging in death-without-dying rituals will keep you grounded and reduce your spiritual loneliness.

July 27: Creative, Sexual Energy

SACRED DANCE

Today, practice the full range of the dance until it becomes familiar to you.

MEDITATION AND PRACTICE

Ancient Greek gods from Chaos to Apollo and Dionysus had their attention on creation, bringing forth worlds, children, and situations through energy generated with sacred dance. There was innocence to the creative act of unification with another being, with the result being beauty and new growth and direction. Eurynome was the first to sense the power of sacred dance in creations of Ophion. As time went on, that innocence vanished when veils emerged because of self-aggrandizing addictions to power, prestige, revenge, and vainglory. Sacred dance also received a certain shroud, as it was twisted to change a loving conversation with the heart of Spirit into a lustful one.

Every human being is on this earth because of a sexual union of some kind; sexual unions of opposing masculine and feminine energies have created many creatures. And, nothing—ideas, new gadgets, ways to grow food, etc.—comes into this world without creative energy. If sexual energy is creative energy, it stands to reason that it should be used appropriately and wisely rather than destructively. It's something to be grateful for, not ashamed of. No one should be hurt by it, including oneself, those here, and Beings who could result from it.

July 28: What of the Irresponsible?

SACRED DANCE

Review the sacred dance given for this week, and begin to memorize the choreography as your own. Improvise, and start to feel the movements.

MEDITATION AND PRACTICE

At times, the gods did ugly acts and caused pain and suffering for those around them. Each act received a reaction, such as when Rhea gave her husband a rock to eat because he was devouring the children she bore due to his fears, or when Ophion challenged Eurynome for the credit for creation of the world, or when Zeus was going with Semele, and his wife told her about Zeus's Spiritual Power. But the powers inherent in each of the gods remained there even with its misuse. That is to say that the power of sacred dance, their Inner Mystic Dancer, remained with them even as they committed these out-of-character acts.

Since at least the times of ancient Greek civilization, people have been hurting others. Today, they harm us and our environments, our communities. Some people claim they have no need for spirituality, or, they say their dogma is the only one that works for humanity. Other people win the prizes and seem to be free of suffering while they continue to drink, smoke, hate, and oppress entire groups of people for no real reason other than skin color or birthplace. And we're told that we need to look at them with compassion and try to understand them. Even worse is when they get away with getting the glory, the money, fame, or otherwise seem to be winning. But so what? You have choices. When you dance your meditation, sure, hold them in the Light and have compassion for them, but also tell them where they can go, and use your choicest words to express your feelings. It's best to put these down in your journal in private or articulate them in the privacy of your Sacred Dance Studio.

July 29: Sacred Dance Responsibility

SACRED DANCE

Review the sacred dance given for this week and embody the choreography, while you add a bit of your own twists.

MEDITATION AND PRACTICE

The ancient Greeks had a deep and abiding connection with Sacred Dance Meditation and freedoms. Gods took over from goddesses perhaps because of the power that was held in the Divine feminine sacred dance. That was evident in their myths and mythos. But the main point to understand from these ancients was that sacred dance itself became hidden and diluted by the gods because they saw the power it yielded. Diluting the sacred led to obscuring the Spirit and confusion of the people—a definite lack of responsibility displayed by certain gods.

Obfuscation of the truth is perhaps a trick of the Divine to have us seek after it harder or by design so that it doesn't fall into the wrong hands. Magick is that way, because if placed into a Soul that has ill will, the power that can be unleashed on to the earth is immeasurable.

Many creation myths talk of the Divine feminine, symbolized with or through a serpent, and all hell breaks loose. It's an explanation of why things are the way they are, why there is chaos from our vantage point.

The power still resides in Sacred Dance Meditation, since it still lives among you. Has sacred dance begun to fulfill its responsibility to you?

July 30: Honor of Responsibility

SACRED DANCE

Today you will trance out the sacred dance done this week, deeply feel the responsibilities and freedoms you have, and sense how these can be expressed through your sacred dance.

MEDITATION AND PRACTICE

Our study of Ancient Greek sacred dance has taken us backward to time eternal and given us the courage to be responsible to look after our thoughts, actions, and Spirits. We have been shown or have discovered the right use of spiritual power. Importantly, we realized from the goddesses and gods that creative energy includes chaos and that nothing remains constant, except that our connections with our Higher Powers and Higher Self lead us.

Review the sacred dances from this week and this month. Write down some of the ways the month's readings and sacred dances have impacted your day-to-day life, if at all. If possible, find someone trustworthy with whom to share what you know, and invite that person to your dance.

July 31: Embodied Responsibility

SACRED DANCE

Review sacred dances from this month. Select one that you'd like to review.

MEDITATION AND PRACTICE

What strikes you the most about our Greek ancestors' practice of the sacred dance?

Know that every human being has the responsibility and the freedom to work on him- or herself internally until achieving a state that reflects spiritual and natural laws and compassion for others. What are the most special moments you remember from your meditation and sacred dance Practice?

AUGUST
Preparing for Harvest

INDIAN SACRED DANCE

A number of bronze, terracotta, and stone figurines of women in dancing poses reveal the presence of dance forms in the Indus Valley Civilization, which was located in what is Pakistan and northwest India today. We find evidence of this culture from around 5500 BCE. And evidence suggests that by 2000 BCE the civilization enjoyed its greatest prosperity.

Sacred dance in India has practically no beginning and a perpetual evolution to support spiritual connection and human wellbeing. Several sacred dance forms that originated and evolved in India use mudras, or hand gestures, which were also used by gods and goddesses. This month we embody their essences and components, particularly with Bharatanatyam, Odissi, Kathakali, and Kuchipudi sacred dance forms, to begin harvesting our intentions.

Dating back to 1000 BCE, Bharatanatyam is a sacred dance from the South Indian state of Tamil Nadu that originated in the Hindu temples of Tamil Nadu and neighboring regions. Individual women performed Bharatanatyam sacred dance, and through it, they expressed Hindu religious themes and spiritual ideas. According to the Hindu Sanskrit, *natyam* means "dance" and *bharata* means "emotion and feelings." The ancient Indian Sanskrit Hindu text Natyashastra references this sacred dance. And, according to lore, Lord Brahma revealed Bharatanatyam to the sage Bharata, who then encoded this sacred dance form in Natyashastra.

Odissi originated within Hindu temples, portraying information from the Hindu scriptures; in other words, it was a religious story-telling dance performed in temple courtyards and village squares in Northern India using the sacred texts as their basis for dance. Odissi dancers related stories and moral tales of gods and god-desses and characters from the Ramayana and Mahabharata. In the Vedic traditions, human history is cyclical in nature, influenced by the evolving and dissolving of the world. Ancient Indian peoples who intermingled with other cultures in the area believed that god delivered the Vedas to them directly, and they were passed on to the next generations by word of mouth. The Vedas, which mean "knowledge" in Sanskrit, are Hinduism's oldest sacred scriptures and could be counted as the world's most ancient religious texts.

Performed by men, Kathakali is a dance from the south Indian state of Kerala. Kathakali dancers wear elaborate makeup, which represents different types of characters. The faces of the Divine are usually green. Characters considered to have an evil streak, such as a demon, have the green makeup marked with red cheeks. Characters who are angry or very evil have red makeup and long, red beards. Women and ascetics are given yellowish faces.

Kuchipudi as a sacred dance originated in a village of the Krishna district of Andhra Pradesh, India. Kuchipudi too became a religious art referenced in the Hindu Sanskrit text Natyashastra. The dance connected with temples and their related spiritual faiths and Practices. Kuchipudi was broadly oriented on Lord Krishna, who is depicted with blue or black skin and considered the Supreme god. This Ancient Indian sacred dance was accompanied by musicians playing instruments, like the mridangam, flute, tambura, and violin.

PREPARATION

For each of the Sacred Dance Meditations this month, you may want to avail yourself of traditional clothing from India as your Sacred Dance Attire. Music referred to in each dance is readily available through your streaming music service. Arrange for incense and oils to be burned safely within your Sacred Dance Studio, and you can think about getting a few Sanskrit letters to remind you that this sacred dance has come down to us through the ages and is worth considering as part of your Practice.

AUGUST 1–7
Harvesting the Spirit (Entry Point)

Sacred is dance—at no time was dance not.

Humanity dances because that is how we are informed, transformed, and transmuted.

Instruments used for Bharatanatyam sacred dance are the mridangam and cymbals. A violin or *ghatam* and flute could also be lovely additions. With or without them, you might consider arranging for authentic India incense and oils to be burned safely within your Sacred Dance Studio.

August 1: Lord Shiva: Lord of the Dance

SACRED DANCE

Imagine you can create and destroy anything with a simple gesture, blink, or expression. Begin standing and facing east, with most of your weight on the left leg, the right leg placed behind the left, and your palms facing upward and held together slightly to the left in front of the hip. Gaze at your palms as you gently reach up to your right. You have a warm smile on your face. Step to the right with the right leg, and bring your arms up high over your head, palms joined. Step the left leg across the front of the right foot, and bring the arms back down to the left hip, palms still joined and facing upward. Your gaze follows the palms. Keeping the palms to your left side, step with the right foot so that the heels of the feet are touching and legs are straight. Then, holding that position, deeply bend your knees. Straighten your knees, and bring the palms up to chest height, with elbows bent. Then, leading with your left elbow, with the left ear leaning toward that left elbow and with the palms upward and fingertips touching, lift the right foot and place it behind you to turn counterclockwise, keeping the elbows out, fingertips touching, and palms facing up. Hold this configuration, and keep stepping behind you as you complete a 360-degree turn.

MEDITATION AND PRACTICE

The Trimurti, or trinity of G-d, was creation, sustainment, and destruction. These were embodied by personifications of Brahma as the Creator, Vishnu as the sustainer and protector, and Shiva as the destroyer or transformer. These three deities all had the meaning of three in One. They were the different forms or manifestations of One entity, the Supreme Being. Brahma *was* the Dharma, the Cosmic Principles, and the Ultimate Reality.

Many ancient Indian peoples carved sculptures of Lord Shiva, also known as Nataraja, in sacred dance poses of the Bharatanatyam into temples. In them, he was remembered as dancing within a circular arch of flames that represented the cosmic fire that both created and consumed everything. The circle represented the cyclical nature of life. The fire also represented the positive and negative aspects of life, the feminine and masculine energies. Shiva is known as the destroyer aspect within the Trimurti, the Hindu trinity, with Brahma and Vishnu. Shiva was one of the supreme beings that created, protected, and transformed the universe. Goddess Shakti was said to provide the energy and creative power of each aspect of the Trimurti. Shakti and Shiva were aware of the power of sacred dance to create, harvest good, and reimagine.

Drawing on deeply rooted knowing and the examples of energy that created the universe, you now know the power you have within your body temple. The ability to change any circumstance you find yourself in, any faulty or limiting beliefs you hold, and any desire to enable your thinking to advance onto higher planes is found within this power. When talking or thinking about something that causes you to consider changing or acknowledging your growth, what comes to mind? How have you changed in your Spirit or your awareness? Of course, please consider everything within a loving and compassionate context appropriate to the circumstances and for the greatest positive impact to enable you to harvest another aspect of your Spirit. You see, harvesting the Spirit is an ongoing process, and that means it's never finished—at least while evolving on earth. It's the proverbial onion that keeps peeling layers. Like

Shakti and Shiva, we seek to dance on that lotus petal of realization. Make some notes in your journal.

August 2: What's in the Guṇas?

SACRED DANCE

As you review yesterday's dance, think carefully about the circumstances that may be holding you in time and space and the path behind you that has led you to this place in your Practice. As you have a sense of complete acceptance, envision the path ahead, loosely and generally. Now, after completing the 360-degree turn, feet are parallel on the floor, knees slightly bent. Reach the palms forward and gently upward. Step forward with the right foot, and bring the left to join it. Slightly bend your knees, keeping the palms out in front of you. Stand straight, then quickly curl back the toes on both feet. Do that stepping sequence again, and then place the right foot way behind you, bending the left knee. The palms now face upward with the elbows close into the body; the torso leans forward, and the head gently bows. Remaining in the lunge, holding the hands with palms up out in front of you, gently lean backward, taking the head back too. Your arms will naturally rise. Then lift the right foot, and cross it to the left of the left foot, keeping it behind; step backward on it, bringing the feet together by moving the left foot back. Simultaneously, bring the arms to a soft curve with palms up, fingertips touching, to return to rest at the left hip.

MEDITATION AND PRACTICE

As depicted in the renderings from ancient India, Lord Shiva's upper-right hand, while in a mudra called *ḍamaru-hasta*, holds a drum, which stands for life and creation. Lord Shiva's upper-left hand holds fire, which is about creation and destruction. A cobra is depicted uncoiling from Lord Shiva's lower-right forearm, and the palm of the lower-right hand is in the *abhaya* mudra, relieving fear and supporting the appropriate use of dharma. The lower-left hand bends downward at the wrist, and the palm faces inward toward his body. It points toward the raised left foot so that it's diametrically opposite to the lower-right arm. He has two eyes, plus a "third eye" on his forehead. His eyes represent the sun and the moon, whereas the open third eye is supposed to be the Inner Eye to wisdom and self-realization. The three eyes together lead to wisdom via the three *guṇas* of *sattva*, *rajas*, and *tamas*. Nataraja dances on a demon, which symbolizes that sacred dance leads to victory over the distractions and delusions of this world. The pleasant face of Shiva represents his calmness despite being immersed in the contrasting forces of Universe and his energetic dance.

Sattva (goodness, constructiveness, harmony), rajas (passion, activity, confusion), and tamas (darkness, destruction, chaos) are present in everyone and everything. It's which of them leads that's different. The combination of these guṇas makes up the character of someone and acts as one's fate. When in right balance, the guṇas are threads woven together, producing the great reality or the composition of the Divine in one's life.

Research the Divine Qualities and see what you find. Which of the three guṇas have you used to harvest your Spirit? Remember that those represented in tamas are Divine Qualities when incorporated to make appropriate change or respond to situations when needed. Which of the Divine Qualities would you like to continue amplifying to harvest the great reality within you or your community?

August 3: Maya and Wakefulness

SACRED DANCE

Review yesterday's sacred dance. Now, gently reach the palms up to your right, and, with a warm smile, gaze at your palms. Step to the right with the right leg, and bring your arms up high over your head, palms joined. Step across the front of the right foot with the left, and bring the arms back down to the left hip, palms still joined and facing upward. Your gaze follows the palms. Do a slight jump onto the right leg, and bring the heels together, forming a *V* on the floor. Bring the upward-facing palms with fingertips touching back to the center chest area. Breathe here for a beat, then step forward on the left foot, turn your head toward the direction in which you're stepping, keeping the fingertips touching. Bring your right foot down behind the left to propel you in a circle counterclockwise with the elbow leading. Repeat, stepping to the left with the right foot behind the left propelling you around until you've turned 360 degrees, and bring the feet back to a *V* shape with the heels touching. Bend your knees, and bring the palms back to the chest center.

MEDITATION AND PRACTICE

With his Sacred Dance Meditation, Shiva destroyed the illusory world of maya and transformed it so that spiritual power and enlightenment were revealed. *Maya* in Sanskrit means "magic" or "illusion," and "originally denoted the magic power with which a god could make human beings believe in … illusion. By extension, it later came to mean the powerful force that creates the cosmic illusion that the phenomenal world is real.… Maya is thus that cosmic force that presents the infinite Brahman (the supreme being)"* as the world we see, touch, smell, and hear. Maya tricks people by hiding their real natures, their Self, from them, which is mistaken for the ego. In reality, the Self is identical with Brahman. The mind tells us we are humans passing through life, rather than immortals. This makes us unable to overcome our limitations.

Consider whether what you see in the space around you is real or illusionary.

The ancients in India taught that maya was perpetuated by giving in to desires that don't lead back to spiritual awareness and wakefulness. Desires for security, wealth, love, fame, and correctness are all among them. Giving in to them creates attachments, which lead to difficulties, keeping the mind in a state of agitation. With a disturbed and unsteady mind, we can't see clearly or discern truth from lie. We become prisoners of our own actions, desires, and

---

* *Encyclopaedia Britannica Online*, s.v. "Maya," accessed July 1, 2020, https://www.britannica.com/topic/maya-Indian-philosophy.

attachments. Freeing ourselves from maya and remaining wakeful is the essence of the spiritual path, regardless of which sacred approach one takes. Yet some remark, "It's all just an illusion, so there's no need to worry." They engage in spiritual bypassing—that is, using spiritual beliefs as a way of escaping and shirking responsibility or deluding themselves.

Do you desire to be deluded? How do you delude yourself?

August 4: Dharma for the Taking

SACRED DANCE

Reflect on yesterday's "Meditation and Practice," and review yesterday's dance if you need to. Reach the palms forward and gently upward. Step forward with the left foot, and bring the right to join it. Take a slight knee bend, keeping the palms out in front of you. Stand straight, then quickly curl back the toes on both feet. Repeat that stepping sequence again, and then shift the weight to the right leg and deeply bend the knee. Rest the ball of the left foot just next to the arch of the right foot; the left knee is also bent. Smiling, tilting your head to the left, and gazing straight ahead, touch your fingertips together and hold your palms toward your chest. Hold this pose for a breath. Then, step on the left foot, and turn your head to the left, keeping the fingertips touching. Bring your right foot down behind the left to propel you in a circle counterclockwise with the elbow leading. Repeat stepping to the left with the right foot behind the left, propelling you around until you've turned 360 degrees. Bring the feet together and, keeping your palms upward and fingertips touching, tap the left foot in front of you, and bring it back to standing. Tap and hold the right foot to your right, resting the ball of the foot on the floor and bending both knees. Turn your head in the direction of the right knee when you put the ball of the foot down. Hold here for a beat, and then bring the feet together. Repeat twice from the point of tapping the left foot forward. Repeat once more, but hold the pose for five beats or so, and tilt the head to the left.

The snake that sits at Nataraja's waist is Kundalini Shakti, which represents the cosmic power that lives in all of us as the representation of Brahman and the opposite of maya. Nataraja's dance wasn't abstract. It was happening in each person, at the atomic level, moment by moment. Lore proposed that the creation of the worlds, their maintenance, and the obscuration and liberation of human Spirit are acts of Nataraja's dance.

Dharma becomes the reflection of maya, with its cosmic law underlying every right action and social order. Dharma refers to *rta*, a power that glues and upholds the Universe and supernatural societies. Dharma is the power that makes us wakeful people and gives us the willingness to pursue and show forth the Divine Qualities. We have the capacity to live from the active Kundalini Shakti, or its equivalent, in our understanding of awakening, and we have the duty to do so to harvest our Spirits.

August 5: Rta and Cosmic Fate

SACRED DANCE

Review the sequences of the sacred dance given on August 4. Shift your weight to both feet, bring the arms up over your head in circular fashion with the palms facing each other, bring them down to your heart chakra area, and bow your head. Keeping the palms held steady, walk, with an exaggerated bending of each knee, counterclockwise in a large 360-degree circle. Lift your head, sweep the arms up and to your sides, palms facing each other to reach over your head and meet at your crown chakra.

MEDITATION AND PRACTICE

Rta is the eternal, cosmic, and moral order. For the peoples who lived in the Indus Valley, rta encompassed the idea that there was basic truth, a harmony, or system of the Universe. That was considered an aspect of being on earth and was a part of Divine order.

In understanding our need to remain wakeful, we can think of rta as representing the eternal and inviolable laws of nature. This includes the precision on which the stars and planets rotate, the assuredness of the sunrise, the way the rivers flow to the oceans, and so on. Rta allows us to see unity in our differences within the cosmic order. By adhering to the basic truths of rta, by practicing harmony and Divine Qualities as eternal and inviolable laws, life on Earth moves in the upward direction. At the same time, the fact that the days come and go on their own and that the natural laws are unchanging allows us to point our attention to that which is eternal inside of us, in our fellow travelers, and in what we manifest in harvesting our Spirits. How do you reconcile rta with maya? Make some notes in your journal.

August 6: Dancing upon Anrta

SACRED DANCE

Combine and practice the sequence of sacred dance choreography given from August 1 to August 5 with the goal of memorizing it. After you have done that, try to consider the leaders of this world (current or previous) who represent Divine Qualities. Hold them in your body-mind as you practice Sacred Dance Meditation today.

MEDITATION AND PRACTICE

Anrta was the opposite of rta for the people of ancient India. For them, anrta represented complete disorder and confusion. The path of anrta goes against the natural laws and causes disease and death. The Lord of the Dance exhibited ways of dealing with this by sacredly dancing on an individual with this energy.

Compound words containing *anrta* point to falsehoods, untruths, deceptions and lies, broken promises, and a temporary body without permanent existence. Because human beings may live in a dualistic reality, the notion of anrta is contrary to rta. If a person chooses to follow a course rife with falsehoods and untruths or deludes another with practices arising from anrta, then that person's life is said to be shrouded with darkness. But we all know that some people on this planet seem to be anrta incarnate. They don't display real care or the nature of Divine Qualities.

What do you say of those individuals? How do you consider them? In terms of what to do about them, how can they be reined in to rta? How do you apply dharma? Jot down some ideas in your journal discussing how you have countered (or will counter) anrta in Spirit harvesting.

August 7: The Divine Cognitive

SACRED DANCE

As we come to the end of the week and close this entry point on harvesting the Spirit, approach your Sacred Dance Studio and Sacred Dance Attire as you embody the principles of wakefulness, dharma, rta, and the Lord of the Dance. As you engage in the full Sacred Dance Meditation from this week, realize that you may experience mental, physical, and spiritual transformation as you destroy old beliefs and create new and more challenging adventures for your Soul.

MEDITATION AND PRACTICE

For the ancients of India, *jnana*, which means "knowledge" in Sanskrit, focused on a cognitive event that couldn't be mistaken. It was described as a total experience with the Supreme Being that set the Soul free from the transmigratory life and the polarities this imposes upon thought. This experience of jnana overcame *ajnana*, or the false understanding of reality, that kept the Soul from seeing clearly. Knowledge, that one's Self was identical with the Ultimate Reality, as acquired through Sacred Dance Meditation, was sought after through Lord Shiva's sacred dance.

Jnana as spiritual knowledge and wisdom denotes knowledge of the Self, an inward experience of the Absolute Reality inseparable from the Divine. It is knowing one need not experience pain or suffering but instead can come from a place of total Awareness. In harvesting our Spirit, we must be diligent in acting from that realization.

The glitz and glam of the world may promise to transform you. In addition, chasing the latest spiritual craze drives many down a dead end. Instead, a calm approach to knowing the truth lies within; a slowing down of activity and a simple inward focus, rather than an outward one, propels you.

❋ ❋ ❋

AUGUST 8–14
Harvesting Wants and Ways of Being (Entry Point)

The Whole World in Your Hands—Yesterday, Today, and Tomorrow

Energy in the body can be collected and harnessed, pointed in the direction you wish to go.

A sari with pleats and a sash around the waist can serve as this week's dance attire, along with jewelry, such as bright earrings, necklaces, and bracelets. You can mark your third eye if you like. Feel free to paint the palms of your feet and hands with a henna dye, if you'd like, in a design or other inspiring mark. An Odissi orchestra includes a *pakhawaj* musician (most often the guru), a singer, a flutist, a sitar or violin musician, and a *manjira* musician. So, you might find music that includes a pakhawaj or barrel drum, a *bansuri* or an Indian flute, a manjira or a set of small cymbals, and a sitar, a long-neck lute. You may wear bells on your ankles too.

August 8: Strike a Pose

SACRED DANCE

Stand facing east. Acknowledge energy radiating out from your chakra energy points, and envision it reaching to the Universe's farthest corners. Bend your knees slightly, and place your left hand on your left hip and your right hand on top of it. This will cause you to twist a bit toward the left side of your body. Look to your left, over your left shoulder; hold this position, and shift your torso left, right, left. Hold the position for four breaths, with your hands still on your hip and looking toward the left. Your face is gently smiling. Blink your eyes five times, then shift only your eyes, looking left, right, left, right. Return to the standing position.

MEDITATION AND PRACTICE

The people of the Indus Valley recorded their sacred dance poses in sculptures within Odissi Hindu temples. An Odissi Sacred Dance Meditation included an invocation, *nritta* (pure dance), *nritya* (expressive dance), *natya* (dance drama), and *moksha*, which portrayed emancipation of the Soul and spiritual release for human beings. This dance used body mudras, which balanced energy and negative behaviors, or directed and activated emotional and spiritual energy created through routine and mature Sacred Dance Meditation. It encompassed one's view of G-d and seeing the Self in relation to G-d.

Hand mudras draw on elemental energies from each finger. The thumb draws upon fire; the index finger draws upon air; the middle finger brings in the power of ethers; the ring finger brings the power of earth; and the pinky finger is representative of water. By combining concentration and activating the elemental forces within our bodies as connected to the Universe, we can therefore create the energy we need to balance ourselves and to harvest our wants and ways of being (explained subsequently). The question is, what do you ultimately want, and how does that relate to your way of being? Before answering, note that some people have said being in a state of wanting isn't equivalent to the state of manifesting; instead, the idea is to imagine having something as the key to receiving. Also, consider that "haves" are never exhausted: the desire for more arises immediately upon receiving, as part of the human condition.

August 9: Have and Be

SACRED DANCE

Review the August 8 entry if needed. Keeping your hands on your hips, shift your weight to the left foot, and drag the ball of the right foot slightly behind you. Tap the floor two times, and then drag the ball of the foot around to your side and then to the front of you, making a large semicircle. When your right foot arrives in front of your body, balance your weight between both feet, and bend both knees. Bring the hands from their position on your hip to the front of your body, crossed at the wrists, left wrist on the bottom. Bring your thumb and ring fingers to slightly touching, with palms facing upward. Try to keep your fingers close together in this mudra. Remain with knees bent in the position for four breaths. The left foot is flat on the floor, and the right foot is resting on the ball of the foot, heel lifted. Tap the right foot on the floor with the ball of your foot, keeping the knees bent and hands in mudra body pose.

MEDITATION AND PRACTICE

The sacred dance used Nritya Hasta or pure dance mudras—full body and hand mudras—to effect spiritual change. At this time in ancient India, the people believed that gods and goddesses danced to express the dynamic energy of life. The image represents Shiva as the Lord of the Dance, choreographing the eternal dance of the Universe. A dance of love and passion filled with the Divine, Odissi was the dance of Lord Shiva.

Indian Sacred Dance Meditation originated from the teachings of the Lord of the Universe. From it came the notion of *bhava*, which is the center of spiritual feelings and affections, as well as the heart and everlasting Soul (the true Self). We can understand bhava as intuition. Attuning to intuition (or hunch, inner voice, calling, or sense of needing something more than surface answers) can provide guidance and insight into what is important and beneficial to the true Self. An example is feeling a deep sense of spiritual wellness through all activities. That means we "have and be" based on listening to and acting on our inner guidance and aligning with Divine Qualities, which evolve over time.

August 10: Attitudinal Focus

SACRED DANCE

Review the entries from earlier this week if you'd like. From the bent-kneed pose you left off in, bring the right foot close to the left foot so that your weight is evenly distributed on both feet and your knees remain bent. Unfurl your wrists, but keep your mudra hands so that the right arm lifts upward and the left arm is brought down and slightly behind your body, with palms facing away from your body. Your gaze is toward the right hand. Hold this position for four breaths. Then stand with your knees slightly bent. Bring your right palm to rest on your right hip, and place your left palm over the right.

MEDITATION AND PRACTICE

The sacred dance in ancient India was built around the *chauka* and the *tribhanga*. The chauka is a masculine stance that equally balances the weight of the body, imitating a square in geometry. The tribhanga is a feminine pose holding the weight on one foot, with bent knees, hips jutted out, and a tilted head. Sacred dancers emphasized the duality of the masculine and the feminine through chauka and tribhanga to praise the gods.

At its core, bhava is having or receiving an attitude of peace, vitality, and wellness. Feeling a deep sense of conscious rest and spiritual peace indicates what is life-giving to the true Self. We also exercise bhava by setting positive and peaceful intentions for Sacred Dance Meditations and for our general focus on our life. It can be difficult to do this with the constant call of the world. Holding the chauka or the tribhanga can address energies that seek to take us off track, to lead us away from our intuitive paths. Harvesting wants and ways of being boils down to feeling more at rest and at peace than agitated, frustrated, or otherwise off balance. It means stepping away from anything that causes us to fall back into delusions about what we are here on earth for. This doesn't mean we can't have tangible goals. It means that the goals are set with the idea of harvesting our wants in relation to the Higher Self and doing our best to know that any wanting arising is an indication of imbalance.

August 11: Release and Liberation

SACRED DANCE

Look to your right, over your right shoulder; hold this position, and then shift your torso right, left, right. Hold the position for four breaths, with your hands still on your hips and looking toward the right. Your face is gently smiling. Blink your eyes five times, then shift only your eyes, looking right, left, right, left. After the eye movement, keeping your hands on your hips, shift your weight to the right foot, and drag the ball of the left foot slightly behind you. Tap the floor two times, and drag the ball of the foot around to your side and then to the front of you, making a large semicircle on the floor. When your left foot arrives in front of your body, balance your weight between both feet and bend both knees. Bring the hands from their position on your hips to the front of your body, crossed at the wrists, right wrist on the bottom. Bring your thumb and ring fingers to slightly touching, with palms facing upward. Try to keep your fingers close together in this mudra. Remain with knees bent in the position for four breaths. The left foot is flat on the floor, and the right foot is resting on the ball of the foot, heel lifted. Tap the left foot on the floor with the ball of your foot, keeping the knees bent and hands in mudra pose.

MEDITATION AND PRACTICE

Chauka means square, which represents a completely stable structure. So, chauka reflects the balanced, all-encompassing, and universal quality of dharma. Body mudras, as we can call them, represent serenity of the Soul. Embodying sacred mudras in ancient India

pointed to having transcended the limitations of life and being elevated to the higher realms of being. The reincarnation cycle was
over, and transcendence was complete.

Moksha is enlightenment and spiritual release for human beings.
It's a harvested result of repetitive Sacred Dance Meditation, being
awakened, and staying awakened through dharma. In this sense,
it's the outcome of aligning wants and ways of being to the point at
which you don't have to think about it anymore.

August 12: Divine Beauty

SACRED DANCE

Now, bring the left foot close to the right foot so that your weight is
evenly distributed on both feet and your knees remain bent. Unfurl
your wrists, but keep your mudra hands, so that the left arm lifts
upward and the right arm is brought down and slightly behind your
body, with palms facing away from your body. Your gaze is toward
the left hand. Hold this position for four breaths. Then stand with
your knees slightly bent. Bring your left palm to rest on your left
hip, and place your right palm over the left.

MEDITATION AND PRACTICE

Rasa referred to emotions or a state of mind that could be affected
through sacred dance. Ancestors from India believed that by using
expressions of the body, sacred dancers gained and provided spiritual insights though movements. Those who were watching them
dance gained insights also. Beauty informed the Higher Self and
was a pathway to Divine ecstasy. Sacred Dance Meditation drew
from notions of sacred beauty to create an empowered aesthetic
experience.

In the Indus Valley, the sole *purpose* of Sacred Dance Meditation
was to use Divine beauty to produce rest and relief for the weary
and exhausted or for those who felt overrun with grief, or for those
heavy with misery, or for people who lost fortunes. It was a vehicle to enlighten and light the path toward a better existence. The

primary *goal* of Sacred Dance Meditation was to create rasa to lift and transport the sacred dancers and people in the temples, into the expression of Ultimate Reality and transcendence.

There are so many beautiful things here on earth, and all of them were Divinely inspired. It's easy to be in the rush of day to day without really allowing beauty into the picture. What do you consider beautiful? How have you arranged beauty in your home and workspace?

August 13: Divine Countenance

SACRED DANCE

Stand in the mudra pose with hands on the left hip, and walk slowly and deliberately forward three steps—left, right, left—then tap twice with the ball of your left foot behind the right foot. Next, drag the ball of your left foot behind you, then to your left side, and then in front of you. This will cause you to turn to your right. Place your hands on your right hip, and repeat the walks—right, left, right— then tap twice with the ball of your right foot directly behind the left foot. Next, drag the ball of your right foot behind you, to your right side, and then in front of you.

MEDITATION AND PRACTICE

Facial expressions in Sacred Dance Meditation in ancient India portrayed love, happiness, compassion, anger, courage, fear, tranquility, and disgust—the entire range of human emotion. The eyes also portrayed emotions, showing sacred dancers as embodying the character of the god or goddess being represented to move people into moksha. Dancers considered the body and eyes as the external and internal manifestations of the same expression. Without the eyes, the sacred dance would be irrelevant.

It's been said that the eyes are the windows to the Spirit, since they can reveal a great deal about what a person is feeling or thinking and how that person is doing. And one's face sends a greeting before anything is said. What a mind is thinking shows up on the face.

You can practice having a neutral facial expression that may be good for certain situations. Yet, your face can become permanently locked in configurations that don't serve you spiritually. Find rest for your face: relax your forehead, relax your jaw, and soften your thoughts. Remember that smiling and laughing are vital for the Soul and Spirit.

August 14: Artistic Beauty Harvest Havings

SACRED DANCE

Practice and trance your sacred dance today. Feel the poses, feel the stance of certainty, and feel your Self secure in knowing that where you stand is in the best possible place.

MEDITATION AND PRACTICE

The quintessence of sacred ancient Indian dance meditation was artistic expression, in every part of the body, to harvest the indwelling Spirit. No feelings were ignored, and no circumstance was demeaned. The people were given a way to celebrate themselves and heal from thinking and ways of acting that diverged from self, while guiding them to seek beauty and artistic forms as a practice toward enlightenment.

Focus on your vibrations in your comings and goings; be awake and aware to receive beauty within your body temple. Share this beauty with other Souls as you dance. You can always be at your peak with the Divine dancing with you. In this way, you harvest your "havings" in the present moment and align them with sacred ways of being.

❋ ❋ ❋

AUGUST 15–21
Harvesting Growth (Entry Point)

Look from whence you came.
The road less traveled is still a traveled road.

Kathakali sacred dance uses a lot of makeup, headdresses, and masks to create an identity. The masks extend the face, making it larger than life. The costumes and makeup elevate the dancers above their human and mundane selves so that they may transport the audience to the higher realms. Music for this sacred dance includes two drums—the *chenda* and the *maddalam*—and cymbals and the *ela taalam*. Using music or bells on your wrists and ankles is a very good idea. Kathakali sacred dance begins at night and finishes at dawn, when "good" conquers "evil," as the story goes.

August 15: Cycles of Change

SACRED DANCE

We focus on the hand mudras in this sacred dance. Face the east, and place the weight of your body evenly on both feet, with the knees bent. Your hands are at about heart chakra level with your elbows pressing outward away from your body. Your face is pleasant, with a slight smile. Place your right palm open with index finger and thumb spread and the remaining fingers cupped together, as if receiving a bottle. Place your left hand with palm facing away from you, index and thumb gently touching each other at the fingertips. The remaining fingers are pointing toward the ceiling and are held together. Keep the elbow pushed away from your body and knees bent. Take three breaths, and alternate mudra poses between hands as you rotate the wrists. Repeat the poses by rotation of the wrists until you get the hang of it. Be patient with yourself!

MEDITATION AND PRACTICE

Sacred dance of Kathakali depicted inner characters of the gods and goddesses, whether saints, animals, demons, or demonesses. The depictions of character were tied to those of the three gunas, as discussed on August 2. The dance also told stories from history. According to ancient Indian beliefs and traditions, human history is cyclical, subject to the world's evolution and dissolution; each cycle forms one yuga. One yuga has four evolutionary levels, which are Satya Yuga, Treta Yuga, Dvapara Yuga, and Kali Yuga. After transiting through the yugas, creation began again, in an endless cycle of evolutions and dissolutions reflecting the spiritual distractions people have the farther they get from the Source.

It's so easy to be inspired at the beginning of a new spiritual Practice and to really get on a course for positive spirals to the Light. Since you began your spiritual journey or revelatory process, do you notice any phasic patterns to your evolution? In your journal, write down three decisions that you think changed the course of your life. Explain why they changed your life. These can be points when you could have gone a different direction. For example, maybe you took a job or joined a church that led you where you are today. Or maybe you listened to or ignored advice from a friend or relative. If you review your spiritual journey map (see March 28), this may help you to remember some events or decision points and get them down on paper.

August 16: Satya Yuga—Ages of Peace

SACRED DANCE

Today you start with the arms at heart-chakra height with the hands in the mudra poses. Feet bear the weight equally and knees are bent. Lift the right heel to touch the left knee, and place it back on the floor. Lift the left heel to touch the right knee, and place it back on the floor. Now, rotate the mudras between hands while alternating your feet to touch your knees. Try to get a rhythm where your lifted foot coordinates with the upward-pointing fingers. That is, if your left foot is tapping the right knee, the left hand has fingers pointing to the ceiling. Practice this until you get the mechanics and can do it without too much thinking.

MEDITATION AND PRACTICE

Lord Brahma, the first deity of the Hindu trinity, was known as the god of creation. He was said to have four faces, which demonstrated complete knowledge, and four hands, which represented four aspects of human consciousness. The mind was his back-right hand, the intellect his left-back hand, the ego the right-front hand, and the empirical the left-front hand. In depictions he carried *mala* beads in the upper-right hand, which symbolized time counted on a complete mala, through which evolution, sustenance, and dissolution occurred. He held the Vedas in the upper-left hand and a water pot in the lower-left hand; Lord Brahma gave grace through his lower-right hand.

The malas, Vedas, water pot, and grace were connected to the Satya Yuga or the golden age of human living, an age of truth and perfection. This yuga had all peace and harmony. The people were awakened; therefore, they weren't seeking spiritual experiences. Human beings were huge and powerful, honest, virtuous, and very intelligent and learned. They were the supremely blessed. There was no need to work, as riches were for the taking. The weather even participated, making everyone feel good and happy. Religion didn't exist, nor did disease, fear, and sadness. And sacred dance wasn't required because everyone was at peace and knew who they were in relation to G-d. Can you imagine such a place and time where there's peace and tranquility among everyone? Just let that sink in and feel what that's like.

August 17: Treta Yuga—Cracks in the System

SACRED DANCE

Review what you've done so far this week. Let's start with the right heel to the inside left knee, followed by the left heel to the inside right knee. Do that three times—right, left, right—then place the right foot down in a wider exaggerated step so you move to your right. With knees still bent, gently stomp in place three times, then repeat on the left. Bring your left heel to your inside right knee, then place the left foot down in a wider exaggerated step so you move to the left. With knees still bent, gently stomp in place three times. Repeat for each side of your body until you get the hang of it. Keep your mudras as you do this, with your elbows pressing away from your body.

MEDITATION AND PRACTICE

Treta Yuga was known as the second Yuga. During this cycle, many emperors rose to dominance and conquered the world. Wars became frequent, and extreme weather, such as floods, tornados, monsoons, and the like, increased. Oceans and deserts were formed. People became slightly agitated compared to their predecessors. They sustained themselves by growing and harvesting through human labor.

The second yuga cycle teaches about another aspect of the Ancient Hindu Trinity: Vishnu, the preserver of life. He was believed to protect lives by adhering to order and truth. He led and encouraged people to be kind and compassionate to all beings.

Vishnu took on many different forms and danced incarnated upon the earth as Rama, Krishna, and Gautama (Siddhartha) Buddha. In paintings and art forms, Vishnu held a lotus flower in his lower-left hand; a mace, which represents the outcomes of action and consequences, in his lower-right hand; a conch shell in his upper-left hand, which spreads the primordial sound of Om; and the Sudarshana chakra discus, the symbol of the wheel of time that stands for a glorious existence, in his upper-right hand.

From the ancients of the Indus Valley, we have an explanation of why the world is a certain way and why we might be going through our experiences. We know that life on earth makes very little sense and doesn't follow our expectations. But we can also think about the cyclic concept of yugas and apply them to our own growth. We can be aware when "a storm's brewing" and prepare for it, standing outside of fear. The only sure thing in life is change. So if we don't hold on too tightly, that will likely lessen the impact when the storm hits. It doesn't mean we don't care; it just means we don't get bantered around by every strong wind. That's easier said than done.

August 18: Dvapara Yuga—
Youthful Mind, Aged Body

SACRED DANCE

Repeat the sacred dance done on August 17. We now add the mudras to the wide steps. When you step to the left and right, rotate your mudras. At each wide sidestep, inhale, and exhale as you do the gentle stomps in place. Focus on your hands as you move, keeping your facial expression light, with a smile on your face, and think of the Supreme Deity.

MEDITATION AND PRACTICE

Dvapara Yuga was the third yuga in the transcending order of the cycle of change. Dvapara meant "two pair" or "after two." In this age, people became tainted with tamasic qualities and weren't as strong as their ancestors; any actions taken without care of consequences or regard for others was considered tamasic. Tamasic people were self-obsessed, dissatisfied with life, and materialistic. Their three guṇas were out of balance. In communities, physical and mental disease spread, and individuals were discontent and at odds with each other. Persons' bodies grew and aged, but their emotional and mental responses and capacity to reason remained childish.

Lord Shiva, the final deity of the ancient Hindu trinity, counterbalances the energy of the third yuga. He helps humanity avoid negative desires like greed and envy and opens the way for people to become enlightened and to break through delusions. He was also considered a destroyer, triggering rebirth. In art forms he was often drawn or cast with a serpent around his neck, which symbolizes Kundalini, or life energy.

The Dvapara Yuga can remind you that what you see in our world is not all that unique. Do you know people who are grown but have childish responses to life? Are you that way? Sacred dance gives you a way to deal with people who are out of balance, including yourself. Aside from engaging in sacred dance, know that there is shelter and protection. You aren't facing the world and its problems alone. But ponder these questions, and make a few notes: How do you protect yourself from conditions across the country and around the world that you really can't do anything about? How do you protect yourself from adults you encounter every day who exhibit childlike reactions?

August 19: Kali Yuga—
The Only Way Is Upward

SACRED DANCE

Bring the sacred dance all together today. Practice all the choreography given this week until you have it comfortably saved on your body and mind.

MEDITATION AND PRACTICE

In the final evolution of the process of change, people entered Kali Yuga, a time of darkness and ignorance. At this point, the ancient Indian people were chained to their passions and couldn't remember who they were in Satya Yuga. Society fell into disuse, and people lied, saying one thing and doing another. Knowledge of the Divine was lost, and scriptures were laughed at. People ate poorly. They had no regard for the environment; water and food were scarce. Their health declined, and families didn't exist anymore. By the end of a Kali Yuga period, the average lifespan was about twenty years.

Perhaps we don't think of our society as going through phases and getting ready for a new start, forgetting, due to manifestations of self-obsession, how wonderful life was supposed to be. Whether one believes that our universe goes through cycles really doesn't matter too much. What does matter is that human beings go through them and that in the darkest moments, sometimes, the Light breaks a cycle. But more than that, spiritual spiraling happens due to an enlightened experience that supersedes the previous ones.

Maybe you've had such an experience but it was so long ago you might not believe it ever happened. Thus you strive to remember and to keep moving upward. You may be lonely on your path, or you may feel like you're not progressing or you shouldn't have come all this way. But you have, and you are! You must believe that you can break the cycle of reincarnation—that is, despite slipping backward and forgetting, staying in a place where your emotions and thinking don't get in the way of being Divine all the time.

August 20: I've Been Dancing for Many Kalpas

SACRED DANCE

Today you'll practice the sacred dance and add some of your own flare, and improvise if you'd like, to make the sacred movements yours.

MEDITATION AND PRACTICE

It was said that a *kalpa* was the period between the creation and re-creation of a world or Universe, being over four billion years long and only one day in Brahma's life. By this measure, the life of Brahma seems fantastic and interminable, but from the viewpoint of eternity it's as brief as a lightning flash. At the end of a yuga, the Supreme Being appeared as the Kalki Avatāra, vanquished the demons, saved his people from their self-obsessions, and thus began the next yuga.

You may feel like you're dancing sacredly in slow motion, and between each spiritual awakening are hundreds of thousands of millions of kalpas. That's the idea behind looking for spiritual progress, not perfection—as is being grateful for the life you have. As you wait for a "new world" to be created in you, focus on your evolution, and celebrate the guidance and direction you've found. How do you feel the integration with your Higher Self is going?

August 21: Pralaya—Period of Rest

SACRED DANCE

Again, repeat what you've learned of the dance this week, and this time try to find yourself in a trance.

MEDITATION AND PRACTICE

Pralaya means "dissolution" or "melting away." It refers to a period when the Universe was in a state of nonexistence, which happened when the three guṇas were in perfect balance. It is a time of repose, or a period of rest between manifestations and was often considered the dormancy between two great life cycles. Pralaya is also a resting place between spiritual leaps. Every living entity shifts between rest and activity, so many types of pralayas exist.

The main point is that more pralayas develop within you as you take each leap upward, helping to propel you further in your spiritual quest, because action follows rest. During pralaya, the old thinking and behaving dissolves, but your memory of your previous self is still there. Aren't you glad you get to rest?

------------------------------ ❊ ❊ ❊ ------------------------------

AUGUST 22–31
Harvesting Joy (Entry Point)

Dedication and devotion bring forth joy.

There is joy in being of service to the Divine and the human beings with whom we encounter.

August 22: Devotion

------------------------------ SACRED DANCE ------------------------------

Enter the Sacred Dance Posture today with your selected Sacred Dance Attire. Stand with your feet about shoulder-width apart and your knees slightly bent. Your heels are near each other, but your big toes are pointing away from each other. Get in touch with your neck and shoulders. While pushing your shoulders down and keeping your mudra held with your elbows pressing outward from your body, slide your head to the right, and hold it there for an inhale and exhale. Slide it back to center, hold it there, and inhale and exhale. Slide it to the left, hold it there, and inhale and exhale. Return to center. The shifting can be very small, almost unnoticeable, or larger as you prefer. When you move your head to the right, shift your eyes to the right, and when you move your head to the left, shift your eyes in that direction. As you inhale think of Spirit; as you exhale think of being in the present moment. Repeat until you have a rhythm.

MEDITATION AND PRACTICE

Kuchipudi sacred dance was done in temples and focused on spiritual beliefs and devotion to the gods and goddesses. Kuchipudi began with an invocation of the goddesses of learning, wealth, and energy. The Sacred Dance Meditation included energizing and sprinkling sacred water and burning incense for purification. Men danced the Kuchipudi, emphasized *bhakti*, and aimed to connect devotees and deities through it. The goal was to invoke immortal joy and salvation.

Devotion is defined as loyalty, dedication, or love for someone or something. We think of it a spiritual path of deep love and commitment to the Divine. We acknowledge it and give it first place in our lives. To our best ability, we acknowledge it in all beings. If we come from this place, we harvest joy. In Sanskrit, this devotion is called bhakti and is expressed through vibrating body mantras and worshiping the Divine through sacred dance. The Bhagavad Gita describes the path of devotion as superior to the paths of knowledge and action. The Bible says we advance because of grace. The Sutras point out that devotion to G-d is pure and egoless. Only when the sacred dancer is free from attachments and focuses fully on liberation and union with the Divine does he or she harvest such joy.

Are you devoted? Are you of a single focus?

August 23: Merging with the Divine via Devotion

SACRED DANCE

Let's repeat the sacred dance choreography from August 22 for eight complete cycles of breaths beginning on your right. Next, bring your left arm up, and open your mudra palm to the sky as if holding a tray with glasses filled with sacred water. Bring your right arm down to slightly behind your right hip, keeping the mudra intact as you do. Now, add the eight complete cycles of breaths, beginning to your right, with head and eye shifts, as you hold your arms in this pose.

Radha and Krishna were known in ancient India as the combined feminine and masculine realities of G-d, being the primeval forms of G-d. It was said that Krishna enchants the world, but Radha "enchants even him." She was the Supreme Goddess. Their sacred dance was considered the highest form of love, symbolizing the Soul seeking Divine love. It's the unique relationship between humans and the Ultimate Reality. Krishna was revered as the Divine, who could only be reached through Radha, or devotion and love. Radha and Krishna were said to exist symbiotically as they were Radha Krishna.

Sacred Dance Meditation is a devotion, an expression of love for the Divine. The dance carries the messages from you to the listening Universe, and from the Universe to you. It is an expressive act that embodies you and your relationship with your Higher Self. Sometimes we don't even realize that we are disconnected to our Higher Self; we just assume it's there and forget about It. The Higher Self in you is the Divine, whom you reach through your increasing awareness of that Indwelling Spirit and allowance of the relationship to flourish. Do you leave your Higher Self? Are you bored with the relationship? If you are, why not try to find some new ways to engage it, such as sacredly dancing in every room of your home or workplace? Or asking a group of people to join you in Sacred Dance Meditation? Perhaps you could learn about a religious Practice that you haven't studied before. Do you express your adoration and devotion to your Higher Self? Do you realize how it loves you unconditionally and your Soul longs for this love? This is the kind of relationship that fills all holes and makes you whole.

August 24: A Sentimental Bhakti

Today revisit the sacred dance choreography given on August 23. After completing the eight head shifts with the left palm up and the right palm slightly behind you, hold the sacred dance position for two breaths. Now lift the right knee to hip level, and hold it for a beat. Then place the foot back on the floor, and do four quick, close-to-the-ground right-left-right-left steps in place. Immediately lift the right knee up to hip level again. The knee lift receives the accent. Repeat this eight times. On the last iteration, close the sacred dance by quickly stepping in place for several breaths.

MEDITATION AND PRACTICE

In ancient India, bhakti was a way to express love for a personal god, goddess, or their representation. In ancient texts *bhakti* meant participation, devotion, and love for any endeavor, while in the Bhagavad Gita, it marks one path of spirituality and toward moksha. Following bhakti, it was believed, led to salvation or nirvana. Bhakti was also a form of devotional, selfless service: in addition to loving and serving a god or deity, one would also love and serve the Divine in everything and through that realize salvation. According to the Bhagavad Gita, a Hindu religious text, the path of bhakti was superior to both the paths of knowledge and of karma. The ancients in India believed that bhakti served as the foundation for all spiritual and sacred paths.

Understanding bhakti allows us to develop, and modify when needed, a consistent process of nurturing ourselves along a chosen path. Members of structured spiritual traditions who believe in their doctrines are sometimes attached to their chosen god or deity and to their Practices. In other cases, people venture in and out of different traditions, taking what they like and leaving the rest. Some people don't believe in deities at all. The point is that your sentimental bhakti is yours. Remember your Self in the process, to be of service to your Highest Good always and to be accepting of all spiritual Practices if they serve the good of all. What do you do when confronted with a spiritual seeker who seems at odds with you and your point of view? How can you harvest any spiritual growth from the situation? Gentleness will go a long way, but you might want to reflect on this question.

August 25: Vishnu's Sacred Dance of Joy

SACRED DANCE

Keeping the mudra position with the left palm open toward the sky and the right palm slightly behind your right hip, step slightly backward with your right foot, and touch the left heel to the inside right knee as we did last week. Place the left foot down on the floor to the side so that you have a wide stance. Keep your left palm facing the ceiling, and touch the right fingertips to the floor. Rotate your body slightly to face the open space between your outstretched leg and your bent right knee. Then bring your palms together in a cupped position. Hold this for a moment, then do four head shifts with the eyes shifting as well, barely perceptible. Bring the palms together, then move them up and above your forehead. Do four head shifts and eye shifts, nearly imperceptibly. Then sweep your palms away from each other, fanning them down the sides of your body to return to a cupped position in front of you. Place them palms together, bring your left foot in as you twist your body and bring your heels together, with the knees bent, and return to standing position, keeping your palms placed together with the fingertips pointing upward. Do eight head and eye shifts.

MEDITATION AND PRACTICE

Our ancient Indian ancestors had one thousand names of Vishnu. Chanting his names was a form of worship and devotion and was a part of the Sacred Dance Meditation. Vishnu sacredly danced creation into existence with three Sacred Dance Meditations. His first and second dances created earth, air, and humanity, and his third created the manifest Universe. Through devoting to his sacred dance, secrets of the Universe and dharma were revealed to people. His wife, Lakshmi, was the goddess of material and spiritual wealth and unlimited abundance; she infused his dances with an active energy. When needed, Vishnu embodied a portion of himself simultaneously at different locations to disrupt and defeat evil and to protect dharma. Vishnu was omnipresent, free from any attachments whenever he was embodied, and equivalent to Brahman, the supreme deity.

Some say that people can be many places at once, embodied in ways that help the cosmos and bring insight to those they are helping. Releasing the Spirit to travel to places can be easily imagined as you pray for your family, loved ones, and community members, seeing them in your mind's eye. If you add the caveat of "not my will but Yours" to your prayers, you can be free from attachment and show your devotion to your Higher Power by trusting in the guidance and results. You can remember what it was like for you when you were younger and imagine what you will be like in the future. Some people believe in past lives. So it's not difficult to imagine that you can be in more than one place at the same time. In the end, the only thing you have control over is devotion to the path and the Divine wisdom of the Universe. How do you devote yourself to your connection to the Divine through prayer? What three sacred dance steps can you align with as you pray?

August 26: Respecting Devotion

SACRED DANCE

Stand in your sacred dance position with palms touching and elbows held away from your body. Knees are slightly bent. Reach your palms over your head, keeping them together, and beginning with the right foot take five steps backward. Open your palms and arms outward away from your body, keeping your arms at shoulder height. Lift the right leg with the knee leading high, and step forward with the right foot then, continuing forward, left, right, left, right. With the right foot, place the weight on the ball of the foot with knees bent. Extend the arm away from the body toward the right, arm at shoulder height. The right hand holds the mudra, with the thumb and forefinger touching and remaining fingers pointing toward the sky. The left palm has the fingers pointing downward to the ground, with the arm held out away from your body, slightly below shoulder level. Hold the pose for a moment, as you head-shift and eye-shift, slightly, eight times. Bring the feet together, and return to the standing position, holding the right hand up with palm facing upward and the left arm down near the back of the left hip with the mudra fingers pointing to the ground. Hold this position.

MEDITATION AND PRACTICE

Goddess Shakti was an integral aspect of every god or goddess, as well as the force energizing the Universe. Every devotional act paid her respect. She was able to summon all primordial cosmic energy to create and change things, people, circumstances, and existences. She was the dynamic Kundalini force thought to move through the entire Universe, liberating those who sought dharma and casting away those who interfered with good. As a living cosmic force, Shakti took on many forms. In addition to being considered the Great Divine Mother, who supplied all Divine feminine power, she was a fierce warrior and the dark goddess of destruction when manifested to destroy demons and restore balance. Knowing that Shakti was there, people were able to feel a sense of joy and sacredly dance in deep devotion.

Devotion allows you to change things. Devotion also requires commitment, which your Higher Self has already given. But you must devote yourself to the path, no matter the circumstances, even when the path gets rough and narrow or when you are depressed, hungry, happy, with people, or alone. Devotion accompanies you in the doubt, darkness, despair, and re-creating, and manifesting. Devotion is an act, but it's also a position, a dance unto itself, with you and the Divine.

August 27: Avatars and Self-Projection

SACRED DANCE

Repeat the same motions you did on August 26, but oriented to the left; so, begin your steps with your left leg, and end with your right hand up.

MEDITATION AND PRACTICE

An avatar was the material appearance or incarnation of a deity on earth. Avatars were true embodiments of spiritual perfection, driven by dharma; they illustrated the divine reality explicitly. Vishnu had avatars who came to both empower the good and defeat evil, thus returning the dharma. Avatars appeared when the Cosmos was in crisis, when evil grew stronger than good, putting the Cosmos out of balance. They restored the balance or moved the Cosmos to the next cycle on the path of re-creation. As stated in the Bhagavad Gita (4.7–4.8), "Whenever righteousness wanes and unrighteousness increases, I send myself forth. For the protection of the good and for the destruction of evil, and for the establishment of righteousness, I come into being age after age."

Wondering whether a savior is coming to help the people of the world live by the Light is missing the point. The savior is within you. Your acts and behaviors save the world. If every human could act, think, and otherwise live from the place of love and wisdom, and not from selfish desires, our avatar would be easily seen as a material manifestation of our Supreme Being.

August 28: A Krishna-Like Consciousness

SACRED DANCE

Please review the Sacred Dance Meditation and choreography given this week. Practice it until you feel comfortable.

MEDITATION AND PRACTICE

Sri Krishna, the Lord of the Dance, was an avatar of Vishnu who was born in northern India around 3228 BCE. Ancient Indians considered Sri Krishna's life to mark a passing into the Kali Yuga. In the Sanskrit language, the word *krishna* means "dark." At that time the color was an expression of the Supreme Consciousness that was unseen by or unknown to those who were unaware. Because of that, in that incarnation Krishna was the dark-faced, flute-playing god, the symbol of pure love, wisdom, and joy. Krishna was said to have transmitted the wisdom of the Bhagavad Gita to one of his earthly worshippers. With that act he was named as the original spiritual master, or the first guru.

Krishna consciousness became a state of awareness in which an individual danced in complete harmony with the Divine or the ultimate reality of Brahman. As a form of bhakti, the purpose of this consciousness was to devote one's thoughts, actions, and worship to unifying with wisdom.

To act with Krishna-like consciousness is to free your Soul from the illusion that it's an individual body and know that all power resides within you. You experience the bliss of your true, eternal nature. Anyone can do this because it's a common natural ability. Sacred Dance Meditation gives you the tools for stepping outside the ego and cultivating a higher consciousness in service to your Spirit. As an avatar of your chosen spiritual path, as fully representational of the Higher Power with committed devotion, this kind of consciousness is achieved. Others who see you observe this. Your Light arrives before you do, and you become able to sacredly dance through all circumstances. Do you want a consciousness like that?

August 29: Getting a Guru

SACRED DANCE

Today is the day to improvise the sacred dance to make it your own. Give it a try so that it becomes you, to deeply communicate with your Higher Self.

MEDITATION AND PRACTICE

In a spiritual sense, a guru was someone moving people forward on their journey to dharma and out of maya. Several levels of spiritual gurus were in ancient India, ranging in expertise from teachers to masters to enlightened masters. Gurus were often sacred dance meditators. Enlightened masters were highly sought after because they were believed to be able to imbue the Spiritual Seeker with sacred dance wisdom written in the ancient Natyashastra texts.

Spiritual gurus show up in our lives as teachers. They can be loving and compassionate or do unimaginable things to get our attention. They may not entertain our delusions and tell us so in no uncertain terms, or they can be professionals who show up in our lives at opportune moments. They help us open and show us what we cannot see in ourselves. The guru reflects a skillful and awakened mind and reveals the same in us. The knowledge from the guru's mind is infused with the Light of experience or of a whole lineage of his prior masters. It has the power to cleanse and transform.

Whether or not you follow a guru, you eventually must be your own guide to Source. You learn that the guru is within. Teachers help you see yourself in this way, to move you from maya to dharma.

August 30: Brahman

SACRED DANCE

Trance-dance the choreography given this week.

MEDITATION AND PRACTICE

In the nonseparate way of contemplating the spiritual path in ancient India, Brahman is identical to the Atman, or Self, which is everywhere and inside each living being. It is genderless, unchangeable, and infinite and is the cause of positive change. A connected spiritual oneness informs and animates all existence. Awareness of Brahman leads to feeling and experiencing moksha, self-realization, joy, and a knowing of inseparability from others. But maya dwells with Brahman. Whereas maya is unconscious, Brahman-Atman is conscious. Maya changes, causes confusion in people, evolves, and dies. Brahman is eternal and unchanging and provides an absolute knowing of consciousness. As a metaphysical construct, it's the unification of everything in the Universe. Within this ideology, humans are faultless, compassionate, and good.

We are connected to Brahman, and Braham allows us to dance with this mystery, helping us to see ourselves as deeply and universally well. With this kind of self-knowledge, we can allow ourselves to shine and devote ourselves to sacredly dancing along our chosen spiritual path.

August 31: Dance in Service to Spiritual Harvest

SACRED DANCE

Review sacred dances given in August, and select one you particularly resonated with. You might want to review the videos and your notes from the week.

MEDITATION AND PRACTICE

Ancient Indians had an extensive and elaborate Sacred Dance Meditation founded on the principles of Brahman and dharma. They considered the human experience and put the sacred dance of Brahman in Lord Shiva and the Sanskrit texts.

Whatever you believe about the way the world or the Cosmos is, know that for years and years, others have had the same puzzles and predicaments, some unimaginable. The world today is really in need of avatars who will dance sacredly in service to bringing Souls across the great divide from delusion to dharma.

Dancing in Truth

EAST ASIAN SACRED DANCE

During September, we rely on East Asian Sacred Dance to further embody notions of truth. So often we're instructed to speak the truth and to know the truth will set you free. A short review of human behavior will almost always tell you this is a myth. Truth is situational. Or perhaps there are Absolute Truths that we need to know and believe in.

What is true for you now? What is no longer true? How does that truth manifest in your life? How do you want to make it manifest in the future?

This month we learn weekly Sacred Dance Meditations drawing on East Asian traditions, culminating in offerings to Spirit to live fully in one's truth. Ancient Korean, Japanese, Chinese, and Mongolian forms give us the basis for our path of truth in connection with Spirit.

KOREAN SHAMAN DANCE

Shamanism is the oldest spiritual Practice of Korean people, originating five thousand years ago, before Confucianism, Daoism, and Buddhism came to Korea. It has influenced many aspects of Korean beliefs, central to which was polytheism and communication with ancestors.

Shamans could be men or women but generally were women, called *mudang* or *mu*. Their role was to act as intermediary between the Spirit realms and humanity to solve problems through *gut*, or spiritual ritual. Sacred Dance Meditation is the central component of gut. During the gut rite, Korean shamans made offerings and sacrifices to gods and ancestors. Besides sacred dance, gut incorporated songs, oracles, and prayers. Through these methods, the shaman asked the gods to intervene, changing people and their situations regarding health, financial needs, spiritual growth, and anything that could be a human being's issue.

Koreans considered the person from a wholistic point of view, taking into consideration environmental factors and the person's temperament. Spirit was known to be the source of breath and life. Illness resulted from a Soul sickness. Mental illness was considered to arise from Spirit evacuation, loss, intrusion, or possession.

The Korean dance Salp'uri is one of Korea's most creative sacred dances. It is based on pauses symbolizing thought that leads to actions, which are shown by snapping the arm and holding a handkerchief. Through movement, the dance expresses looking within to Spirit, rather than outside, for truths.

The dance was used in Korean shamanism for two purposes. The first was to rid someone of evil spirits. The shaman removed *sal*, or negative energy, from the person by taking it into herself. She released the sal from her own psyche after that. The second purpose was to soothe the spirits of the dead and lead them to heaven. The shaman was particularly involved in helping the living with grief, especially helping women come to a peaceful place after the death of their mate.

JAPANESE KAGURA

Kagura is the oldest sacred dance in Japan, dating back to the prehistoric Jōmon era from about 14,000 to 1000 BCE, when female shamans and priestesses went into trances and communed with spirits. From their trance state, the women conveyed gods' words to the people.

The original kagura dances were called *mikagura*, which were performed in several sacred places, like sanctuaries and Shinto shrines. A *miko* was a shaman who took care of religious duties in shrines and served as spiritual mediums and sacred dancers.

The dance conveyed animism, shamanism, and love of nature and fertility. The word *kagura* literally means "seat of the deity"; the sacred dance was a ritual to elicit help from the gods.

Kagura dances had two main parts. First, purification rituals invoked the gods, as certain deeds created impurities that should be cleansed. One's peace of mind and good fortune resulted from removing impurity, leaving the human as a perfect Spirit. In the second part, movements honored the invoked spirits. Every aspect of the dance pointed to the crucial need to encourage the *kami* to come down and dance.

The word *kami* had several nuances. It meant "spirits," "essences," or "gods," and in some contexts it referred to the energy that produced these unseen elements. But kami could also be embedded as sacred essences in nature, locations, and people. Such essences were also able to control the power of phenomena that inspired a sense of wonder and awe, affirming the divinity within people, places, and living things. Kami lived in everything, but at particular locations people and kami interfaced, mostly in nature spots believed to be imbued with sacred spirits, such as mountains, waterfalls, rivers, and trees.

In this sacred dance, you'll wear your Sacred Dance Attire overlain with a white garment, and you will want to wear white socks. You will need a large handheld fan, a red scarf, and percussive bells on a wooden stick.

CHINESE SLEEVE DANCE

Sacred dancing with long sleeves started long before the Zhou dynasty. Ancient Chinese people engaged in the sleeve dance from at least 1045 BCE to 256 BCE, yet sacred dance was recorded in Chinese before 2000 BCE on bronze implements, we're told. During the late Zhou dynasty, *wu* referred to "female shaman." That was when the gods of nature dominated and heaven worship was the spiritual culture of the ancient Chinese people. The world and the gods were a holistic formation of the Cosmos; known as Tiān, the formation was the highest power and the ancient Chinese term for heaven. G-d was manifested as the northern culmen and starry vault, regulating nature from the stars and constellations of the Little and Big Dippers (a.k.a. the Gate of Heaven and the Pivot of Heaven, sometimes referred to together as the celestial clock).

From there, the gods directed life and existence on earth and generated beings as their successors. The ancestors were venerated as the equivalent of heaven on earth. Because shamans went between humans and the gods of heaven, they were highly respected. The ancient Chinese thought "the Universe create[d] itself out of a primary chaos of material energy."* From the principle that everything came from one source, the forces organized as yin and yang, which characterized everything. Creation was therefore a continuous ordering, not a onetime event as other cultures tended to lean toward. Yin and yang constituted duality, which couldn't be escaped. The principle of yin and yang underpinned the yearly seasons, the movement of the sun, males and females, and disorder and order in everything and every situation.

The gods themselves were also subject to that principle. As the yin forces of expansion, they were expanding gods or spirits. As yang forces of contraction, they were demons or ghosts. People were *hun*, or more yang, or *po*, or more yin. Yin and yang formed two layers of the Soul, that of the rational and of the emotional. Together, yin and yang created a twofold operation of the god of Heaven, which pointed back to the northern culmen and starry

---

* Stephen Feuchtwang, "Chinese Religions," in *Religions in the Modern World*, 3rd ed., ed. Linda Woodhead, Paul Fletcher, Hiroko Kawanami, and David Smith (London: Routledge, 2002), 150.

vault. That then merged to what was known as *shen*, or Spirit. People and their ancestors had a part to play in ongoing creation and evolution. They influenced the god of Heaven and the formation of heaven itself. Thus, each creature was also creator, and life on earth consequently was not only a fixed constituent of truth but also a promoter and author of it. Because the wu went between the earth and sky, they were highly revered, as they carried information between the two and influenced the balance of creation and creator. The Sacred Dance Meditation of water sleeves allowed flow of life's truths to be made available to all beings.

MONGOLIAN SHAMAN DANCE

Mongolia is situated between Russia to the north and China to the south. The ancient Mongolian animistic and shamanic ethnic religion of Mongolia, including Buryatia and Inner Mongolia, had been practiced since the age of recorded history. Mongolian shamanism was centered on the worship of Tengri, or blue-sky god, and the Highest Tengri, or Qormusta Tengri. Tengrists existed and thrived within the eternal blue sky, the earth Spirit of fertility called Eje, and the Holy Spirit that governed the heavens. They believed that their needs were provided for by nature spirits, ancestors, heaven, and earth. Furthermore, they thought that by living a respectful and upright life, they kept their lives in balance so they could perfect their personal Spirit, or what they called Wind Horse.

For the ancient Mongolians, beings went to an underworld where they couldn't breathe. It was darker than earth and contained modified forests, rivers, and inhabited spaces. Like the Egyptian ancestors, they believed in Shadow Souls and different names and attributes of the human Soul. For the ancient Mongolians, the heavens above were like earth but had a pastoral feel, with no human negativity. Beings who dwelt there were considered perfect. Shamans were said to have often visited these realms.

Shamans entered altered states of consciousness through dancing, drumming, chanting, and so forth. The altered state produced an out-of-body experience, Soul travel, or Spirit possession. Being a shaman wasn't a choice—one was selected by a message sent from the Spirit world. Like the shamans in other cultures discussed this month, a shaman was chosen because of serious illness or hallucination. During such an event, a qualified shaman was called in to evaluate the sick person to see whether the person had been chosen to be a shaman. If that was the case, the person was verified and initiated to use magic formulas, songs, and sacred dances to do the work of healing and warding off evil.

After initiation, the new shaman received a staff, which had a horse's head carved on the handle with the base shaped like the horse hoof. After a few years, the shaman received a sacred drum. These sacred implements protected the shaman from negative forces. The shaman wore head coverings too, which represented the power of animal spirits. For instance, a covering with eagle feathers gave the shaman strength, and owl feathers gave the power of nocturnal vision.

PREPARATION

Sacred Dance Attire differs for each week and is described at the "Entry Points." If you'd like to use music you may. Arrange for incense and oils to be burned safely within your Sacred Dance Studio, and you can also remind yourself that these sacred dances have come down to you through the ages and are worth adding as part of your regular Practice.

Please visit www.cswalter.org/sacreddancemeditations for video demonstrations. They are not intended to be step-by-step instructions but are meant to give you a view of the sacred dance.

SEPTEMBER 1–7
Dancing in Truth (Entry Point)

The body shows forth Truth.

Slow the body to determine which way to go, to hear the voice of Spirit leading, to realize the Truth of your Being.

The Sacred Dance Attire for this week is a white overlay long enough to touch the floor. Your face holds a very pensive affect, and your focus is downward. This dance's hand gestures symbolize worshipping the sky, while the footsteps move downward to worship the earth. You engage with Salp'uri Sacred Dance Meditation this week. It builds energy through very slow repetition of the choreography to allow internal focusing and thereby enhancing spiritual connection with G-d.

September 1: The Body of Truth

SACRED DANCE

Stand with your feet close together, with your left palm on the front of your hip and your right palm holding the white handkerchief in the back of your right-hip area. Bring the right arm out, and hold it parallel to the floor, keeping the handkerchief or scarf held loosely. Bend slightly forward, and rise and lower your body for eight breaths, using the balls of your feet. The movement is very slow. Hold your left elbow away from your body with your hand on the hip as you do the movement. Gently rise and lower the right wrist with the scarf or handkerchief as you rise and lower. Return to the starting position, then bend the knees as if you were going to sit. Hold the position for eight breaths, keeping the arms in their place. Return to the beginning position with the handkerchief behind you.

MEDITATION AND PRACTICE

The ancient Indigenous Korean shamanistic tradition, called Muism, began five thousand years ago, eventually connecting Korea with Central Asia, Siberia, and northern Scandinavia. Its rituals involved a shaman contacting the Spirit world, Soul travel, and ecstatic trance. Ancient Koreans worshipped the sky, through a gut, or ritual, called *jecheonuirye*. Shamans moved into and out of trances at will and, during them, their followers believed the Spirit left the body and traveled to other realms. In these realms, other spirits help the Shaman perform spiritual, psychological, and physical healing. The sacred dance we perform this week, a ritual worshipping with one's own body, was the original form of jecheonuirye.

Some say the body knows and shows the truth, even when the person doesn't see it. Truth is characterized as fact: honesty, reality, knowing. The important part is to slow down to hear it, to silence the incessant thoughts. Stillness comes from focusing inward while being in motion.

As you slow your thoughts and focus inward, note what arises for you. As you quiet your thinking and focus on moving, see what kind of worship your body-mind experiences. When you complete the sacred dance, note what arose in you that might be a truth you were unaware of or didn't want to face.

September 2: *When to Tell the Truth*

SACRED DANCE

Repeat what you did on September 1. When you return to center, extend your right arm parallel to the floor as you're on the balls of your feet. If your Sacred Dance Attire is very long and touching the floor, use the left hand to gently raise it so you won't trip. Gently hold the scarf away from your body. Imagine the scarf is leading you around as you turn around in a clockwise circle where you're standing, very slowly. Repeat for four breaths. Return to resting.

MEDITATION AND PRACTICE

The role and reverence for the mu was based on how the shaman connected with seekers. Mu maintained a holistic view of a person, considering the individual's interaction with inner and outer worlds. The Spirit was considered the source of life's breath, and any physical illness related to spiritual sickness. Ancient Koreans also believed that illness of the mind was due to loss of the Spirit by intrusion or possession by malevolent spirits.

When the body tells us something isn't right, that could be because it's absorbed negativity or held on to fear. In our lives, we often encounter people who are mean, angry, resentful, selfish, prideful, greedy, or otherwise demonstrating ego-driven behaviors. Sometimes these people seem to get more out of life than we do and cause considerable pain to whole societies. They can be from any walk of life, religion or spirituality, gender, age—liars are everywhere! But everyone lies. One of the first lies some people tell every day is that they are doing fine. We say we're fine because people don't really want to know how we're doing. We either maintain the polite interchange among strangers, or we don't want to truly engage with others. Other lies are deeper, such as remaining in denial when we can't face the truth, remaining silent or inactive when we see injustices, or not taking responsibility for problems we've caused. We all lie about something. So, when do you tell the truth? Sometimes the truth is elusive because of the lenses we use.

But one truth is that your Inner Mystic Dancer longs to commune with the sacred. Another is that being with the sacred and listening to what the body-mind is saying can help you decipher your truth and find the courage to say and do what you need to in every situation.

September 3: Knowing

SACRED DANCE

Review the dance on September 2. Repeat that, and after the four breaths, bend your body slightly forward, and do several deep contractions from your midsection, with the scarf held out and away from you, for six breaths. After the contractions, deeply bend your knees, and bring the scarf slowly across your body toward your left shoulder. As you do that, slowly look upward toward the sky. Bring the scarf in slightly in front of your face. Then bring the scarf directly in front of you and stand up, slowly, keeping the scarf in front of you, with your arm slightly bent, holding it lightly.

A person became a shaman by either being born into the practice though matrilineal inheritance, having experienced an illness, or being "chosen" by the gods. Those who had become ill had a spiritual experience known as *shinbyeong*, sometimes known as the divine or shaman illness. It entailed being possessed by a Spirit, called a *momju*, and a loss of self. The chosen had symptoms of physical pain and mental illness. Believers asserted these symptoms could be cured only when the possessed accepted a full communion with the Spirit. The possessed then underwent the *naerim-gut*, a ritual that, when completed, healed the sickness and formally established the person as a shaman. During this ceremony, the shaman-to-be predicted future events in other people's lives.

We know many people—perhaps even us—who are constantly persuaded to do things and buy things to activate change, when those same promises for years have effected no change for others. Laws protect us from being swindled, but we still fall prey. So many times, we know the truth but don't want to face it, so we tell ourselves stories. But lying undermines trust of ourselves and others. Trusting is based on a desire for certainty, which there is none of, really. That's where the adage "trust but verify" comes in.

You can channel the Spirit to give you courage to hear what you know and to respond from your Inner Mystic Dancer. What would your world be like if people were spiritually, mentally, and emotionally healthy and acted from that stance? How many people can you influence by lovingly dancing in truth?

September 4: Reality or Realities?

To add to this week's dance thus far, after standing up with the scarf in front of you, slowly crouch down to brush the floor with the scarf, and flick your wrists between brushes. Repeat this for several breaths. Return to standing with your hand on your hip and the scarf held out in front of you.

MEDITATION AND PRACTICE

Shamanism has been a sacred method for millennia and is the longest surviving spiritual Practice. A shaman has been called a medical worker, diviner, mystic, and magician and can move at will into trances. While in a trance, the shaman's Soul was said to leave its body to travel into the spiritual realms, where she encountered all kinds of spirits—helpful and not. Shamans try to help defeat evil spirits and prevent them from hurting people. They heal individuals, tribes, and communities on physical, spiritual, and emotional levels.

So many spiritual Practices existed before the advent of our popular and now global religions, suggesting spiritual intervention is part of the human condition and that people look for spiritual answers to their situations. Concepts from shamanism—misapplied later—informed some of the world's major religions. Evil spirits, spiritual warfare, demon possession, and ghosts—these were wrangled out of benign shamanism. Yet the notion of healers and saviors also come from it. Maybe evil spirits are what we are when we have difficulty facing reality or the truth of our existence. We can think of spiritual Practices as ways to help us, and we get to the point of seeing Reality. It's also nice to have a facilitator, such as a shaman, to lovingly but firmly help us to see or to intervene on our behalf.

Are you willing to be a shaman? Are you called by the Divine to help people acknowledge their realities and thereby see Reality?

September 5: Authentic Truths

SACRED DANCE

Today, practice what you have learned so far this week. Try to get comfortable with all the moves, and get into a flow.

MEDITATION AND PRACTICE

The first goal of a *kangshinmu*, or someone who has undergone the naerim-gut, was to unite as one with G-d as part of the ceremony with the purpose of helping members of the community. During the ceremony, the candidate became one of two types of shaman.

One was the mudang; the other was *myŏngdu*. The myŏngdu conducted ceremonies for families of people who died and brought the deceased person's Spirit to a shrine in her dwelling for their safe passage to the next world.

When we go against our Selves, we sometimes wind up feeling ill. So many times, we put everything else before aligning with our Higher Self. We don't have time to prepare healthy meals, visit friends or fellowship, or see a therapist. We don't have time to do Sacred Dance Meditation or other spiritual work, which has been shown over and over to cause healing in the mind-body. We don't take time to understand the relationship between our mind-body and Spirit. Our society is so focused on the quick fix, taking medicines rather than herbs, rather than foods, rather than spiritual direction.

This is not to condemn any medical solution but to encourage forward movement and sacred dance. Listen to what you're hearing from your authentic depths when you dance. If you feel inclined, you could add a shaman to your team of well-being practitioners. If you've made promises to yourself or set intentional directions, please keep them, claiming your forward movement.

September 6: Wholeness and Truth

SACRED DANCE

Review and repeat what you did on September 5, and get this sacred dance into your body, finding ways to improvise and own the choreography.

MEDITATION AND PRACTICE

Shamanism in ancient Korea wasn't a religion, and there were no priests, texts, and dogma to adhere to. But shamans understood the Universe to be complex. The ancient Koreans believed in the Shaman's Tree, by which the shaman traveled from one world level to another.

The Shaman's Tree included an immovable central pole of creation and the primary gateway to worlds beyond the physical dimension. It provided a path between three main worlds: the upper, with Father Sky/Light; the middle, where humanity dwells; and the lower, where hidden things dwell. The tree represented the interconnectedness of truth of the earth, of humans, and of nonordinary reality within the Great Mystery.

Sometimes going to other realms helps us to find wholeness in our truth. We accept that help is available to us when we need it. It can be found on many different planes. We seek it, we need it, to continue our sacred dance of truth.

September 7: Slowly Revealed Truths

SACRED DANCE

Understand the Salp'uri Sacred Dance Meditation as a trance. Imagine yourself as you saw yourself yesterday. Recall your desire to know the truth, to recall the truths you know now, and slowly incorporate them into your body as you move. You can think of yourself traveling on the *axis mundi* (earth's axis), freely able to move between the realms.

MEDITATION AND PRACTICE

Shinbyeong meant "Spirit sickness" and was the central feature of a shaman's initiation. The symptoms of the shinbyeong could last from several years to up to thirty. Legends say that extreme cases of Spirit sickness prompted mudang to leave their homes and wander through mountains and rice fields. In the tradition of Muism, ancient Koreans considered the shinbyeong process a structured spiritual experience and awakening. Shinbyeong eventually caused the shaman to become one with G-d. Then, the shaman disassociated from secular life and embodied a higher form of consciousness.

For some of us, truth must be revealed slowly; we need to be convinced over time, like the ancient Koreans. Some truths are so revealing that they can at first cause us to feel unsure, a little ill, and desirous to be alone to digest them. We may reject them, only to return to them later—tomorrow or thirty years after. But by embracing the revealed truths slowly, thoughtfully, and deliberately, we can be assured that we are on the right path. We hear the call of Spirit and follow it so more can be revealed.

※　※　※

Tricks of Truth (Entry Point)

Ring the bells of truth.

There are many ways to entice the truth into being.

In this week's sacred dance, wear your Sacred Dance Attire over-lain with a white garment, and you will want to wear white socks. Remember the fan, scarf, and percussive bells, as discussed earlier.

September 8: Move Slowly toward the Truth

SACRED DANCE

Lift your arms up and in front of your face and cross the wrists with the left hand in front of the right. Hold the position for a few breaths, with knees slightly bent and your reverence toward the sky. Slowly and gently shake the bells, keeping them in place with the fan. The bells and fan should be directly in front of your face. Continue to gently shake the bells for several breaths.

MEDITATION AND PRACTICE

Kami were spirits worshipped in Shinto, the Japanese religion, as early as 1000 BCE. Spiritual powers and spirits existed in the natural world and were part of the landscape, forces of nature, and beings and their demeanors. Kami were also sometimes the spirits of venerated dead persons and had good and evil, positive and negative characteristics. They were manifestations of *musubi*, or what was considered the interconnecting energy of the Universe, and were role models for the people. Although hidden from this world, kami nevertheless inhabited a complementary existence mirroring embodied life.

Sometimes we seek truth, but often it seeks us. It's not clear which way the flow goes. Sometimes it may feel very elusive, as if it's trickery, like a neon light drawing us down a path with an unpleasant, unexpected turn.

Are there some people, places, or things you want to shake your bell at, either in gratitude or chastisement for tricking you? Have you considered yourself on the right course only to encounter a dead end? Have you experienced dashed expectations that required you to regroup? Or, due to an unforeseen shift in your consciousness, have you found yourself on a great, though unsmooth, path? Did you feel like you were tricked? These are kami moments, allowing us to learn and see. How did you reconcile these kami moments? Honor the bringing of the truth into being. When you have such a realization, make a note in your journal or calendar to memorialize it.

September 9: Truth in Love

SACRED DANCE

Inhale, bend your knees, and gaze toward the earth. Bend slowly forward from your waist and exhale, keeping the wrists in place and shaking the bells. Rise to a standing position, and inhale. Repeat this for six breaths—inhale at standing, and exhale when you bend forward. Return to the standing position with the bells and the fan held in front of your face, and focus your gaze above your head.

MEDITATION AND PRACTICE

Kami could nurture and love when they were treated well or cause destruction and disharmony when they weren't. They had to be appeased to gain their favor and avoid their wrath. Kami had a gentle nature, an assertive nature, a happy nature, and a mysterious nature. They were invisible to humans and inhabited sacred places, natural spaces, or people during Sacred Dance Meditations. Moreover, they were mobile and could visit places of worship and stay however long they liked; they often didn't stay too long at any one place. Many different varieties of kami existed, typically linked to natural and physical features, such as the kami of wind, kami of entryways, and kami of roads. Kami served the people and the areas around them. The exchange was reciprocal between them and every other imaginable being or essence.

Ancient Japanese kami philosophy does not place absolutes on truth; it takes the complexity of life into consideration. It marks the reciprocity between being human and Divine and paints a picture of balanced emotional states. We all have swings in our moods, and that often colors our ability to see the truth or interpret others. We also can be easy-going, but other times we must be assertive. Telling truth in love requires us to use the best aspects of our multifaceted humanity to help others, but sometimes we are on the receiving end of that. Some people need a good shove, and others need coddling to grasp a truth. Sometimes we need a shove or extra care to help us stay on track.

Was there a time when you were startled by something someone lovingly said or when a circumstance allowed you to see something you didn't really like? Or a time when you lovingly urged someone to see a truth? What about those occasions that you now wish someone *would have* told you the truth in love? Are people in your life now whom you should speak to about a truth?

September 10: Truth as Tough Love

SACRED DANCE

Slowly open the arms so that your elbows remain bent and held away from your body; the fan is held open as if you were going to fan yourself but is slightly away from your body. Hold the position for two breaths. Now smile gently as you step to the right with your right foot. Place the bells in front of you as you bend your knees and bend forward slightly from the waist, and shake the bells and nod your head forward, keeping the fan steady. Rise, and walk slowly in two clockwise circles, shaking the bells as you do so. Return to center. Hold there, and breathe.

MEDITATION AND PRACTICE

In Ancient Japan, Ame-no-Uzume was the goddess of dawn, and Amaterasu was the goddess of the sun. Amaterasu was created by a divine union of Izanagi and Izanami, who grew from the originator of the Universe, Amenominakanushi. Amaterasu was responsible for keeping balance and harmony within the earthly realm. She had two brothers: Susano'o, the god of storms and the sea, and Tsukuyomi, the god of the moon. Amaterasu developed a beautiful worldly landscape with her siblings when she created ancient Japan. One day she got fed up with her brother Susano'o for his ongoing disrespectful acts and sayings toward her. She added up the resentments from when he destroyed her rice fields, threw a dead horse at her loom, killed one of her attendants after a fight, damned her creation, and claimed she wasn't good at being a goddess. She expelled him from the heavens. Full of grief and anguish from his nonsense, she hid inside the Ama-no-Iwato, the "heavenly rock cave." When she did that, the earth went dark, and chaos ensued.

Sometimes, we must practice tough love when we give feedback, to say when enough is enough. And our feedback can have consequences for them, others, and ourselves. Like Amaterasu, many of us have retreated into "a cave" from time to time when we needed to, not responding to calls or texts or going where hurtful people are. At that stage, we've reached the breaking point. For most, that's way down the line after years of being silent or trying to turn the other cheek, as they say. Saying no is powerful and helps others recognize how far astray they've wandered.

When you set a boundary, you also need Divine encouragement and support to keep your resolve. In the end, your tough love is for your benefit as well as theirs. Do you need to exercise tough love with someone? Have you ever done so?

September 11: Laughing in Response to Truth

SACRED DANCE

Smile gently as you step to the left with your left foot. Place the bells in front of you as you bend your knees and bend forward slightly from the waist, and shake the bells while nodding your head

forward, keeping the fan steady. Rise, and walk slowly in one counterclockwise circle, shaking the bells as you do so. Return to center.
Hold the position, and breathe.

─────────── MEDITATION AND PRACTICE ───────────

As Amaterasu hid in her cave, the clever goddess Uzume turned
over a tub and started dancing on it near the cave entrance where
Amaterasu was, ripping her clothing off as she did so. The other
deities watched her and laughed with pleasure so much so that
the entire Universe shook. But before she turned over the tub,
Uzume had hung up a bronze mirror and a beautiful jewel of
polished jade outside the cave. When Amaterasu heard all the
laughing and felt the Universe jolt, she looked out to see what
was happening. She saw the jewel and her glorious reflection in
that mirror. Amaterasu slowly came out. At that moment, the
god Ame-no-Tajikarao ran forward and closed the cave behind
Amaterasu, keeping her from retreating inside it. A different god
tied a magic *shimenawa*, a rice-straw rope, across the entrance.
The deities Ame-no-Koyane and Ame-no-Futodama invited Amaterasu to come back to her Divine place. When she acquiesced,
the earth once again had light.

It's amazing that so many people care about us and want to help
us—if only we would recognize them. When we see the truth and
act upon it, our supporters could be very happy that we finally saw
the Light. We all have loving people in our lives who will "dance
upon an overturned tub," make a commotion of sorts, and bring
happy people with them, to motivate us. Prayer groups, meditation
gatherings, satsang, sangha, recovery groups, grief circles, writers'
groups, choirs, adventurer groups—support groups are everywhere.
Some are available by virtual connection.

Do you have support groups in your life? Do you let them see
you or help you when you have cave experiences? If you don't,
please plan to get into at least one group that will welcome you and
miss your Light if you're away too long.

September 12: The Mirror of Truth

SACRED DANCE

Keeping the bells shaking, slowly bring the fan and bells in front of your face, with the right wrist in front of the left so the bells are closer to your face. Open your arms and hold the fan and bell away from your body with your elbows bent. Step backward, beginning with your left foot, for four steps. Bring the fan and bells in front of your face, and hold the position for two breaths. Then step backward on the left foot, and turn and walk in a clockwise direction, moving the fan and the bells in front of and away from your face. After completing the circle, step forward on the right foot, and take four steps. Bring the fan and the bells to cover your face once again, and slightly bend the knees while bending slightly forward from the waist. Continue to shake the bells for two breaths.

MEDITATION AND PRACTICE

Miko, descended directly from the goddess Uzume, were female shamans. They were spiritual mediums and performed religious duties at shrines. Miko traditions date back to the prehistoric Jōmon period of Japan, when female shamans experienced trances. From them they would deliver messages from the Divine to the people they served.

In ancient Japanese times, someone could become a shaman by generational passage, through voluntary training, or by being tasked with it by a community leader. As with ancient Koreans, the appointee had to display several characteristics: neuroses, hallucinations, unusual behavior, and hysteria. These were known as shamanistic sickness.

Look in a mirror today, and see yourself as you really are. Stand there for several minutes, and look into your eyes. Don't groom or primp—just look. Tell yourself that you love yourself and that your Higher Power loves you too. Make some notes in your journal about your experience.

September 13: Good Fortune and Truth

SACRED DANCE

Practice, and improvise what you've done this week so far.

MEDITATION AND PRACTICE

Shamans underwent intensive training and rituals, passed down from an older female shaman. The candidate would learn to become possessed, to communicate with kami and other spirits. All the preparation and initiation were achieved by sacred dances, songs, chants, and magical formulas. Up to seven years were needed to become initiated into shamanic work. Her mentor, other elders, and fellow shamans witnessed the mystical ceremony. The initiate wore a white shroud symbolizing the end of her previous life.

A Shinto shrine, whose main purpose was to house one or more kami, was a place for connection with the Divine. Since there was no structured dogma or worship of an individual god, its most important building was used for the safekeeping of sacred objects. Kami were enshrined in the sanctuary. The sanctuary, however, might be the natural area around the shrine, such as when the shrine stands on a sacred mountain to which it is dedicated and that is worshipped directly, or when nearby altar-like structures believed capable of attracting spirits can serve as a direct bond to a kami.

Think about what's right for you, how to practice hearing, and moving in directions in which you feel called. It's a good idea to hear and see the many aspects and affirmations that Spirit provides for you. When you're in tune with everything—rocks, streams, people, and "interconnecting" guides—sometimes the way is made clear.

September 14: Sounding Truth

SACRED DANCE

Today, as in previous dance meditations, find your way into the trance of this dance. Let go, ring your bells, bow, walk in circles, dance forward and backward, move the fan so that you look into your imaginary mirror, and bring your kami out into the world for all to see.

MEDITATION AND PRACTICE

Kagura suzu was the ritual tool of twelve bells used in kagura Sacred Dance Meditation. It had three tiers of bells suspended by coiled brass wires from a central handle: two bells on the top tier, four bells in the middle, and six bells for the bottom tier. The shape was inspired from the fruits of the *ogatama* tree. The bells repelled negative energy and brought forth positive energies. A larger form of suzu was hung from a rafter in front of a Shinto shrine. People pulled on ribbons to get them to sound. These too, when rung, summoned kami, allowing one to acquire positive power and authority, and disbursed bad vibes and energy. The ribbons were made of silk and were colored in purple, white, red, yellow, and green. Symbolically they represented the spiritual power of kagura Sacred Dance Meditation to touch aspects of the Self and reverberate throughout the Universe.

We have a mission in life that's important to know and fulfill. The truth needs to be sounded loudly in your Soul. And while many would consider that we only utilize the positive side of us, our negative, or Shadow, side is just as useful in hearing our own truths and making them visible for others. Align with your calling so that you will enjoy balance. Wear colored clothing that reminds you to sound your bells!

❋ ❋ ❋

SEPTEMBER 15–21
Flowing with Truth (Entry Point)

Truth flows from the edges of the Universe.

Truth is circular in that it produces power to revise, establish a deep involvement with revision, and create beauty, all while leaving the Ultimate Reality intact.

This week, your Sacred Dance Attire can include either long, flowing sleeves or scarves that you hold in your hands. If you use scarves, please hold them loosely in your hands, being sure to have one end of them between your fingertips, gathered so that they won't touch the floor.

They don't have to be anything special, but they should be long, light-weight, and narrow. Male energy may choose to use objects representing swords, but these should be plastic or other material that does no harm. The sword blade should always face away from the body. You're to imagine that you embody power and cosmic energy and you're a conduit for pulling it from the earth and the edge of the Cosmos.

September 15: The Balance of Truth

SACRED DANCE

Begin by standing at a farthest corner of your Sacred Dance Studio, facing the northeast corner (a little to the left of where the sun rises), with your knees slightly bent and your head down. Your arms are crossed in front of you as if you're making the edges of a square, and your scarves are cinched in your hands. Slowly pivot to the right, gaze toward the sky, and face the center of your Sacred Dance Studio. Then pivot to the left, back to your starting position, and then turn to the left, and gaze toward the sky. Face the center of your Sacred Dance Studio. Bring your feet together. Repeat this for eight breaths: inhale on the turn toward the center of the space, exhale on the return to the corner.

MEDITATION AND PRACTICE

The Chinese word *wu* means "wizard or shaman," describing a person who could mediate with the Spirits and had god-level powers to generate creation. Wu were viewed as bridges between their communities and the spiritual world. During their trances in Sacred Dance Meditations, shaman sought intervention from the heavens to cure the sick, ensure a good bounty, bring rain, give people some insight into the future, or talk with deceased ancestors. Rituals led by shamans were done in people's homes, on top of mountains, and in shrines. In trances, shamans received visions and messages and initiated out-of-body experiences to travel to other worlds.

The important aspect about truth is balance. Upon first hearing a truth or something that challenges our beliefs, the first response is typically resistance. We feel dismayed, confused, or victimized. Or we may dig in our heels to show we are right. For example, technology has evolved, product quality has been changing, and prices seem to keep going up. We may see fewer people at worship or spiritual-support centers. Surrounded by so much change, people may be depressed or even may live in the past all the time. But if we follow the ancient Chinese approach, we'll understand that change is a form of creation and happens all the time.

The issue is finding wu and allowing it to flow through your life without trying to stop it. It requires going between the heavens and earth to find a new way, a bridge, to nurture yourself while recognizing your connection to the Higher Power.

September 16: Respecting Truth

SACRED DANCE

Repeat what was given on September 15. After returning to the opening position, fling the scarves from both hands by raising your arms up and behind your head and away from your ears, leaning your torso backward and looking up to the sky while you hold the end of the scarves. Bring your arms around to the front of your body in a circle at chest height, and slip the right hand up over your head, and bring the left hand around to the center of the right side of your body. Move the scarves so that they don't touch the floor. Repeat this arm movement, continuing to face the northeast corner of the studio. Play with the movement of the scarves for sixteen breaths, sending energy, love, and healing truths through the scarves out to the earth. Let your gaze follow the scarves in motion. After you have completed this, bring the scarves to rest by draping them over your shoulders—right hand to left shoulder, and left hand to right shoulder—bow your head, and bend your knees slightly.

MEDITATION AND PRACTICE

The oldest Chinese character dictionary, the Shuowen Jiezi (121 CE), defined *wu* as "a sacrifice; a prayer master; an invoker; or a priestess."

The character depicts a person in a dance pose with two very long sleeves. Wu was Sacred Dance Meditation embodied, with one woman or two women together, invoking the spiritual or the Divine. The female dancer was an invoker or priest who was able to render herself invisible and invoke gods to come down to earth. She was able to make rain, interpret the meaning of dreams, heal the sick, precisely predict futures of fortune or scarcity, or death and destruction, and transform communities. The wu were greatly feared and respected.

If we disrespect truth or try to stop it or change its flow, we wind up miserable or run out of time. We get sick or depressed. Perhaps that is the path to the shaman's world: affliction makes us say we've had enough, and we start moving with some urgency to attend to this life.

What truth do you still deny? The best way to recognize your truth is not only to be connected to the Divine but also to pray to your Higher Self or Higher Power to transform your thinking so that you can see clearly. You must invoke your true nature so that you can dance along the path clearly. You cannot allow yourself to be deceived. You don't have a great deal of time. Spiritual calm and realization come from practice, so be patient, and don't abdicate your power. Respect the way the truth leads you, and use every avenue and every minute to understand what you're being led to do. Dance alone if you must.

September 17: Heaven Is Where Truth Is

SACRED DANCE

Today, start in your Sacred Dance Attire and with your scarves cinched in your hands. Face the northeast corner of your Sacred Dance Studio, and turn to the right. Pose with your right foot extended, and sweep your left scarf in front of your body, then step with the left foot, and sweep your right scarf in front of your body. Repeat this pattern, alternating the steps. The standing leg is slightly bent, and your head is tilted toward the standing leg. Try to keep the scarves from touching the floor. This means that the inactive arm must be held up over your head. These are slow exaggerated moves as you swirl the energy in front of you. You're moving your scarves with your upper arms from the shoulder joints, not the wrists. Repeat for eight breaths on each side of the body, with an inhale and exhale for each step. When you complete the last exhale, bring your feet together, and drape the scarf in the right hand over the left shoulder and the scarf in the left hand over the right shoulder.

MEDITATION AND PRACTICE

Wu were known to interact with their revered ancestors, who resided in the heavens, Tiān, after death, and they brought back the truths they gathered to the people in their communities. Heaven was considered a continuum, with the Supreme Deity on the far end, and nature or earth on the near end. For them, heaven saw, heard, and guided everyone. Heaven was simultaneously affected by what people did and, having a personality like people did, was happy or angry with them. Heaven blessed those who pleased it and sent calamities upon those who offend it.

What is heaven? Most people say it's in the sky, at the end of a rainbow, or somewhere only accessible to people in altered states or in an afterlife. All cultures have some sort of imaginary place where life is better and more beautiful than what can be experienced on earth. But heaven is where truth is, which is inside us. The idea that heaven is separate from our Inner Mystic Dancer leaves us feeling disconnected, alone, and dependent. Heaven is a state of mind, where we can live without delusions and still enjoy the beauty we see every day, no matter how miniscule that vision may seem. The truth is that some of us pass beauty every day and don't see it. Some hear truths every day and refuse to abide by them. That's human nature, most likely.

Where's heaven for you, or is there such a place? What is your conception of heaven? What happens if you perceive it differently or consider that your idea of heaven isn't the only one or that it's not real? If you don't think heaven exists, consider how you might embrace such a concept, where people and things are nice and easy, and you manifest it lovingly for others in your day-to-day interactions.

September 18: Truth Depends on the Question

SACRED DANCE

Flick your left wrist with the scarf in front eight times, until your left arm cannot move any farther, and quickly bring the right arm out to flick the scarf with your right wrist, as you quickly drape the left scarf over the right shoulder. Repeat on each side, keeping your knees slightly bent. Have your gaze follow your scarf. When you reach the end, bring the wrists together by a circular motion, right over left. Bend your body so that the scarves touch the floor.

MEDITATION AND PRACTICE

Ancient Chinese practitioners had two methods to contact Divine ancestors. The first was the mystical wu, involving dances and trances. With rituals using supernatural powers, they entered sacred unions with the Divine. Thus, some sacred dancers were able to communicate directly with nature, travel deep into the earth, or visit far-off galaxies. Their duties included presiding at formal ceremonies, calling down the invited gods and ancestors, performing exorcisms, dancing at sacrifices for rain, healing the sick, and averting diseases and natural disasters.

The second method was using oracle bones, or a rational way to get to the Spirit realms. Used for divination, Oracle bones were made from the cleaned shoulder blades of oxen or the flat underside of a turtle's shell. The process began with someone asking the wu a question about any area of life, including family issues, weather, farming, and politics. Wu answered questions for people on any topic.

A wu carved symbols regarding the questions being asked on the bones of the ox or the turtle shell. She heated the bone or shell with hot implements until it formed fractures and fissures in the surfaces. She then interpreted the direction of the cracks to answer the questions and predict the future. Spirits would communicate with wu through the oracle bones. Shamans were consulted by people at all levels of society, from field workers to royalty.

The question asked causes the answer to manifest. Depending on how you enter search terms in a search engine, you get different internet answers. The same is true when asking for guidance. If you ask, "Why am I here on earth?" you'll get a set of answers. But if you ask, "What is the Divine will for my life?" you may hear something different. As is said, "The answers will come if your house is in order." That means you must have a clear channel, know the questions to ask, and be receptive before taking the appropriate actions.

September 19: Answers as Revealed Truths

SACRED DANCE

Practice each section of the choreography given this week. Bring the sections together into a flow, and allow yourself to fully learn it and feel it in your body.

MEDITATION AND PRACTICE

Wu of the Zhou dynasty from 1046 to around 226 BCE used oracle bones as the rational side of the Sacred Dance Meditation. Divination using shoulder bones is known as scapulimancy; divination using the turtle's shell, or plastron, is known as plastromancy; and divination through fire is known as pyromancy. During the Zhou dynasty, divination was grounded in cleromancy, or selecting answers from an array of seemingly random numbers to determine Divine intent. A formation of an array of cracks and lines would be considered random outside the wu's practice. But during her trance, they were believed to reveal the will of G-d or other supernatural entities and ancestors. Seekers and wu interacted in a prescribed process with the wu, making notes on the bones before and after the divination and sacred trance dance, such as the following:

- Who asked the question and when?

- What was the main concern posed and the general category? For example, a general category could be farming and the specific question would be about whether to plant a field.

- The shaman could note what the spirits revealed in the answer, and how the wu interpreted it through the cracks in the shell or bones, such as whether to plant.

- The wu could later note confirming outcomes—that is, whether the prophecy turned out to be true and what happened to the person who asked the question, after, for example, the field was or wasn't planted.

From our perspective, it may seem strange to use ancient Chinese methods to get questions answered. Today some people have prayer journals and G-d boxes that allow them to write down their needs and see what answers they get and when. They light candles and seek answers by listening to the Divine and overhearing words from people's conversations. They get guidance from words heard in what seem to be randomly played songs, or through what seem to be opening and closing doors to opportunity. People go to psychics and other mediums. People have their dreams interpreted. Whatever our belief system, we all seek answers to something. The key is to remain open to hearing the answers to requests and prayers and responding appropriately to them. So many times, guidance comes as a clear signal, but we ignore it, or worse, second-guess it. Just know that revealed truths are made manifest, and it's up to us to follow them, not resist them.

September 20: One Flow after Another

───────────────── SACRED DANCE ─────────────────

Today, practice the sacred dance given this week. Find ways to improvise, and add your own scarf and body flow. Add a few breaths to extend the sacred vision of power being drawn into your body.

───────────── MEDITATION AND PRACTICE ─────────────

According to ancient Chinese legends, the Universe at the beginning contained nothing but formless chaos. As with other ancient belief systems, the formless chaos gathered into a cosmic egg. It contained the principles of yin and yang, and from it Pangu, believed to be the first living being and the creator of all, originated. Pangu created Hua Hsu, who divined a twin brother and sister, Fu Xi and Nüwa; both had the body of a snake and face of a human. They created offspring from clay and infused them with the Divine. Fu Xi then created life on earth: the family as a way of connecting, along with everything else, including wu. Fu Xi learned from the wu that "everything could be reduced to eight trigrams, each composed of three stacked solid or broken lines, reflecting the yin and yang, the duality that drives the universe."* The trigrams pointed to tendencies in movement, certain processes in nature corresponding with their inherent character, and an interconnectivity consisting of the energies associated with father, mother, three sons, and three daughters and their functions. This information that Fu Xi gathered came to make up the important book of divination that we know as the I Ching.

Dancing through change is a part of our function, and that makes people seek guidance. That, in turn, moves people to an active participatory state, communing with truth and avoiding passivity. Over a lifetime, or even over a day, we have a continual flow of questions, and many answers that can take us into myriad directions. We must be open to flowing in multiple directions at once. Each direction has attributes, and each attribute is a part of us. We rely on directions to move us, speak to us, and give us truths, one after another.

Can you identify one or two sacred directions you're being called toward? Or do you feel any sort of randomness along with an order to the directions? Can you hold these two ideas in your mind and body as you navigate through your path? Start by slowly reading the meanings of each symbol and see if any of them cause you to feel something or react. List them in your

---

* Eliot Weinberger, "What Is the I Ching?" *ChinaFile*, February 25, 2016, https://www.chinafile.com/library/nyrb-china-archive/what-i-ching.

journal, and then connect the associated attributes. Where in your life do you find yourself needing to use the attributes? Take a few moments to write about this.

September 21: Truth Is Medicine

SACRED DANCE

Fully trance the sacred dance from the week.

MEDITATION AND PRACTICE

A wu was consulted to determine reasons for illnesses, and she told her patients what sorts of sacrifices were needed to heal and recover. She received the ability to garner Divine power and ensure long life via sacrifices to Shang Di, or the Divine, and she mediated between people and spirits in other worlds. The shaman petitioned for her clients according to the three aspects integral to living, called *shen*, *jing*, and *qi*. Shen was the emotional, mental, supernatural, and spiritual aspect of a human being. Jing was the body's physical make up. Qi was the Life Force all humans embodied.

Illness arose from imbalance or a misalignment of the three aspects of living, according to the worldview. When people were given a clear picture of the truth as it affects those aspects and took corrective prescriptive actions, many recovered. The stories show they relied on the truth of wu for spiritual, mental, emotional, and physical healing and support.

From archeological evidence, we know that wu Sacred Dance Meditation truths underlay not only the foundations of I Ching but also Chinese medicine. The important point is that truth gives us the medicine we need to dance forward on our paths. Many who have danced before our time knew that, though it be obscured for a time, truth supplies the nutrients we need to balance our mind, body, and Soul.

❋ ❋ ❋

Bringing Truth to Others (Entry Point)

Be still my wandering Soul.

Waking dreams and sleeping dreams are both Soul travels that bring me truths.

You need a small stone or other marker such as a crystal or an implement to act as an altar at the center of your Sacred Dance Studio. Please note that this week's dance contains movements that bring you from standing to the floor on your knees. A yoga mat or pillow might help reduce any knee pain, or you may choose to squat instead.

September 22: Spiritual Visualization

SACRED DANCE

Face east, with your feet slightly wider than shoulder-width apart. Rest your arms at your sides, with hands cupped. Vigorously bat your right arm across your body while holding your left hand slightly behind you, then come to a full stop. Then do the same with the left arm. As you move, imagine you are pushing planets and rearranging the galaxy. You'll naturally feel your shoulders move and sway with the batting of your arms. Repeat this motion until you enter a trance, and if you feel inclined, you can make a guttural sound. Take steps around the altar, moving in a clockwise direction as you move your arms. When you return to your starting point, slowly drop on your knees or in a squatting position.

MEDITATION AND PRACTICE

Ancient Mongolian shamanism, Tengrism, focused on the worship of Mother Earth and Eternal Heaven, along with other spirits of nature and their ancestors. A shaman made spiritual connections, found ways into the afterlife, and interacted with spirits on people's behalf through Sacred Dance Meditation. The shaman's small sacred dance space, called a *ger*, represented the relationship between people and the Universe. Importantly, the ancient Mongolian shaman dance invoked the ability to Soul travel, to go between the present and other worlds to find answers to quandaries of life through a body of Light.

Different beliefs circulate today regarding Soul or Spirit travel, or what we refer to in this book as spiritual visualization, which includes astral projection and other out-of-body experiences. For our purposes, spiritual visualization is an awareness that feels as if you're freed from the confines of the body and as if you receive information from a deep sense of knowing. When spiritual visualization is perfected, we can consider ourselves multidimensional and see and feel things in the environment from a different perspective. Creative ideas are generated, and solutions arise. Through spiritual visualizations, we learn to use our imaginations to the full extent. Imagination is powerful and can create miracles of movement. For example, we can sit quietly, or lie down just before going to sleep, and imagine standing outside ourselves to see what we look like and what our temperament is. If we're in the flow, we can apply what we see to ourselves as new truths and then set new intentions. We can also see what we'd like the future to be.

September 23: The September Southern Equinox

SACRED DANCE

Revisit the sacred dance given on September 22 to refresh your memory. Begin on your knees, facing east with the altar as your focus. Being in a kneeling position evokes humility, as you remember your power is to be used for leading people to truths. On your knees, repeat the arm movements you learned on September 22. Lean forward as you do them, until your forehead touches the floor in front of you, or as close as you can go, so your arms are held at your sides. Pause here for several breaths, and offer your healing truth to all beings. Slightly raise and lower your torso, with your arms outstretched to your sides, for four breaths. Then, repeat this raising and lowering of your torso with the arms outstretched and palms cupped, to your left, back to center, and then to your right. Then, you raise your head and lean backward, with the arms outstretched to your sides. Repeat this sequence until you enter a trance. End today's dance meditation kneeling with your forehead touching the floor and your arms outstretched.

MEDITATION AND PRACTICE

Rituals have marked the transition between seasons since the beginning of human history. Equinoxes and solstices are sacred times of the year. The ancient Mongols visualized the Universe as spherical, which included time. Circular motion informed everything and tracked time passing. The path of the sun, the seasons, and the cycle of the living along with the cycle of death were cyclical. Cyclical movement overlapped in the four earthly directions, over the axis of the earth, through the galaxies, and down into the lower worlds. Shamans honored the earth moving around the sun and celebrated Spirit in several dimensions and directions, knowing that the sun split time.

The autumnal equinox occurs when the sun is directly above Earth and crosses the celestial equator going south. Pause to remember it today as you engage in spiritual visualization.

September 24: Magick Numbers of Truth

SACRED DANCE

Begin today's dance kneeling or sitting on a pillow or mat. Bring your palms together in a cupped position in front of your heart chakra. Swing the right arm out away from your body, up, and then across your eyes. Bring it back to the starting position and then use the left arm to do the same thing. Alternate flowing the arms and covering the face for sixteen inhales and exhales. Then, bring the palms in front of your face, and sway to the left and right sixteen breaths. After this, raise the palms to the ceiling and continue the swaying for sixteen breaths. Slowly bring the palms back to a cupped position in front of the heart chakra. Pause there for eight breaths. Raise the palms toward the ceiling, and bring your palms back and forth over your head. As you gaze into the palms, lean backward as far as is comfortable for you, and then return to the upright position while remaining in the kneeling stance. Repeat this for sixteen breaths. After the last repetition, place your forehead on the floor, with your arms outstretched.

MEDITATION AND PRACTICE

A core concept of Buryat shamanism was the tripling of the physical and spiritual world. Three main spirits presided over each of the heavens, earthly plane, and underworld. Similarly, people were believed to have three parts: the physical body, the breath and life or Divine Spirit, and the Soul. The Soul also had three elements. The first Soul was in the physical skeleton; damage to the skeleton also damaged the Soul. Practitioners of Buryat shamanism took great care to avoid damaging the bones of animals during ritual animal sacrifices. The second Soul, housed in the organs, was believed to have the ability to leave the body and transform into other beings. The third Soul was connected to the Breath of Life. It was very similar to the second Soul, except that its absence meant the end of one's life.

The number *three* is often the most magical number in many traditions. It is the first odd prime number, which gives it the power of indivisibility, and it is the first number used in sacred geometry. *Three* forms the understanding of time spent on earth. In all cases, the concept of the triumvirate mother, father, and child exists in creation stories. We have seen this as we have considered various Sacred Dance Meditations from our ancestors. *Three* is sacred in all ancient cultures. When we consider that the Universe may be constructed mathematically—everything we know about ourselves and our environment points to such a form—how do we consider it magick? Breath is life, but it can be described through mathematics. Mathematical interactions make up our body's cells.

What are your beliefs around numerology? Let *three* as a magickal number vibrate in your spiritual visualization today.

September 25: Dreaming Truths

SACRED DANCE

Today, practice the combined choreography from September 22 and September 23, until you feel it in a fully embodied way.

MEDITATION AND PRACTICE

Ancient Mongol shamans were said to have power dreams, which meant that they traveled while asleep over a rainbow to the upper world. Different dream states could open a door for Spirit communication. Some people have dreams about future events that come to pass; others have moments between sleep and wakefulness when spirits visit them or offer visions. And then sometimes dreamers know they're dreaming and work something out, solve a problem, or get answers to a situation or question.

Everything that happens during our lives—interactions, hopes, fears, past, present, future—is working the background in our dreams. In dreams, consciousness helps us to understand situations and to create new attitudes and perceptions. Whether awake or asleep, we are in the state of dreaming truths when we open ourselves to that kind of assistance. But we must not take the dream as gospel. We've all experienced dreams that seemed so real that we awoke deeply disturbed.

What do you think dreams mean? Do you remember your dreams? Be careful about whom you share dreams with. Psychologists such as Carl Jung, Calvin Hall, and Sigmund Freud theorized that your subconscious is amplified while you dream and that dream information is pretty revealing. Whatever you believe, dreams have messages regarding simple perceptions or actions, such as getting your tires replaced, making a call to a distant relative, or recognizing an aspect of yourself that needs attention. Yet, dreams do come true, sometimes.

September 26: Soul Loss

SACRED DANCE

After you're fully in your Sacred Dance Attire, repeat the dance from September 25, and memorize the choreography. Practice it until you have it firmly in your memory.

MEDITATION AND PRACTICE

The concept of Soul loss is found in many cultures, including ancient Mongolia. Soul retrieval, the solution, had two forms: the levels of Soul and Spirit. They were both redeeming. The first was getting the Soul, the core of a person, back. The second was refreshing the Life Force, which maintained the functions of the mind and body. These Soul retrieval techniques were separate rites used by the shamans in their communications with the gods, while going between dreams, and during travels on the rainbow. In the shamanic worldview, power and health are one and the same. If the body is full of power, there is no room for Soul loss.

You can be a lost Soul, and you can have Soul loss. Maybe a trauma is buried in the recesses of the mind or one that is front and center giving you trouble. It's easier to see in others than in yourself. People with Soul loss feel like the never fit in; they watch life go by and avoid getting involved with anything. Sometimes they say they can't remember things or feel out of touch. Maybe they don't like being around people. They're scared and maybe a little paranoid or may experience chronic illness. The symptoms show that they have allowed the Life Force to drain. Trauma can do that, especially if people have too many traumatic events or have one major event that permeates their consciousness and that they may not even know is there.

Make a list in your journal of people in your life who you perceive to have Soul loss.

September 27: Sacred Dance of Soul Retrieval

SACRED DANCE

Today, practice the sacred dance in its entirety, combining what you learned September 22–24. Begin to feel comfortable with each motion.

MEDITATION AND PRACTICE

Shamans in ancient Mongolia didn't dwell on past events; there was only a vast, awesome, ever-moving, moment of now. During a Soul-retrieval session, people brought their traumas, often in the form of illnesses, and sought relief from them. A practitioner journeyed outside the human conception of time to go to the place where a traumatic event was still occurring for a person, to locate that person's pretrauma Soul. The shamans would create a space in the Soul where the ever-occurring event ended, therefore removing its power over the person. When completed, the Soul was retrieved, and the trauma couldn't influence the person anymore in the present, or hinder the individual in the future. The shamanic healer located the lost Soul parts in the Lower, Middle, or Upper Worlds of the Spirit World and then brought them together and returned them, so that the person could function without illness.

Often Soul loss happens when we're unable to process an experience and therefore are unaware of its impact. One type of Soul loss happens during childhood when we might not even remember the incident.

To heal, you must be open to experiencing the trauma of losing a piece of you. So, the first thing to do is to write about what you see as patterns in your life. If you listen, you can get at every trauma that lies within. You could also engage the help of a spiritual professional you align with. After you determine what behaviors or events have affected you from childhood, reenact the first trauma in your mind but then rewrite the story in your imagination and in your journal. What would it have been like if it were different? Who would have been there to make sure the trauma didn't occur? How would the environment feel or be different? Sometimes the pieces of you reside with individuals you held dear and considered safe, such as your grandmother or grandfather. After writing and imagining the alternate scenario, do sacred dance, and feel and embody the revision. Commit to repeating the dance of Soul retrieval on a regular basis for a given period.

September 28: Nothing Quick

SACRED DANCE

Repeat the sacred dance from September 27, practicing it and getting it into your body memory. As always, set up your Sacred Dance Studio, and wear your Sacred Dance Attire.

MEDITATION AND PRACTICE

Shamans in ancient Mongolia had a steady line of people who sought them out and trusted their cures because they worked. However, everyone expected the change to be slow because it took a while for people to realize they needed help. Lost Soul fragments were scattered throughout the ends of the Cosmos. They had to be coerced to return to make the Soul whole. In their travel to the spirits, Shaman weighed and heard the petitioner's sincerity in their request for healing.

Trauma and Soul loss can come in many forms, and the effects are unique to each person. Losing a job, living in a narcissistic environment, being poor, being wealthy, having to face a change with a partner, dealing with adult offspring unable to stand on their own two feet, dealing with race and class issues, and many other events and situations can cause Soul loss. We know we have the loss or losses, but we can't see the magnitude of its negative impacts. We need the courage to learn how to retrieve our lost Soul pieces and place them in a Life Force frame.

Be specific and measured about it: for example, because of your job loss, you may have a need to relocate. Often, you may look back at a decision that led to trauma and feel regret, shame, guilt, or self-denigration. Your lost Soul parts are living in them. You must ask those feelings and thoughts to let pieces of your Soul return to your Life Force.

When you have finished writing about your experiences, commit to engaging a Sacred Dance Meditation mantra, such as a sweep of your hand, a swaying of your torso, or a cupping of your palms in front of your heart chakra each time you hear or feel messages of trauma. You might want to develop several of them and create a repertoire you can call upon from your body memory. Feel the pieces of you begin to reintegrate.

September 29: Partner with Truth

SACRED DANCE

Fully engage in the sacred dance from this week, as you have thus far toward the end of weekly dances in this book. Find ways to improvise, and incorporate what you felt the last two days with Soul retrieval.

MEDITATION AND PRACTICE

Ancient shamans in Mongolia living on the cold and harsh mountainous steppes came to the aid of so many, in tiny *ger* spaces. They went on Soul travels to retrieve lost fragments of people, healed the sick, and caused change in their communities. They believed in the people they lived with and would do anything in their power to help. They partnered with truth, the different aspects of the heavens, earth, and underworld to ease life's cares.

It takes commitment to be a partner with truth. Following the spiritual path requires that commitment, though. Being of service to others, to be their shaman, is the main point. As with shamans, you must heal your own trauma first. Then truth is your partner too.

September 30: Being a Dancing Shaman of Truth

SACRED DANCE

Trance your dance today.

MEDITATION AND PRACTICE

Asian shamans taught the way forward with dance, such as the Korean Salp'uri Dance, the Japanese Kagura, and the Chinese Water Sleeve Dance. In Mongolia, the shamans showed the way with a shaman's dance. After first feeling the call of Spirit and wrestling with their own traumas, our ancient shaman ancestors agreed to bring people across to commune more directly with the Divine. But a shaman wasn't in service if there weren't people in need.

Plenty of shamans exist in the world today, and many of them originate from the same essential belief system. They have come through the ages to speak to us now, to encourage us to be Sacred Dance Meditation shamans as we travel through our own lives. You must share the truth, as well as continue to discover new truths. Many people need to dance sacredly with you, and you need them.

OCTOBER
Sowing Seeds

ANDEAN SACRED DANCE

Vegetable gardeners utilize late-season planting of cold-weather crops in anticipation of the following-year season. The seeds stay in the soil in a type of hibernation, only to sprout when the time is right, pushing through toward the light. Planting spiritual seeds is much the same.

To aid us in this spiritual work, we look toward South America for our sacred dances this month. People traveled to South America by crossing the Bering Strait about fifteen thousand years ago from Russia. They came south through North America and then on to South America via the Isthmus of Panama. Evidence places the first people in South America at around 9000 BCE. They prospered through food cultivation in the Amazon basin, and by 2000 BCE many people settled in the Andes and the surrounding regions. Irrigation systems developed and helped manifest greatness.

The Andes, or Andes Mountains, stretches along the West Coast of South America to the area that includes the coastal deserts to the west and into the tropical jungles to the east. Our sacred dances for this month draw upon the Practices of ancient people there, the Quechua of the Incan Empire in Central Andes. The Incas built an empire at Tawantinsuyu with no animals or technology. They didn't write, but they used quipu, a system of knotted and colored strings, to convey information. The quipu dates back possibly to Peruvian civilization of Norte Chico during the third millennium BCE. The Incan Empire stretched from modern-day Argentina to southern

Colombia and was divided into four areas, which intersected in Cuzco. Machu Picchu lay between the Andes Mountains of Peru and the Amazon basin and is one of the Inca's worship sites. Incan Andean geopolitical states are in present-day Colombia, Venezuela, Ecuador, Peru, and Bolivia.

The Norte Chico civilization of Peru, which dates to 3200 BCE, is the oldest civilization in the Americas. The civilization included numerous cities and flourished between the fourth and second millennia BCE, with the establishment of Huaricanga in the Fortaleza area. This complex society of Norte Chico arose contemporaneously with that of our Egyptian ancestors, and predated the Mesoamerican Olmec by nearly two millennia.

Ancient Peruvians engaged in public sacred ceremonies and observed the seasons with festivities. They danced sacredly to Inca music during their rituals. Dances were intended for agricultural protection and plenty and for rain. Dance also mimicked the origins of Incan society and the culture's reverence for animals.

The main ceremonial dance of the Quechuan people of the southcentral highlands of the Peruvian Andes was called *supaypa wasin tusuq*, known as la Danza de Tijeras, or the Scissors Dance, by the Spanish colonizers. It portrayed many nuances of the creation and the ways in which the gods supported planting and harvesting.

Mapuche sacred dance was a ritual of worship acknowledging Divinity through a healing ceremony in pre-Columbian Chile. A deep and abiding aspect of the Mapuche belief was the role of the *machi*, or shaman, whom we'll learn more about this month. The Sacred Dance Meditations of the Mapuche were accompanied by the *kultrun*, a magic drum with sacred symbols drawn or carved into it and filled with sacred objects.

PREPARATION

The Incan word *taqui* described dance, music, and singing—one word expressed their interconnectedness. Sacred dancers wore multicolored Sacred Dance Attire that incorporated elements of nature and honored the spirits they worshipped. The clothing was decorated with gold fringes, colorful sequins, and small mirrors and was embroidered with the Spirit names of the dancers as well as different elements of nature. The dancers' headdresses were large with detailed decoration; they seemed otherworldly.

If you're led to do so by Spirit, get some Andean or Chilean music and instruments, including shells, bells, and hand and wrist percussive instruments. A tambourine and a set of bells are helpful to have. For this month, you can use colorful clothing of red, orange, yellow, green, or purple for Sacred Dance Attire. Dancing with others would be fantastic but isn't required. Just let go, and receive the bountiful feeling of the sacred.

Please visit www.cswalter.org/sacreddancemeditations for video demonstrations. They are not intended to be step-by-step instructions but rather, are meant to give you a view of the sacred dance.

OCTOBER 1–7
Sowing Seeds of Abundance (Entry Point)

Sacred Soil

Flowers bloom from sacred soil, first prepared before any seed sprouts.

October 1: Sacred Huacas

───────────────── SACRED DANCE ─────────────────

If you want to incorporate music into this week's dance, consider flutes and harps.

Stand facing east, barefoot, placing your hands on your hips, and slightly bend your knees. Imagine you are standing on a high plain in the Andes mountains, feeling the warmth of the earth on your feet and the sun on your skin. Inhale, and bend your left knee as you slowly slide your right foot sideways to your right and back in. Place the weight on both feet as you face forward with knees just slightly bent. Pause and inhale. Lift your face to the sun, and now bend your right knee and slide your left foot out sideways toward the left and back in to return with knees slightly bent. Inhale.

───────────────── MEDITATION AND PRACTICE ─────────────────

The spiritual Practices of our Incan Ancestors included a sacred *huaca*, a multilevel phenomenon that was said to have a Spirit or god within. Huacas—gods, spirits, and ancestors—manifested on earth in the form of nature, such as mountain peaks (*apu* means mountain Spirit), rivers, springs, caves, rocky outcrops, and stones. The people believed every object or being had a physical presence and two spirits. And without them, the object or being couldn't function.

Huacas were also a special initiated group of sacred dancers who drew the ancestors and Spirit to earth, entering ecstatic states of Spirit possession. They specialized in taquis, a singing Sacred Dance Meditation that praised ancestral deities and linked ancient gods with the *ayllu*, or clan. For the ayllu, religious beliefs were practical, related to living an abundant life and conquering interference. The people were in sync with the agricultural cycle, so masked huacas danced in cleansing rituals ahead of ceremonies and the ritual cleaning of agricultural aqueducts, often for five days or more.

To plant, you must first prepare the soil, which needs fertilization, water, and turning over to prevent compacting. Anything put on compacted, unhealthy, or dry soil will either blow away with the wind or be eaten by critters who don't have any inkling of the seed beyond the immediate value of avoiding starvation. Spiritually speaking, you must prepare the mind for the fragile seedlings of ideas that lie in your subconscious or even unconscious self. What ideas would you like to cultivate that are lying so deep within you that you have nearly forgotten or given up on them? What prevents you from cultivating them? Please write these in your journal.

October 2: Bloom in the Now

SACRED DANCE

Repeat the choreography from October 1 several times on the right and left. Alternate this sequence: right, left, right, left. Find your breath so that you inhale just before you bend your knees and exhale when you slide the foot away from your body. Coordinate looking to the sky and looking forward with sliding your foot out (look up) and in (face forward). Keep your hands gently resting on your hips, and be mindful of your Sacred Dance Posture.

MEDITATION AND PRACTICE

Huacas could be places used for astronomical observations. An intriguing Incan huaca was the Intihuatana, at the highest point of Machu Picchu. Intihuatana, carved from a slab, had jutting stone on top and four sides, each aligned with the cardinal directions. It had astronomic markers aligned with relevant dates in the Inca calendar. Like other sacred sites erected by other ancestors in disparate areas of the earth, they showed the rise and fall of celestial bodies in their ecliptic. During the two equinoxes, the sun stood directly above the Intihuatana without casting a shadow. Through its high elevation, the ancients connected to the different levels of the Spirit world—earthly existence and the underworld in one precise point. By touching the sacred stone or placing one's forehand against the stone at Intihuatana, after performing a Sacred Dance Meditation and prayer ritual, a person could open a vision to the spiritual world.

Like the sacred dancers resting their heads on the mountaintop praying for support, your spiritual seeds represent potential—surrounded by Light but waiting in darkness. They must be placed in the fertile soil and then pressed down so that they might develop roots. What prevents you from pressing your idea seeds into sacred soil? What can you do that eliminates any barriers to germinating your ideas? What substitutes can you think of that will give you the same or close to the same imagined satisfaction? Write down a few substitutes for each idea you wrote yesterday. If these are brought into the sacred soil, can you help them bloom?

October 3: Lakes of Wisdom

SACRED DANCE

Review what you practiced in yesterday's sacred dance, and practice until you've achieved a pattern. Keep your hands gently resting on your hips and be mindful of your Sacred Dance Posture. Repeat the sequence for eight breaths, and then allow your arms to drop to your sides. Then, keeping your gaze forward, closing your palms to make a loose fist with both hands, swing your arms in the opposite direction with the movements of your feet sliding, allowing your upper body to flow with the movement of your arms. When your right foot slides away from your body, your right arm, bent at the elbow, swings across your body to the left. When the left foot slides away from your body, the left arm, bent at the elbow, swings across your body to the right. Repeat the choreography with your arms swinging for sixteen breaths.

MEDITATION AND PRACTICE

According to the ancient people of Inca, Viracocha, the supreme god of the Incas, created the world at Lake Titicaca during the time of darkness. He created the sun, moon, and stars and brought Light into the world. He is said to have created heavenly bodies and giant people from stones. When he was finished and satisfied with his idea creations, Viracocha wanted to share his knowledge of creation around the world. So, he traveled as a beggar in disguise. He headed west across the Pacific, not seen again in the ancient city or near Lake Titicaca. Lore indicated he promised he'd return one day.

When in full nurturance, with water, security, and Light, idea seeds come up beautifully, and give rise to new seeds that will have potential. From the wisdom of your Soul and Spirit you have a vast area filled with idea seeds, just waiting for you to plant them. Some people are bored with life or get bored with their spiritual journey. You may be bored in your career or with your family life. Here is a solution. The mind-body-Spirit is filled with new possibilities, new hopes, new dreams, and new ways to be of service. Perhaps you have wanted to serve the poor, work with people who are suffering from addictions, or teach children to read. You can use your idea seeds several ways to bring yourself upward and bring others with you, too, without seeking recognition. Make some notes about how you can voluntarily bring Light to those in need of what you have to offer.

October 4: It's in the Trying, Waiting, Contemplating That Spirit Dwells

SACRED DANCE

For several repetitions, repeat the right-left-right-left sequence with your arms swinging to your sides. You'll notice a slight bobbing begins with your body. Now, with palms closed, when you swing the right arm across the front of your body, allow it to stop just in front of your pelvic area, and deliberately swing the left arm to the back of your body, stopping it just at the lower part of your back, just above the tailbone. Repeat this sequence with the slightly closed fists for sixteen breaths. Then return to standing with your hands resting on your hips.

The ancient Incans viewed themselves as descendants from Viracocha, being aligned with him through any *curaca*, or divine king. When a curaca died, his mummified remains became huaca that linked the ancient past of creation to the present life of the community. The way this occurred was through expecting new life to follow through the abundant seedlings planted from Viracocha. With the soil prepared and the seedlings resting in their troughs, it was beautiful. Yet, nothing grew without the sacred rain that sacred dancers petitioned for.

All your idea seeds are sitting in their beautiful troughs, pressed into the sacred soil. Your ideas come from your Inner Mystic Dancer, and you have created them to serve others, to help them see more of the Light, to be of service, without seeking recognition. The sacred rain that falls upon them is your continued efforts to be willing to serve your Higher Self in whatever way you're led. Sometimes you may feel impelled to work with children, only to find that it's different than what you expected. That's okay: just keep generating ideas and trying new things. Being this way keeps you from turning into whitewashed sepultures.

October 5: Stepping Back and Evaluating

SACRED DANCE

Repeat the sequence first described on October 4. Then do that sequence as you walk in a circle, first clockwise and then counterclockwise. Then return to your standing position. Allow your hands to drop to your sides, and bow your head forward.

MEDITATION AND PRACTICE

Viracocha made mankind by breathing into stones. But his first humans were giants who displeased him. So, he destroyed them with a flood called Unu Pachakuti that is said to have lasted sixty days and nights. From the flood he saved two beings to bring civilization to the rest of the world. They were Manco Cápac, whose name meant "splendid foundation" and who was the first king of the Incans, and Mama Ocllo, which meant "mother fertility." These two founded the Inca civilization and carried a rod, the golden *tapac-yauri*. After that, he created better humans from clay. He gave them gifts; among them were agriculture and sacred dance.

When seeds are planted, some of them produce and some don't. Some aren't planted deep enough into the soil, or some have expired before planting. Or some just can't grow in the conditions they were planted in. We must be able to regroup when we see things aren't going the way we'd hoped. This is part of the process of creation.

The challenge is to understand how to evaluate ideas that seemed good but didn't live up to expectation. It's like an experiment that goes awry—it needs refining. What to do then? Gather data, and laugh, and then ask your Higher Self for guidance. Be grateful that you had the idea. Use the knowledge for the next experiment, and embrace the humility that comes with it. Find a way to bring your idea to fruition in a different way.

October 6: Germinating and Dormancy

SACRED DANCE

Practice the sacred dance given this week, and make it yours. Improvise, and feel the movements to place them in your memory.

MEDITATION AND PRACTICE

Viracocha had two daughters, Mama Killa and Pachamama. Mama Killa, a beautiful woman who cried tears of silver, was the goddess of the moon and regulated time and the Incan calendar by the moon's movements. She often warned of impending danger through eclipses. In her temples were dedicated priestesses to speak wonders to her and keep the night safe. Viracocha also had two sons, Imaymana Viracocha and Tocapo Viracocha. They named all the trees, flowers, fruits, and herbs and taught the people which were edible, which had medicinal properties, and which were poisonous.

Imagine that an eclipse happens when an idea is temporarily hidden, either because the shadow of another body obscures it or another body comes between it and you. These blockages can cause fear and sometimes sadness to the point of tears. Yet maybe you should think of personal eclipses as hibernation, where things are taking shape, where the Divine is guiding you with what seems to be a detour. You can be excited about an idea that has been refined, only to find that it needs time to develop and grow. Relying on the Divine timing and refining to germinate your idea seeds is key. Let them hibernate in the cool of the dark fertile sacred soil. Furthermore, you need to know which of your idea seeds are going to further the Divine will and not cause any negative consequences in the community. Your sacred dance and manifestations of your ideas are to bring the highest level of healing to the people you interact with.

October 7: Pushing Upward with Pachamama

SACRED DANCE

Practice the sacred dance you've done this week to see if you can enter a trance. Find ways to improvise, and move around in your Sacred Dance Studio. You can perform this dance in wide or tight circles while thinking of sacred seedlings.

MEDITATION AND PRACTICE

Pachamama, or World Mother, was a fertility goddess who presided over planting and harvesting and sustained life on earth. Her shrines were hallowed rocks or the hollows of trees. The four cosmological Quechua principles of water, earth, sun, and moon originated with Pachamama. The principle of water stemmed from Lake Titicaca, where all creation began, from the idea seeds of Viracocha. The principle stated that people were connected through water, just as the principle of earth stated that earth was where the beauty of human life was to be carried out and creation to flourish. The sun provided the needed physical light, and the moon regulated time and indicated the right moments to plant. The *ayni* was the reciprocal system of giving and receiving help with others, supported by the four principles. Sowing seeds responsibly and with the huacas was an integral part of the ayni, which arose from Pachamama's sacred considerations.

It's monumental to bring idea seeds forward, and even more so to nurture them to materialization. Pushing through all the blockages, doubts, and fears requires support from the community, which you often must create. There are others who bring ideas forth with whom we can confide, collaborate, and commiserate when needed. You can find them where your idea seeds lead you; they are kindred Spirits. Sprouts develop with the intervention of the Divine.

※　※　※

OCTOBER 8–14
Sowing Seeds in the Sun (Entry Point)

Everything depends on the Light.

We should dance in the Light everywhere at all times.

October 8: Surface Pressure

SACRED DANCE

Imagine a line drawn on your floor that you will dance upon, moving along it, that runs the length of your space. You'll need enough space to take twelve small steps and to turn around in.

This week, please avail yourself of a tambourine and a set of bells if you chose to use them. Holding a tambourine in your right hand and bells in your left, stand facing east, and inhale and exhale several times. To begin, walk forward in ten to twelve small steps, bringing your hands above your head as you walk and shaking the instruments. You look toward the sky as you stretch your arms upward. Feel the sun on your body; feel yourself in relation to the size of the Universe. At the end of the walks forward, hold your arms outstretched for a few breaths. Lower your arms and head.

Inti, known as the sun god, was the most important Incan god. His worshippers aspired to be welcomed into his home of splendor at the end of their earthly life. It was achievable for those who lived good lives while here. The people revered him so much that they built a statue of Inti called Punchao, standing at Temple of the Sun in the sacred complex at Cuzco; the temple and statue were made of thirty thousand pounds of gold. The statue represented Inti as a child and was believed to contain the Spirit of Inti. The statue was wheeled out into the sun in the morning and returned to inside the temple in the evening. The sacred dancers meditated upon his power and wisdom, and the people put their trust in him unconditionally.

On earth, we rely on the sun for our lives. Everything we do, the food we eat, healthy water, and oxygenated air require the life-producing elements of warmth and light. Plants instinctively lean toward its warmth as they grow. Every new idea, great thought, and new direction relies on warmth and light to be able to sprout and push through surface pressures. Self-doubt, criticism, feelings of inadequacy, and feelings of being left behind and left out can be examples of surface pressures.

What are some of your surface pressures? Make some notes.

October 9: Into G-d's Hands

As you arrive at the last of the small steps forward, you will turn 180 degrees to face the opposite direction. Raising the right knee to propel you around, pivot on the left foot, leaning toward your left side and holding the instruments above your head. When you're facing the point you started from, bow your head, and lower your arms to your sides. Breathe here for a few beats, then take ten to twelve small steps back to your starting point, bringing the instruments over your head and looking to the sky. Then turn clockwise 180 degrees, raising the left knee to propel you forward and pivoting on the right foot; lean toward your right side, lower the arms, and bow your head. Repeat this sequence four complete times.

MEDITATION AND PRACTICE

The well-being of the Inca Empire, its people, and the guarantee of a good harvest were in the hands of Inti. High Priest Willaq Umu, considered the most senior religious figure in the Incan world, was his attendant. A team of newly ordained priests supported the work of the high priest. Each major Incan town had a temple for Inti and many resources devoted to worshipping him. Incans reserved large areas of land and entire herds of animals for Inti; much of the area near Lake Titicaca was used to worship and remember him. Everything and everyone were connected in some way to Inti.

Once we have prepared the soil in troughs to cuddle the seeds, next we press the seeds into their base. We water. We hope to sustain temperatures for optimal growth. Then we wait. It's not up to us to make the seeds do anything. They have their own connection to the Divine. For our idea seeds, we do the same thing.

You do the footwork, reducing surface pressure, trusting that the idea has its own inherent good because it came from a thought or impulse originating from your connection to the Divine mind. Now, leave the rest up to the Higher Power, placing whatever comes in the Hands of G-d, and continue to act on the next forward-leading steps.

October 10: Meet the Disturbances

SACRED DANCE

Now, you will quicken the pace, using only four steps to move forward; when turning, you will make a slight hop on the pivoting foot, bringing your arms down toward the ground with each pivot, and up toward the sky with each set of steps and hops. You look toward the sky with your arms up and bow your head when you bring your arms down. Alternate your turns—first counterclockwise, then clockwise. Repeat this for four complete cycles.

───────── MEDITATION AND PRACTICE ─────────

In the Quechua language, *pacha* referred to both the whole Cosmos and the present moment. Incan ancients revered three levels of the Sacred: *hanan pacha, kay pacha,* and *ukhu pacha.* The upper realm, which included the sky, or the entire astronomical constellation, was hanan pacha, where masculine sun god Inti and Mama Killa, the feminine moon goddess, lived. Kay pacha was the invisible world, where people, animals, and plants lived. Those in kay pacha often struggled between doing what was honored in hanan pacha and what was being directed in one's inner world, ukhu pacha. As the place of new creation, ukhu pacha was associated with harvesting and Pachamama, the fertility goddess. Human disruptions of the ukhu pacha were sacred on this inner level, and in the present moment. Sacred Dance Meditations were often associated with disturbances. In Incan Practices, during the time of turning and aerating fields, the soil was purposely and purposefully disturbed and accompanied by sacred rituals.

When earthquakes, floods, fires, hurricanes, tornados, tsunamis, heat waves, and cold freezes occur, even with warnings, they can destroy much of human life and keep seeds from growing. Little disturbances also occur, like when it rains the day you planned for a picnic or an outdoor wedding. These kinds of disturbances can set you back, but the drive to live usually pushes forward and generates ways to deal with life's external disturbances.

But what of your inner disturbances? You have been led to be of service to your community and take guidance from the Higher Power, which sometimes comes in a revelatory moment or with deep prayer and meditation. So, you set out. Then someone laughs at you or avoids you because the person thinks you're crazy because of your chosen path. Or your mind will manufacture doubts, forgetfulness, laziness, anger, should-haves, would-haves, could-haves, and what-ifs. These are disturbances. Make a few notes in your journal about the inner disturbances you face. How can you practice a sacred dance movement from this week to remind you to focus on today and your many blessings?

October 11: Maturing Seeds as Spirit Descendants

SACRED DANCE

After the four cycles of pivots with hops, now you move forward by stepping on the right foot and tapping with the right, then stepping on the left foot and tapping with the left. You swing your arms slightly in front of you with each tap; your arms swing to the opposite side of the tapping foot.

MEDITATION AND PRACTICE

An ancient Incan story tells of Punchao, a child's Spirit dancing inside a sacred waterfall. A boy from the pueblo saw Punchao dancing in the waterfall, and he taught the boy how to dance sacredly. This came to be how supaypa wasin tusuq was communicated, from child to child, throughout the country, for the rest of time. The sacred dancer as Punchao held a golden rod in his right hand as he danced in the waterfall. The boys who learned the sacred dance grew up in Quechua villages. The Sacred Dance Meditation was a prayer done by men celebrating the Andean divinities tied to nature, such as the sun god Inti and the moon goddess Mama Killa. No two dances were identical because of a portrayal of sacredness and originality. The sacred dance then passed through hereditary lines, from father to son.

We are descendants from our Higher Power, and so we are instinctively led to return to It. We are deeply curious, which keeps us wanting to experience new things and bring forth new creations. But we typically imagine failure before trying something new, or we've become disillusioned from past failure. Some of us are hampered by social structures and financial constraints. We may ask ourselves, *What's the use? Why bother?* These are great questions to pose to the Universe. Just remember that you're a mature descendant of the Divine. With that knowledge you can ask to be returned to a sane and a more curious state and to be freed from self-imposed limitations. You have a limited amount of time on earth but an unlimited connection to Source, and your unique idea seeds need to be nurtured to maturity, precisely because of the inclination to feelings of failure that we humans can succumb to if we're not careful.

October 12: Seeds That Latch On to You

SACRED DANCE

Keep that same sequence of stepping, tapping, and swinging of the arms from yesterday, repeating five times. Then turn counter-clockwise 180 degrees to return to your starting point, repeat the sequence five times, then turn clockwise. Repeat this sequence for four complete cycles. Conclude the choreography by standing in your original position, facing east.

MEDITATION AND PRACTICE

High priests in the ancient Incan world danced sacredly in medita-tion to generate supernatural vision, during which time Pariacaca, god of water, rainstorms, and creation, who was born a falcon but later became human, spoke to them. Priests were the protectors and guards of calendrical information. With it, and in their shamanic consultation with the water god, they were able to tell the villagers when to conduct plantings and harvestings. In addition, *huacasa*, or leaders of song and dance, danced sacredly in support of bringing clarity to the high priest's visions.

Have you ever been taken over by an idea that seemed to come out of nowhere? It's as if the Spirit chose you to do something, and you're possessed and obsessed! Maybe it's an intuitive thought, or exposure to a message from a friend going through change, or some other communication that prompted you to do something out of the norm. Or you have an idea that you present to your Higher Power, and you follow it down roads you never thought you would travel. In these instances, your ability to rely on G-d's leading is demon-strated, and you allow yourself to flow with it. For those of us who like to imagine we're in control, this can be scary! But there is no need to fear. Just let go, and allow the Divine to steer. Express your gratitude whenever you aren't in control, and understand that the Divine plan is greater than you can imagine, benefits beings, and can lead to a greater positive vibration across the planet and the Universe. What are some ideas that have overtaken you? Jot down a few notes.

October 13: Seeds That Bring Wealth

SACRED DANCE

Practice the sacred dance so that you develop bodily memory and know it; embellish and improvise as you wish. Take it into yourself, as you do each week with your sacred dances.

MEDITATION AND PRACTICE

The sacred and societal center of Incan life was Sacsahuaman, a fortress outside Cuzco. The ancients considered it the "navel of the world," the home of the Inca Lord and site of the sacred Temple of the Sun. The immense wealth of the Inca was displayed in gold and silver, decorating every piece and crevice. Priests held large community gatherings for ceremonial Practices and Sacred Dance Meditations here. Sacsahuaman was a huaca, or revered place.

In the United States, money plays a huge role in our social structure. Living and thriving without it can be a challenge, and many young people follow paths based on how much money they can make. We single out certain individuals as successful based on financial gain. While there's nothing exactly wrong with money and wealth accumulation, those who dedicated their lives to learning from a Higher Power don't often find such large sums of money. Yet, we must think of wealth as more than money. We can redefine wealth as the ability to keep on the path less traveled, avoid delusion, remain awake and curious, and generate ideas that contain Light for the good of all.

What are your thoughts and feelings on wealth?

October 14: Seeing Seeds with the Divine Lens

SACRED DANCE

Perform the dance from this week until you feel in a trance. Feel how wonderful it is to dance sacredly in the sun.

MEDITATION AND PRACTICE

Supay Wasi refers to specific mountain caves that acted as entrances to ukhu pacha, the interior world of the Ancient Incans where supaypa wasin tusuq (scissors dance) took place. In supaypa wasin tusuq, the man who danced played the role of the mediator between Mother Earth and the Andes, managing the connection between them. The sacred dancers were descendants of the *tusuq laykas*, Ancient Incan priests, fortune tellers, healers, and shamans. The main musical instrument for the Sacred Dance Meditation during ancient Incan times was flat stones clapped together. The sacred dance ritual called on the gods of hanan pacha, kay pacha, and ukhu pacha to bless the community's seed plantings and bring the power of Pachamama to the fore.

All humans have the seed of the Divine within them, whether they realize it or not. The notion of an internal Divine seed that can keep us germinating new ideas, being hopeful, expressing pleasantness is easy to embrace. Most of the time we can control our reactions to situations if we can't control anything else. Those reactions are learned behaviors. We try to see every situation, person, event, and circumstance from the Divine lens, from a higher perspective. We endeavor to see ourselves as the Universe sees us: wonderful beautiful creations that have the potential to continuously evolve into beautiful expressions of the Divine. Each idea we have comes from that perspective and keeps us pushing forward on our path.

❊   ❊   ❊

Raining Creativity (Entry Point)

Creativity is part and parcel of humanity.

Exposure to enthusiasm and handling split milk both get creative juices going.

October 15: It's the Little Things

Your Sacred Dance Attire for this week may include feathers, rattles worn on your body, and a staff. A staff can be anything you bless (or "charge" as they say) as such, so a branch or a bamboo stick, or similar lightweight object qualifies. Once you use it for this purpose, regard it as sacred. The staff may be adorned as well, with feathers, leather wrappings, markings, or other types of sacred items that will remain on the staff as you move it. Make sure you can hold the staff comfortably as you move.

SACRED DANCE

Begin today kneeling, facing east, head bowed, and staff in your right hand, with feathers in your left hand. Bow forward. Slowly wipe your left hand along the floor or earth from right to left, making a large semicircle in front of you and to the side. Move the staff in front of you and up over your head with your right hand; if you aren't using a staff, you may simply hold your right arm up. Switch the staff to the other hand and make a large semi-circle with the right hand, and again lift the staff up over your head with the opposite hand. Repeat four times on each side. You will rise up and down on your knees as you nurture the earth in preparation to receive holy waters from heaven. On your last reverence for the earth, bring your palms out to your sides, away from your body, keeping your head bowed and arching your back. Then raise your arms up and open to shoulder width, and press up on the right leg, holding your upward gaze, and find your way to a standing position with all your weight on the right leg.

In October, ancient Incans held the Festival of Water. The people prayed for rain, knowing crops would fail without it. In Incan times, October was known for Uma Raymi Killa, or the moon of the celebration of water. During it, some llamas, which were signs of wealth in those days, were sacrificed in honor of the deities, while some were taken out to the open plaza to encourage the rains to fall. Over several days, people engaged in sacred celebrations of gratitude for the food and gifts they manifested.

Spirit consciousness imbued in the Ancient Peruvians the idea of the Creator being capable of evolving matter out of nothingness.

We can think of creativity as the ability to view the world in a different way from others and find new and innovative solutions to problems by spotting patterns and connecting seemingly unrelated things. When lost in a creative endeavor, no matter how big or small, calmness sometimes comes from being in oneness with the Divine. The creators feel safe and nurtured, shielded from the day-to-day noise and pressures from the world. Creativity often begins with gratitude for prayers and intentions that were fulfilled in ways unimagined. We can "pray for rain" by praying for more creative energy to be manifested, seen in the small daily work we do, which sometimes translates a great big flood of new idea seeds. Making room for them requires a sacrifice—namely that we give up praying for specific outcomes while we send our Spirits up to commune in faith with the Ultimate Reality.

What thoughts will you sacrifice to develop your creative instincts more fully?

October 16: Spiritual Musings

Stand facing east, with your Sacred Dance Attire, instruments and adornments, and staff. Picking up where you left off on October 15, take a step forward on your left foot, turn with your right foot to start clockwise circle, bringing your arms down so they are parallel to the floor. As your right foot touches the floor, double tap the floor with the ball of the foot and then step forward on it while leaning down. Then tap the left foot twice in the same way, and step forward on it. Continue to complete the circle. Practice a few times until you feel comfortable with the dance choreography. Include alternating moving the arms so that the rattle and your staff move with the steps.

MEDITATION AND PRACTICE

Tiahuanaco sat on the south portion of Lake Titicaca, which was thirteen thousand feet above sea level. Constructed on a half-acre, the city was made from trachytic rock. Its entry gate was guarded by a huge doorway made from a single block of rock one-and-a-half feet thick, seven feet high, and one hundred thirty-one feet wide. The door had carvings of Inti, with its head surrounded with solar rays. It depicted him with wands in each hand. On each side of Inti were kneeling winged creatures that also held wands in their hands.

The Incas built roads, adorned their temples with gold, and installed a great system of underground pipes with hot and cold water passing through. Incan people lived a life of comfort and luxury. They used unknown powers to manipulate huge blocks of stone to build great statues and monoliths. The people were enlightened and engaged in arts and science to move their communities forward.

Creativity comes about from the interplay between environments, people, personality, serendipity, and the quest for spiritual muses, which are those objects, people, and activities that spark ideas and awe or inspire us. The writings of a guru, architecture of a temple, and a natural phenomenon are examples. Creative thinking involves making new connections in our minds. That's the result of cultivating imagination and deliberately exposing ourselves to new experiences that push us to learn, translate our awe, and gain new power and strength. Some exposure comes from being in places where we can be allowed to think new thoughts or hear thoughts or experiences from spiritually enlightened people. Spiritual muses show up in other places too, like museums, in travel, or in lectures. Clinical psychologists sometimes encourage us to use artistic expression that arises from spiritual muses to develop creative ways to handle problems and difficult feelings.

October 17: Create the Valuable

SACRED DANCE

Once you're comfortable with the choreography given yesterday, resume by making a complete circle, then step backward on the right foot and spin around twice, clockwise. Then step forward on the right foot and turn counterclockwise. Repeat stepping backward, turning three times clockwise, and then stepping forward and turning counterclockwise three times. After the last turn, begin double-tapping the right foot, stepping on it, then double-tapping on the left foot. Move around the room in a large counterclockwise circle, that way, alternating the right and left feet. Allow your body to freely flow with the tapping.

MEDITATION AND PRACTICE

Many of the Ancient sacred dances in Peruvian society were Aboriginal meditations on agriculture and worship of the gods. One of the dances was Huayñucuni, a private ritual ceremony in honor of Mother Earth. It included the apus praying and exhaling a deep breath while throwing *koca kintu* (six perfect coca leaves each as a group of three) into the air. People understood that act was to seek permission to use the land and provide sacrifices so that there was an abundance. People practiced the Huanca dance to ensure a good harvest. The Sara Kutipay was a Sacred Dance Meditation honoring Aboriginal peoples who gathered and planted food. That Sacred Dance Meditation brought the discipline and consistency that underpinned the entire spiritual fabric.

Many people would have us believe in a return on investment, that is, what we gain from something must be at least equal to what we put into it. We can take the idea of investment and apply it to our creative spiritual revenues, the deposits we make with it into our Divine bank, and the way we manifest ourselves in our lives. When we consciously create, it gives us something new and valuable for ourselves and our families, friends, and associates and shows the Universe partnering with us. Creativity and its yields are sacred gifts from our Higher Power; they imply a contract of sorts in which we are obligated to use our creativity to make things better. When we create, we thank the Divine for giving us aspects of Spirit and using our Higher Self to bring the Divine into view for others to see. Some people think only artists are creative, but everyone has gifts to join the Divine in cocreation of the Universe.

October 18: A Spiritual Creativity Process

SACRED DANCE

Review the choreography given so far this week for the sacred rain dance. After you have made one complete rotation around the room in a counterclockwise direction, add in another sequence of the clockwise and counterclockwise spins, stepping backward and forward. Repeat the choreography several times until you feel comfortable. After your last clockwise spin, you'll step with double taps to your starting position. When you have finished, return to your Sacred Dance Posture.

MEDITATION AND PRACTICE

The number *three* was sacred in ancient Peru, corresponding to three distinct levels of the human being, including the physical, energetic, and spiritual bodies. The three major energy centers of the body were *yanqai*, *munay*, and *yanchai*, or belly, heart, and mind.

The people made kintu bundles out of three leaves, which also represented their belief in three worlds: the lower world of ukhu pacha, the middle world of kay pacha, and the upper world called hanan pacha. The leaves of the kintu bundle were imbued with loving energy before being placed into service of the shamans.

Alto misayoq were shamans who had powers to predict the future and possessed the ability to communicate directly with the apus, or Spirits of the sacred mountains and Pachamama. Once their kintu bundle was arranged with the leaves, these shamans used it to hover over each of the three energy centers, beginning with the belly, then the heart, and then the mind, for healing and transformation. The alto misayoq petitioned apus for blessings through Koca kintu prayer rituals with sacred dance, which included walking and kneeling with the eyes closed.

The ceremony aimed to reinforce the sacred philosophy of giving and sharing. The people gave to Mother Earth and received from Father Sky (the Universe); they shared within community.

Some of us think that creativity just happens, and it may be that way for some, or even could be for all of us if we're open. But to access the Spirit and bring value to our lives and those around us in a predictable and sustainable manner, we need to act to fuel our creativity.

Write down everything you've done that was creative, no matter how large or small. Then, make an outline of places you'll go or things you will do each month to see or hear something new and different that you normally wouldn't. These can be museums, churches, concerts in the park, free lectures, TED talks, a child's game or recital, or any number of activities. Make them part of your Creativity Plan. The point is to fuse disparate experiences and activities to receive inspiration from the Universe.

October 19: Peering Inside

SACRED DANCE

After you return to your starting position, face east, as you do regularly. Raise the staff and shells over your head with both hands and gaze upward. Make sure you don't drop the shells. Hold them steady, kneel, and then bow forward, bringing your arms down as you do. Breathe, then return to holding the staff and shells over your head. Then bow forward again, shift the staff into the right hand, and wipe the floor in front of you to create a large semicircle on the floor. Swipe from right to left and back, then leave the shells on the floor in front of you as you hold the staff with both hands in the center. Bring the staff up over your head, making the elbows taut and looking up. Bow forward, and then bring the staff up, then bow forward and hold for a few breaths to end.

MEDITATION AND PRACTICE

The apus of the ancient Andes Mountains were superior Spirits that protected people, brought blessings, and responded favorably to offerings. The people believed the apus didn't talk to human beings—they embodied them. Through their invocations, giving, Sacred Dance Meditations, and prayers, they asked the apus for protection.

We may perhaps consider creativity as fun and spirituality as boring, routine, or onerous. As a result, sometimes we seek excitement from external events, discussed in other meditations. But when those secular events also become routine, something feels missing. And we repeat the cycle of feeling unfulfilled. That's why we use our Creativity Plan to get inspiration.

Creativity occurs inside you as you assimilate new experiences into your connection to the Divine. You take input from your experiences and filter it through the Divine lens to see what you want to create.

October 20: Practice New Ways to Respond, New Ways to Act

SACRED DANCE

Practice and improvise today so that you're able to move sacredly from your memory of the choreography from this week.

MEDITATION AND PRACTICE

Ancients in the Andean societies prayed when they planted a seed. Placing a seed *was* prayer, and prayer *was* a seed.

When we are connected to our Higher Self, knowing that we are creative, knowing that we are nurtured through our spiritual muses, we can practice new ways to respond to challenges and changes. We respond by creating positive thoughts, words, and actions in varied situations and by giving. Instead of thinking that an event will be mundane, think of what you can bring to it. Also, think of the people who will be there and what they need from your connection to the Source of creativity. Realize that no event, situation, or request is about you. Give love and acceptance while you acknowledge that the flow of life is transient. Creative ideas come; some take root, and some don't. But they are there to make our lives more interesting and to get us to cocreate with G-d. They help us relate to and connect with our fellow travelers. Think of spirituality as creative energy, and by accessing it you will always be guided to respond in creative, albeit appropriate, ways.

✳ ✳ ✳

OCTOBER 21
Psycho-Spiritual Mystical Text Chat

SACRED DANCE

Trance the sacred dance today, and lose yourself to Spirit.

MEDITATION AND PRACTICE

The sacred dances of the spiritual Andean peoples were aligned with harvest, planting, and dialogue with Great Spirits. They were connected in multiple ways to the past and future, with the present being a dialogue with their spiritual ancestors.

Jungian analyst and author Marion Woodman tells us the creative process diminishes if we're not talking to Spirit constantly. That chat, and the creativity that comes from it, makes our lives rich and light.

Creativity arises out of a mystical union with the Divine. A lot of people talk all the time about the Creator but seldom see Spirit as an artist. Seek, then, to form a creative alliance, artist to artist, with your Great Creator. How might you consider your Higher Self as an artist?

※ ※ ※

Faith in the Unseen, Unimagined Creative Places (Entry Point)

Idea Seeds in TW (Three Worlds)

The Unseen gives us idea seeds to sow on many sacred levels.

For this week's Sacred Dance Meditations, we move again along an imaginary line that connects us to the central cord of the Universe. The starting point moves you through the three worlds, as you plant and nurture seeds in three areas of creation. You may use your Sacred Dance Attire if you like or add colorful additions to it. There are no handheld instruments in this week's dance, but you can use flutes, drums, or recorders to accentuate your work. The choreography and movements aren't fast, but they aren't too slow either. They are meant to be pensive and allow you to think about what you may create in different worlds.

October 22: Earthly Levels

SACRED DANCE

Begin facing east in your Sacred Dance Attire. Clap your hands vigorously and loudly six times. Then let them drop to your sides. Step forward on the right foot, turning to the side, and skip forward twice. (You'll actually skip sideways; the direction will be forward relative to your original standing position.) Then swing around, and step on the left, turning to the side, and skip forward twice. You hold your arms down at your sides as you gently pinch your

Sacred Dance Attire between your thumb and forefingers, as if you are cinching it up from the floor. Alternate skipping and twisting to each side for eight breaths. Swing the left foot around so your body turns in a clockwise direction 180 degrees to face your starting point. Repeat the moves until you reach your starting point, then turn 180 degrees again.

MEDITATION AND PRACTICE

Mapuche sacred dance was a worshipping and healing Practice found in pre-Columbian Chile. In the *guillatún*, an important Mapuche celebrative ceremony, the Sacred Dance Meditation petitioned the spiritual world for prosperity when carrying out new and creative endeavors. Guillatún, meaning to pray, was a major communal event of extreme spiritual and social importance. During the ceremony, dances and prayers were offered in which the participants asked for plentiful harvests, good health, and abundance. Participants often made an offering of a lamb to carry through their principle of asking and giving.

Situations must be worked out, but they process on levels we can't contemplate with our minds alone. We must be open to the concept that what manifests on earth comes out of other dimensions. That's not too much of a leap considering that our expanding physical universe contains multiple solar systems and reaching them takes light-years. We're dancing on a cord that connects us to these other worlds; we're a part of a multidimensional universe, from which we receive creative idea seeds to sow.

October 23: Creative Worlds

SACRED DANCE

Begin with the sacred dance choreography given on October 22. When you have returned to the starting position and swung the left leg around, after the 180-degree rotation, repeat the steps for four breaths, alternating sides. Then with the right foot, step forward, swing the arms left, then step on the left, and swing the arms right.

Bend forward slightly, and look down as you do this. Repeat for eight breaths. Then turn clockwise 180 degrees by swinging your left foot around. Then step forward with the left foot, and gently walk forward once again, swinging your arms in the opposite direction of the stepping foot. Bend slightly forward, and gaze to the floor. There is a definite swaying to your moves and a bit of a punctual moment with each arm swing. Repeat this sequence until you reach your starting point, and swing the left leg around in a clockwise direction so you turn 180 degrees.

MEDITATION AND PRACTICE

The role the machi (shaman) played in the Sacred Dance Meditation was inseparable from the ceremony. Shamans were usually women who gained their roles following an apprenticeship with an older machi. Machis had knowledge of regional medicinal herbs, sacred stones, and sacred animals. They were responsible for *machitún*, or healing ceremony, during which ancestors were invoked who, in the Mapuche belief, had left the underworld, lived in the spiritual world, and controlled the art of diagnosing evils and diseases. They watched over the machis and assisted in their treatments. Prayers were offered to Ngen, the spirits of nature, through *kemukemu*, the sacred altar that connected the disparate distant worlds above and below the earth. The presence of a machi was required for the sacred dances, as she was the only intermediary between people and the unseen worlds.

You can use your imagination to visit, as well as create, different worlds. Some people have places they go to listen to angelic singing to receive inspiration, such as an enormous celestial villa they create in their minds, with angels and helper spirits, friends, or other supportive beings there to greet them. Or they imagine they're inside of the Louvre, in the Taj Mahal gazing at art or talking with famous but not embodied artists, or visiting Mecca doing their bows with millions of people. Or they visit healers and psychics by imagining a purely healthy physical and mental body and removal of any residual past connections to ailments that manifest in aches or pains. The

Spirit and the mental energy we have are nearly limitless. Accessing and directing it is critical and requires daily attention.

October 24: *Shamanic Travel*

SACRED DANCE

Step forward on the right foot, and simultaneously turn your body to face the side. Skip forward (in relation to your original starting position) twice, then swing around, and step on the left. Turn your body to face that side, and skip forward twice. Repeat for several breaths as you dance sacredly along your line. Hold your arms down at your sides. Skip forward with your right foot; then with your weight on it, bend forward from the waist, and swing your right arm down in front of you. Step and skip on the left foot, swinging the left arm down, then with the right foot. Step forward, and bend forward from the waist with all your weight on the left. Repeat this sequence four times, then swing your left foot around to take you counterclockwise to face the direction you came from, at 180 degrees.

MEDITATION AND PRACTICE

Sacred Dance Meditations were held in a ramada, an open area made with tree branches, constructed by the participants.

A ritual ceremony called Ngeykurewen was performed for a machi initiate. There she received a wooden staff spiritually charged with sacred energies into a sacred *rewe*, which was sculpted artistically to reflect the four main sacred levels. At the top of the staff, a human head was carved into the wood to represent the human spirits involved in machitún or guillatún ceremonies. Using the rewe gave the machi ability to transport themselves to Wenu Mapu, far above the sky where the deities lived, so they could maintain communication with the sacred spirits. During ceremonies, the shaman's rewe was positioned in the center of the space and surrounded by the other members of the community. When not involved in ceremonies, the rewe was placed outside the machi's home as a sign that a shaman lived there.

While it may not be our calling to engage in shamanic travel as the ancient Andeans did, leaving the earth for unseen dwellings on other planes, we can act like a shaman in real life and bring creative energy to people we interact with. This can be deliberate without being intrusive. People sought after shamans for answers during ancient times, and even today people go to shamans for answers and healing; you're sought out all the time as well.

Go to people and events or meetings with the idea that you're there to help them in their situation. Bring a few ideas for them to use on their journey. Everyone we know has something they need a solution for.

October 25: Underworlds

SACRED DANCE

Repeat the sequence from October 24 involving skipping and swinging your arms in front of you.

MEDITATION AND PRACTICE

The Ancient Mapuche believed in a creator called Ngenechen, who was embodied as an older man, an older woman, a young man, and a young woman. According to the Mapuche, Ngenechen designed three worlds that influenced life in the community: Wenu Mapu (above), where the beneficial deities and the old ancestors lived; Nag Mapu (on earth), where all the living, both good and bad, dwelt; and Minche Mapu (below) where some good and deceived spirits dwelt.

Often, modern spirituality centers on being good and avoiding evil, and its practitioners characterize people as good or bad. Perhaps it's better to talk about underworlds, or places where people go when they can't connect with the beauty of life, and from that space they can receive new ideas or remain in darkness. Every one of our ancient cultures talks about an underworld or a place where there's confusion and delusion, where beings go when they don't want to be informed or live in the Light. The idea is that they can be in a contained environment or space where they can't cause disturbances to the enlightened. But can deluded beings, embodied or disembodied, be sectioned off so that they don't impact you? It's up to you to find creative ways to keep negativity and delusion from taking you to the underworld.

October 26: Psychological Reconditioning

SACRED DANCE

Step forward on the right foot as you turn your body sideways, and skip forward twice. Then swing around, step on the left foot, turn your body to face that side, and skip forward twice. Repeat for several breaths as you dance sacredly along your line for several breaths. Hold your arms down at your side. When you have finished this segment, stand with feet together, and clap your hands loudly five times.

MEDITATION AND PRACTICE

The Ancient Mapuche believed in four types of spiritual beings. There were Pillan and Wangulen, male and female ancestral spirits that lived in the Wenu Mapu, a spiritual world of good. The Ngen were spirits that lived in nature. Lastly, the Wekufes were spirits who dwelt in Mapu, the world of deception, placed there because they broke the *admapu*, the perfect harmony of the Wenu Mapu.

We simultaneously live in the world of good, the world of nature, and the world of deception. When we're balanced, the creative ideas coming to us are inexhaustible and constant. There are so many of them that we must choose which of them we will pursue. Yet many times deception tells us that we can't do one or more of them due to constraints. We forget the way that the Divine has the power to do anything if we partner with it. If we don't want to pursue a creative direction given to us by the unseen, that's a choice, but it's best not to be deluded into thinking it's impossible. To get to that realization, we need to see the world in a more unstructured way. A bit of harmony is in seeming chaos.

October 27: The Body's Seeds of Faith

SACRED DANCE

Review and repeat the choreography from October 21 to 23 so you have a body memory of it, and establish a personal rhythm. Feel yourself being transported along the central cord of the universe, connecting to its different levels.

MEDITATION AND PRACTICE

The Mapuche people considered the machi both a sacred dancer and vocalist. The messages brought back by the machi were accompanied by the rhythmic cadence of the kultrun, a magic drum decorated with sacred icons and filled with sacred objects. The Mapu, or land, was always the central core of Mapuche life and beliefs. This view is represented in the kultrun, which each machi designed according to the knowledge and spiritual strength given to them by Ngenechen.

We can adorn our bodies with sacred symbols and emblems, either by temporary or permanent means. Our insides can be adorned too. Inside of us dwells the essence of our thoughts; what we focus on becomes who we are. These also become our body's seeds of faith, where we plant the ideas that come to us from the outer world, which work their way through our Spirits, and we feel a leading deep in our belly.

October 28: Creating Faith at the Crossing

SACRED DANCE

Review and repeat the choreography you learned on October 24–26, until you can feel it and know it in your body and mind.

MEDITATION AND PRACTICE

In the ancient ancestor's Practice, the circular shape of the kultrun drum represented the worlds and the infinite spiritual creative space they found themselves in. The drum skin was painted with two lines that crossed in the center of the drum to depict four natural and spiritual positive and negative strengths that corresponded to the sacred powers from the earth and the stars, earth's waters, the cardinal directions, and the winds.

As we become adults sometimes creativity dwindles. Children are full of creative ideas and are often unafraid to share them with anyone who'll listen! To get back to that free-flowing way of being and connection, we align at the crossing of our inner worlds formed with our mind-body-Spirit.

You can imagine the line that runs from your head to your toes, and one that intersects it at your solar plexus. At that crossing you can place your finger and think about what the mind can do to lead you to delusion or truth, what the body does to sustain your life, and how Spirit calls you to higher awareness.

At this central point, we constantly re-create our faith in our creativity and our recollection of what the Divine intervener can do in our lives; from that intersection, we interact with others. Our interactions are also our seeds, our plantings placed along our paths.

October 29: Dormant and Yet to Be Imagined—Clearing the Channel

SACRED DANCE

Practice bringing the entire sacred dance together, getting it into your body memory.

MEDITATION AND PRACTICE

The center of the kultrun drum represented the power that brought balance and stability to Wenu Mapu, where positive gods and ancestors dwelt. It resonated with Nag Mapu, or earth where all the living were. And by connecting Minche Mapu, the land underneath, the drum drew from the good that negative spirits indirectly produced by their interference. The drum symbolized an unending connection to Spirit and stability and referenced the ability to create, vibrate, and emerge with vigor alongside the deluded.

Generally, making noise causes disturbance. Beating a drum, clapping hands, stamping the feet, and such vibrational changes move the energies. So does chanting sacred words or humming or singing.

We live here with interferences and intruders, which can be external, such as unexpected shifts in health, family circumstances, and livelihood, or internal, such as responding differently to people and situations and encouraging ourselves to stay on a course. Disturbances can just arise simply from inappropriate self-talk that knocks us over.

October 30: Cleaning Up Creative Mess

SACRED DANCE

As you often do, please make the sacred dance choreography from this week yours, as you allow yourself to move from memory. Apply and acknowledge the ways in which your mind-body facilitates creativity.

MEDITATION AND PRACTICE

The ancient ancestors were free to create and try new things. But sometimes, the creation wasn't exactly what was envisioned, such as when Viracocha created the giants at Lake Titicaca but later wiped them from the earth. The act demonstrated a need to change courses or clean up the outgrowth of the idea seed.

In creating new worlds, it's important to understand that not all idea seeds bloom into greatness. Some things turn out to be duds. They don't produce too much and may even cause us to have to spend energy getting things straightened out. Some creative ideas stick, and others may not. What sticks is using the energy to make us better people, more loving, kind, open, and compassionate. All of it is okay because the point is in the trying, the effort, and the planting. Thank your Higher Power for the creative ideas and the energy you had to carry it out. When things go awry, you ask for more ideas.

October 31: Remaining Childlike

SACRED DANCE

Review all the sacred dances for the month. Combine them, or take parts of them as you feel inclined, and make new dances of your own.

MEDITATION AND PRACTICE

Our Incan ancestors were on the planet at the same time as our Egyptian ancestors, and they share the creativity of building pyramids and social orders, extreme abundance, and realization of their connection to the Cosmos. Their ideas were unlimited, and their application of technology exceedingly advanced. They planted seeds of abundance, sacredly danced upon them, and believed that the seeds would produce and provide what they needed to enjoy and sustain life. They sacredly danced before the Divine in this assurance.

Remain forever curious; to keep that sense of knowing, you only must hold your hands under the spring to produce what you need. Keeping a childlike freedom to play and create helps to ensure that we sow idea seeds planted from love and faith.

NOVEMBER

Thankful Deeds

ANCIENT PERSIAN
SACRED DANCE

Like many of the cultures discussed over the course of the year up to this point, ancient Persians celebrated and mourned and moved through transitions and change with Sacred Dance Meditation since as early as 6000 BCE. In 500 BCE, the Persian empire ruled over numerous nations, from Egypt in North Africa to the edges of India in the Far East. Iran is one of the ancient world's empires that believed in the power of sacred dance.

Zoroastrianism, dating from the fifth century BCE, is one of the world's oldest spiritual traditions. It was the religion of the pre-Islamic Iranian empires for over a millennium.

Zoroaster was a spiritual guru who taught a philosophy of self-realization and realization of the Divine; exactly when he lived is unclear. Zoroaster emphasized the freedom of the individual to make choices and individual's total responsibility for one's deeds.

Ahead of Zoroaster, though, was the cult of Mithra dating back to about 2000 BCE. Mithraism began in Persia, where many gods were worshipped, including Ahura Mazda, god of the skies, and Ahriman, god of darkness. Mithra was the most important of the gods, as the Iranian god of the sun, justice, and war. In Persia, Mithra protected tribal society. Persian sacred dance was an integral part of Persia's sun and light god reverence. In worshipping Mithra, people participated in celebratory, sacrificial, and offering ceremonies. These included sacred dances, but they were only performed by men. Sacred dance was the first ancient Iranian dance and the origin of the dance of magic. Mehrgan was one such celebration that took place at Persepolis, during which people from different parts of the Persian Empire brought gifts that marked their prosperity and gave homage to the king and contributed to the celebrations. It was customary for people to send or give their king, and each other, gifts. Sadeh was another festival that dates to the first Persian Empire, Achaemenid Empire. Sadeh marked the point when a hundred days remained until spring began. Sadeh honored fire and triumph over the forces of darkness, frost, and cold.

In the sixth and seventh century BCE, Zoroaster reformed the Mithran deities. By the mid-fifth century BCE, the Zoroastrians had dominated the sacred dance world and worshipped under the open sky, ascending mounds to light fires. This fire festival lasted for three days, with dancing and music and much food to eat. These fire festivals represented the light of god (Ahura Mazda) as well as the illuminated mind. They began to keep the fires burning all the time, never extinguishing them. No Zoroastrian ritual or ceremony occurred without the presence of a sacred fire.

PREPARATION

You may want to wear a sleeveless overlay to your Sacred Dance Attire, a head covering of some sort that will keep your hair from getting in your way from swirling and turning, and a sash around your waist. All of these are options. You can download flute music from your favorite music provider if you like, or you can simply dance in silence for this month's Sacred Dance Meditations. There are also preparations for each week's sacred dance, which you may attend to as you wish.

Please visit www.cswalter.org/sacreddancemeditations for video demonstrations. They are not intended to be step-by-step instructions but rather are meant to give you a view of the sacred dance.

NOVEMBER 1–7
Thankful Heart, Thankful Deeds (Entry Point)

Fire, an Ancient Symbol

The element of fire reminds us to be pure in our thinking and acting and to acknowledge the flame we carry.

Fire is an important symbol in the Zoroastrian tradition, illuminating the path to enlightenment and giving rise to the ability to choose good thoughts and acts. Flame is an agent of ritual purity from which insight and wisdom are gained; it's the perfect element to light up the thankful heart. Because of that, you could also use some incense of frankincense or myrrh to evoke a spiritual connection. For the Sacred Dance Attire, you may want to add a cover for your head with a cap or scarf, as is the tradition for this Sacred Dance Meditation. You will want to use small battery-powered lights to hold loosely in your hands.

November 1: Thankful Heart

SACRED DANCE

Begin by facing east, holding the battery-powered candles (turned on) in the palms of your hands, arms at your sides. Begin walking slowly clockwise to the left to complete two circles large enough to encompass your space. Your steps are slow, and you pause between each of them. Your knees are slightly bent, as if you're dipping with each step. Once you have returned to your starting point, place your wrists at your hips with your palms cupped upward to hold the light.

MEDITATION AND PRACTICE

Zoroastrians regarded the existence of negativity as necessary for good or positive energy to triumph but thought that people needed to push or resist against it. They believed that Ahura Mazada was the god of Light, and Ahriman the god of chaos and darkness. People could freely choose to follow a path of good, with a clean and pure heart.

A thankful heart is one that doesn't feel entitled to or owed anything but one that acknowledges that blessings and grace are the ways in which we accrue. A thankful heart looks for the good in others, in all situations. In having a thankful heart, we acknowledge life as a gift and live it to the fullest in fun, laughter, and communion with the Divine in all its manifestations. Sometimes a thankful heart shows up as not speaking ill of anyone or criticizing what we receive through grace. It sometimes requires us to shrug off certain moments when we could complain.

If you have been accustomed to finding fault, a thankful heart may be cultivated by letting faults lie, without even bringing them up to anyone, and just saying to your Higher Power that you'd like to point out the errors but today you won't. A thankful heart remains free from judging people. But none of these precludes you from taking good responsibility for your well-being and spiritual growth. A thankful heart is a catalyst and a multiplier of good. How do you exhibit your thankful heart?

November 2: What Are Deeds?

SACRED DANCE

Begin facing east as you gently kneel to the floor, and again place your wrists at your hips with the palms facing outward. Then, keeping your hands cupped so that you keep the light facing outward, raise your arms up, and bend them so that you can just see the palms of your hands above your head. Sweep the right arm outward to the right and backward over your head, and over to your left side and around to the front of your body. Your gaze follows your moving palm, while the left wrist rests at your left hip. You'll naturally lean backward and around to the left with your arm movement. Repeat this twice on the right, then return the right wrist to the right hip. Now do the same on the left.

MEDITATION AND PRACTICE

The conflict between the positive Spirit Spenta Mainyu and the negative Spirit Angra Mainyu, both offspring of Ahura Mazda, represented the battle humans must undergo in making positive and negative choices, or living in truth or in lies. Through deeds, people could redeem themselves because they were one hundred percent responsible for their lives, Souls, and fate. What happened to them when they died was believed to be influenced by what they did in life. After death, a person had to cross over the Bridge of the Requiter, which separated the living from the dead. For people with mostly bad deeds, the bridge narrowed so much that when crossing the individual fell into a place ruled by Ahriman. People who performed mostly good deeds crossed the bridge to a garden paradise near the sun.

Deeds are actions to make things better without expecting or asking for anything in return or for acknowledgement. It's giving without any ego attachment. Some people have a practice of doing one good thing to help another human being every day without anyone knowing of it, including the recipient of the deed. Try to make a habit out of doing one thing for someone else every day without letting anyone know. You can let the person behind you in line go ahead of you, pay the toll for the car behind you, send an anonymous inspirational note to a colleague or friend—the list is inexhaustible! Go over your daily routine to see where you can add a deed to it, and then write some ideas down in your journal. Or make a list of reminders on your mobile device so you can have it handy.

November 3: Good Deeds Do Go Unpunished

SACRED DANCE

Review the choreography given so far this week. Facing eastward, bring both wrists to rest at your hips with the palms facing the sky so the lights are visible. Raise the right palm toward the sky, keeping your elbow softly bent, then slowly move it forward and backward, making imaginary waved lines at your right side as you bring your wrist back to your waist. Repeat on the left. Then repeat on both sides, right and left. Your gaze follows your palm, and the movements are slow and deliberate. You may think about the relationship between your good thoughts and the light you bring into the world by thinking them, in addition to the light you bring to your own healing and sense of safety and well-being.

MEDITATION AND PRACTICE

According to the ancient Zoroastrians, the Soul is made up of nine total parts. The physical body is made of matter and sensation, the physical frame and nervous system, and the skeleton and muscles; life energy, the astral body, and the ethereal substance; and lastly the spiritual essence, which links the Spirit, Inner Soul, and Divine spark. During life, the nine elements work together on three planes. After death the first two main parts dissipate, leaving only Spirit, which through good deeds, unites with the Creator.

Some say that good deeds are always punished, meaning, the good intentions are always met with resistance. Good deeds aren't punishable. They have no strings attached, no desires to get any ego recognition from the outside world. You don't tell people about your good deeds either; otherwise, you'd let your ego lead. But when you do something such as donate to a food pantry and the pantry rejects your donation for whatever set of reasons, that could be considered a good deed just because you did it. You can't hang on to the outcome. Just do the good deeds, and leave the rest up to your Higher Power.

November 4: What Is Gratitude?

SACRED DANCE

Begin by reviewing and repeating the sacred dance given on November 3. When you have returned both wrists to your hip area, slowly reach the palms forward away from your body, then up over your head with the palms facing upward, just in front of your forehead.

To your ability, keep your arms stable above your head and lean your torso backward. The leaning doesn't have to be far, just slight. Allow your head to go as far as you're comfortable with, but watch for letting it fall all the way backward. Bring the wrists back to your hips with the palms facing upward. Repeat the leaning three times, and remember to breathe.

MEDITATION AND PRACTICE

Zoroastrians engaged in the sacred fire dance as a symbol of purity, truth, and divine grace and as a gift to Ahura Mazda. They believed there was divinity, or *atar*, in flames. Because of that, a sacred fire burned constantly in the temple areas and in the village homes. Fire was treasured because of what it enabled humanity to do, such as prepare food and keep warm, and because through it people could acknowledge the heavens. At sacred ceremonies, priests made offerings, and people recited prayers and danced sacredly around open fires. Sacred fire was present at every ritual and ceremony. Frankincense and sandalwood were offered in thanksgiving for what had been given to them and what they could give to each other and to their Supreme Being.

Gratitude comes when we accept that we have opportunities, goods, services, and health and we don't take them for granted. We express humility in situations that relieve our identification with lack or the tendency to be shortsighted. This isn't to say that we leave reality. Sometimes we have devastating losses and grief. We don't ignore them or push the feelings down. But at the same time, gratitude through a mind-body-Spirit point of view gives us the ability to heal and grow and to note that our circumstances always have a glimmer of Light in them.

November 5: The Ultimate Gratitude List

SACRED DANCE

After reviewing and repeating what you did on November 4, return to standing, and again move your arms up over your head and follow your palms with your gaze. Walk forward three steps and then backward three steps, then backward three more steps and forward three steps. Extend your right arm with palm upward just above your ear and your left arm downward just to your waist, with palms facing up. Then bring the left palm up and the right one down. The feeling is one of flowing, so take your time. Repeat four times on each side. Bring the wrists back to the hips to rest. Bring the arms again up over your head, with the gaze directed at them. Bring them down in front of your body, and cross your wrists with the palms facing up so that the right wrist is resting on the left. Repeat four times. Then repeat four times with the left wrist resting on the right. Keep your elbows held away from your body. Now bring your arms up over your head with the palms facing upward. Turn slowly in a clockwise direction, then turn in a counterclockwise direction. Upon return to the center, place the wrists at your hips and then find a kneeling position, and hold the palms in front of you.

MEDITATION AND PRACTICE

Ahura meant "lord," and *mazda* meant "wisdom." Therefore, Ahura Mazda was the Zoroastrian idea of a Supreme Being with much sacred wisdom, who created the worlds. The ancients believed that Ahura Mazda provided guided pathways to enlightenment to people who spoke and acted from truth and that the sacred fire would illuminate the way.

Talk of being grateful for our health, property, and friends almost seems perfunctory. Those of us who have made a gratitude list may have gotten bored. I challenge you to develop a gratitude list every night before you go to bed that goes beyond the routine, the surface, and the boring. Are you grateful for being able to think? To be able to make choices? To say no, or yes, or maybe? Are you grateful for the air you breathe or the ability to walk? Are you grateful you can practice your own brand of spirituality? If you have limitations, what supports do you have that you can look toward for gratitude? Keep a gratitude journal beside your bed at night and make a list. Include the deeds you did over the course of the day. In the morning when you arise, think about the day ahead and how you're grateful to have another day to do deeds in service to your fellow travelers.

November 6: Thankful Heart as Practice

SACRED DANCE

Practice and embellish the sacred dance given this week. Make the choreography yours, and embody the feeling of giving and doing. Understand that your giving creates energy, a thankful heart, and gratitude.

MEDITATION AND PRACTICE

Ahura Mazda created both Mithra, the sun god, and Anahita, a water goddess of fertility, healing, and wisdom. Ahura Mazda also created the Angra Mainyu, the destructive Spirit of darkness, and Spenta Meynu, the creative Spirit. Both the ancients in Persia and the Zoroastrians believed in a conflict between positive and negative energies, but humanity would prevail each time because of the ultimate connection to the Creator. That was evident through the sacred dances and festivals to which people presented gifts to the Supreme Deity and the community on earth. Everyone was expected to give freely and with happiness. The people believed that giving was an expression of Ahura Mazda.

As part of Sacred Dance Meditation, it's appropriate to incorporate a thankful heart, which lends itself to a sense of humility. Some people lose their way or have experiences that cause them to become disenchanted with life, even after a long and arduous spiritual journey. The ultimate thankful heart helps us understand that we can only live in the moment. Any blessings that come our way—material, emotional, mental, or spiritual—have been given to us by the Divine and our will to cocreate with G-d.

November 7: Energy from Gratitude

SACRED DANCE

Today, repeat the sacred dance from the week and lose yourself in it. Think of all the wonderful deeds you have done and will do, your thankful heart, and the energy you create from being extremely grateful in your life. By doing this, you bless and free others to feel good about themselves.

MEDITATION AND PRACTICE

When the gods and myths of the ancients in Persia merged, much of the essence of the Persian worldview was taken up by Zoroastrians. With their sacred fire dance meditations, they brought sacred energy into the mind, body, and Spirit. The people were empowered to be responsible for their lives, and there was an acknowledgment of choice in all endeavors. People believed in the power of gratitude and the energy it created. They were used to thinking about abundance and tried to steer clear of negative energy.

Can you thank your Higher Power or whatever energy or Spirit you recognize? Can you vibrate that in your body through your voice? Can you sing it? Can you whisper it? The funny thing is that you don't have to believe it! Just saying it, vibrating it, creates positive energy. The more gratitude you can express, the more positive energy you create. You get angels, ions, and electrons moving around you. You attract others who are generating the same positive energy, which leads to even more. Say what you're grateful for. Take a few items off your nightly list, and shout them out! Find a place, be it in your car or out on a walk, where you can let your mind-body know you're a walking expression of Spirit and for that you're grateful.

※ ※ ※

Thankful Oneness with the Divine (Entry Point)

Give and Receive

There is nothing noble in giving with a string and nothing valuable in diminishing the giver. Giving and receiving are Divine deeds.

Spins and gestures in ancient Persian sacred dance cleared the spiritual channels and actualized dance as the power of life and a means for becoming one with the Divine. If you have them available, gather your small handheld LED candles or lights for this week. They need to be small, so they can be cupped in the palms as if you're holding water, not grasped by the fingers as if you're picking up a pen. Covering your head with a veil or cap would augment your Sacred Dance Attire.

November 8: Connecting Thinking with a Grateful Heart

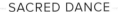

SACRED DANCE

Start facing east, as you have all year. Pull your elbows in at your waist, and cup your palms together. Raise your left palm to extend your arm just above your left ear as you extend your right arm away from your right hip. Palms are turned upward. Imagine you create a diagonal line from your left fingertips and your right fingertips, which traverses your torso. Hold your back strong so that you remain in the Sacred Dance Posture. Your gaze is toward your left palm. Now, using your shoulders so your arms remain straight with a slight curve, move both arms so that your right palm is upward and your left palm downward, away from your left hip. Alternate these four times on each side, keeping the palms facing upward so you won't drop the light and turning your head so your gaze follows the palm that is above your head. Return to center, standing with feet shoulder-width apart, knees slightly bent, with your palms cupped in front of your waist.

<hr>

MEDITATION AND PRACTICE

In ancient Persia, Zurvan was a neutral, omnipotent creator deity who solved cosmic conflicts between faith and doubt. Zurvan was the god of infinite time and space, existing before anything or anyone. Legends recount how Zurvan desired children or heirs to his creation, and, for a thousand years, he tried to manifest them. Toward the end of the period, Zurvan began to doubt whether he could bring them forth, and he felt depressed. But he realized his need to be whole and let go of his doubt; then, his two heirs, Ohrmuzd and Ahriman, were conceived.

A thankful heart connected to thinking is the ultimate way to connect mind, body, and Spirit. If we have a heart full of love and faith, and a head full of doubt, we're lost. We must let our hearts dominate until the brain can catch up. We must let the brain lose its lifelong, learned attachment to ego and self, which can feel like a thousand-year process. When the heart and mind are connected, though, decisions and choices are made from a basis of compassion. We can be thankful in our behaviors, which are driven by our thoughts and our hearts. We come from a place of fullness and share that fullness in our daily interactions.

November 9: Dancing into Right Thinking

<hr>

SACRED DANCE

Reach your right foot out and away from your body with the leg straight so that you touch the tip of your big toe to the floor. Your weight remains on your slightly bent standing left leg. Lift your left palm upward in a semicircle, as you circle your right palm inward toward your body and then outward away from the body toward the right. In this pose your right elbow and cupped palm, still holding the light, are both facing upward and away from your body. Bring the right palm back to center by rotating the wrist; as you do so, bring the right foot back to center. Knees are slightly bent. Now bring the left palm back through the semicircle so that you return to center with the palms cupped in front of you at your waist.

<hr/>

MEDITATION AND PRACTICE

Zurvan was, according to the ancient Persians, the center of the universe, the axis mundi. As the god of finite and infinite time, he was the ruler of all actions and interpreted them in relation to eternity. He danced sacredly with spiritual growth and maturity and led people away from decay.

When we want to think differently, it's sometimes easier to first act differently. We may have a goal of getting up at four in the morning for Sacred Dance Meditation. But we don't do it because it's dark outside, we didn't sleep well, or we doubt deep down that getting up early will make a difference. So, we lie in bed. The way to get out of this trap is through taking the body so the mind will follow. Dancing your way into right thinking is what that's called. It's impossible to decide about a theoretical situation. You must experience it. The same is true for thankful thinking. You must practice it. Take action to move yourself into a place where your thoughts focus on the positive. That means you must pay attention to your thoughts and replace any negative or less-than-pleasant thought with a positive one—but also utilize a sacred dance movement to help bring you to it.

November 10: Listening to Guidance

<hr/>

SACRED DANCE

Review and then repeat November 9's sacred dance movements, on the left and then right side. Alternate this portion of the dance eight times, four on each side. When you have completed the repetitions, return to center with the palms just at your waist, facing upward. Repeat this a few times until it comes naturally to you.

Because Zurvan controlled infinite time, his sacred dance took place across infinite realms of space, wisdom, and power. That produced an unlimited potentiality of giving life to contingent beings, those that could give rise to different outcomes.

We must know ourselves and our Higher Power to access the space of wisdom and power. When we seek guidance about having a thankful heart or taking an action based on gratitude, in relation to the whole of the Universe, there is the opportunity to recognize multiplicity. We have unlimited creative power inside, and manifesting is contingent upon first asking and then hearing and acting on Divine direction provided. The outcomes we manifest might have occurred differently if we acted differently or accessed guidance in a timelier fashion or in a different manner. Therefore, it's critical to be very careful about what the heart and head focus on, what we say, and what we do. You can get to a point where your Inner Mystic Dancer is leading all the time and is in constant communication, receiving Divine guidance. But getting there requires that you listen carefully all the time. In other words, at no time should you be checked out from your Higher Self.

November 11: Using Affirmations to Develop Good Thoughts

Reach up with the right palm facing upward and then away from your body to the right, and as you do so twist the palm and reach behind your head so that the palm now is above your crown chakra with the palm facing the sky, your light still in your palm. Much of this movement is in the shoulder so that you don't drop the light. Bring the left palm forward first, away from your body at the waist level, then circle it away from your body to the left, then circle the upward-facing palm inward toward the left waist and then move the arm to allow the upward-facing palm to rest just at the small of your spine, near Kundalini. Keep the light cupped in the left hand. Now, place the right foot just behind the left heel and with a step on the right, step on the left sort of rhythm, turn in a clockwise direction four breaths.

<hr>

MEDITATION AND PRACTICE

As god of finite time, Zurvan was known to provide strength, stamina, and energy and facilitated positive change. These were key aspects connecting Sacred Dance Meditation thinking with actions. He created positive contingent beings that facilitated forward motion for their lives. During finite time, these made for communities of people who danced with good thoughts. They therefore contributed to formation of positive infinite time, over the course of which people matured into certainty of connection with their Higher Power.

Affirmations are phrases and movements we repeat to ourselves. They are usually important in reprogramming or rewiring our reactions, particularly negative ones.

Consider a driver who disrespects someone in another car because of what feels like a delay from sitting in traffic. The driver may yell or think up some negative outcome. Though that driver can't be heard in the next car, the driver hears his or her own yelling. That creates negative energies in the spaces. It reinforces the behavior of impatience. And conjuring negative outcomes causes stress, which produces negative energy in the body and mind.

Rather than being irritated with another driver and imagining catastrophes, you can affirm that there's enough time, space, and resource to get where you're going and that people will understand if there is a delay in arriving. The energy will be at least neutral. So, you want to use affirmations to develop thoughts that will serve you and others. In the situation with the driver, it's easy to just remember that time is irrelevant to Spirit; it is a human construct. You are not controlled by it, and, in fact, you can stop time.

If you have the inclination, please write down some affirmations that you can use to develop good thoughts. They can be simple, such as "I have compassion for myself and others." "I believe I am Divinely directed." "I'm guided by Divine thought." "My thoughts create warmth and love." "I believe in humanity's creativity." "I know all is in Divine order." Once you have some written down, memorize one to use for today. Then memorize a few more so you can pull from them when your thinking challenges your faith.

November 12: Thinking and Gratitude

SACRED DANCE

Review and repeat the choreography given on November 11. After doing so, bring the left palm cupped and facing upward in toward your waist, circle it out away from your body on the left, and bring it to your waist. Circle your right palm gently behind your head and bring the right upward-facing palm to your waist. Stand with knees slightly bent.

MEDITATION AND PRACTICE

Zurvan was associated with Atar, the god of fire. The ancient Iranians didn't cast images of their deities or build temples. Instead they worshipped in the open at festivals and ceremonies, or *yasnas*. Sacred dance and worship were integral to frequent yasnas. Their purpose was to allow people to commune with the Divine for an outcome, for general well-being, or to show gratitude and piousness.

Sometimes it seems that human nature is to find fault and complain. Focusing on what's wrong or how we weren't treated fairly and then recounting the incidents in our heads contributes to negativity and lack. It also produces unproductive anger, which causes stress, grief, and sadness in our bodies. Collectively, we create angry communities if we all follow human nature. In a world where we are so focused on the negative—though it's not healthy or appropriate to ignore or accept poor treatment—sometimes we get what we expect.

So, expect good, and focus your thinking on what you can be grateful for. Just hold it in the front of your mind, along with your affirmation. Make a commitment to yourself that you will do that for thirty days and see how your energy changes and see if you attract new responses from people. Practice thinking and speaking only gratitude, even if you have an actual reason to complain or criticize. Write the date in your journal, and put a notation on your calendar for the conclusion of thirty days. Each time you find yourself criticizing or complaining about someone, something, or a situation, just switch your thinking and speaking to something you're grateful for. Since you've been writing down your gratitude lists, you can select one of those items or find a new one.

November 13: Giving as Receiving

SACRED DANCE

Today you'll bring all elements of the sacred dance together and practice. You might do a few swirls that you create, and then feel the dance in your body, as you try to do each week. Make the dance as much yours as you can.

MEDITATION AND PRACTICE

In ancient Iran, Atar acted as an intermediary; he represented fire, which was considered a sacred element. Burned offerings did not exist at that time. Even outside of yasnas, fire was always treated with utmost care as a sacred element and, above all, was never permitted to go out. Underpinning this relationship with fire was the idea that time understood action and over time people came closer to their deity.

At a few places around the world, this time of year is full of gift-giving, preceded by or in conjunction with reflection on deeds and accomplishments. So much of what we hear is about how the giver receives many blessings from the act of giving, which was discussed in April's entries.

Receiving is being in the state of mind and body where you can accept someone's appreciation of you. You give the giver that satisfaction by thankfully receiving the offering. You probably know people who receive a material gift and discount it—it's too much or too expensive—or criticize it—it's not good enough. And it's true that some gifts are given with strings attached, which you're free to reject—for example, if someone decides to give your children a puppy or if you get a large piece of jewelry with an implication attached to it. But otherwise, receive material gifts graciously without the unspoken expectation of having to reciprocate or commit to something. Do you have any hesitation in receiving material gifts?

November 14: Your Thinking Heart

SACRED DANCE

Let's trance this sacred dance out today.

MEDITATION AND PRACTICE

Ancient Persians believed that Spirit guided the mind-body and gave it consciousness. They also believed the world was guided by a world Spirit, comprised of a collective consciousness.

Yesterday's discussion centered on material gifts and being a gracious receiver. But what of nonmaterial gifts? Are you gracious when a soft, kind word is spoken to you from a partner or friend given in recognition of a contribution to a project, or offered about your attire or new glasses? Do you readily receive these gifts? Or do you dismiss them with a wave of your hand? Notice how you receive these gifts, and give the giver your gift of acceptance. And perhaps you can find ways to give at least one nonmaterial gift each day to someone, to practice your heartfelt thinking. The world would be transformed if everyone did that.

※ ※ ※

NOVEMBER 15–21
Thoughts and Deeds
Change Perceptions (Entry Point)

Seeing What We Want to See

In strength we can see reality, and we create reality in what we do.

November 15: Thoughts, Words, Deeds Create Us

SACRED DANCE

Begin standing with your fingertips touching, arms held down in front of your body, with the palms facing upward just below your navel. Breathe for a few beats, and, with your right foot leading, step clockwise to the right to complete a circle in four steps. Next, breathe, slightly bend your knees, and then step counterclockwise. Breathe, and slightly bend your knees when you return to center, holding the position with your fingertips and arms.

MEDITATION AND PRACTICE

Ritual or spiritual dancers in ancient Persia were called dervishes. Men were the only ones who could engage in sacred dances, which were referred to as *sama* and *dhikr*. Sama was the spiritual Practice of listening to and achieving unity with the Divine. Dhikr were mantras and prayers repeated and vibrated in the mind-body. With dhikr, people used prayer beads and often recited names of gods. Sama, performed while reciting mantras and using prayer beads, was a mystical journey. The dervish deliberately sought to hear the truth and endeavored to change himself through self-compassion and love. To do this, he had to let go of self. When he returned from this spiritual journey, he was changed a little. He expressed gratitude for his spiritual connection to the Divine each time he entered the dance.

We already know that the Practice of Sacred Dance Meditation changes us. We also know that we can re-create ourselves by our thoughts, what we dwell on, and what we do. It's difficult to set aside the ego, prioritize being in communication with the Divine, and be self-compassionate when we fall short. We are taught so much of the opposite that we need to ask ourselves what we are doing, saying, and thinking. But most important, we must ask ourselves why. So much fear surrounds letting go of the self as defined by social structures that doing so requires gradual change, with small moments of listening and repeating mantras that gradually dominate our lives. In this way, our actions align with a higher purpose, and we can let ourselves truly believe we are not influenced by what other people need us to be.

November 16: Energy

SACRED DANCE

Start facing the center with your fingertips touching. Repeat the two turns to the right and left, adding in the knee bends as you return to the center, as instructed for November 15. Now, as you step to the right for the clockwise turn, you circle your right arm out and away from your body and hold your upward-facing palm out in front of you. With the next step on your left to continue the clockwise turn, bring your left arm over your head, palm facing downward. With the next step on the right to continue the clockwise turn, bring your left palm to meet your right with the fingertips touching, arms held slightly away from your body just below your navel.

MEDITATION AND PRACTICE

Sama was a means of meditating on G-d through sacred music that accompanied sacred dancing. It brought out the love of G-d, purified the Soul, and was a way of becoming one with G-d. This Practice allowed all of one's doubt about devotion and place in the world to be eliminated. The Soul and Spirit communicated directly with G-d, through a trancelike state where one whirled off the self and only allowed the Spirit to indwell and take center stage of one's life.

We can all create a daily ceremony aimed at achieving oneness with G-d. Looking at ancient Persians; we can learn from them to bring the energy needed to our daily Practice. We can also prioritize our lives so that we have the energy and time to spend with G-d and to be grateful for another opportunity to do so. After meeting with the Higher Power every day and letting ourselves be healed by the compassion coming to us, we get to the point where we really love the time spent and it's difficult to pull ourselves away. But the key is to take the love of the Divine with us to show others the way.

November 17: Habits Broken

SACRED DANCE

Review the dance choreography from the prior days this week, and repeat it. Picking up where you left off on November 16, now step on the left to complete a counterclockwise turn, and hold the fingertips so they are just touching. Bend your knees slightly, and take a breath after concluding the turn. Repeat on the right. Don't worry about perfection. The idea is to step around in a circle and move the arms as you do so. Repeat clockwise and then counterclockwise turn, four times.

MEDITATION AND PRACTICE

According to lore, dervishes turned down money and material comforts and only sought the unconditional love from being with their Higher Power. Importantly, they transmitted that love to the earth and the people on it, hoping to help accelerate a global level of enlightenment. They were human beings born into the world just like you and me, complete with distractions of all kinds and paths leading to all sorts of places. Yet they learned to turn away from the world, to break habits of self-aggrandizement and delusion, and instead practiced connecting their inner most Selves with the love of the Unseen.

We too need to break habits, learn new ways of being, and practice a focus and presence in the here and now—although we don't have to be paupers. The most difficult habits to break are those we aren't aware of and engage in automatically. It's difficult to remain open, inviting, and accepting of love when we have these habits. Little by little we can break automatic responses by thinking through responses and taking our time. With practice we can look immediately at our thoughts and options, dismiss those that aren't supporting, and apply an internal love to them upon letting them go. Eventually they no longer arise.

November 18: New Practices Established

SACRED DANCE

Review and repeat what was given on November 17, and speed up your turns as you get more comfortable. Think about the energy field you're creating along your spine and with your sweeping arms. Return to center, and place your palms facing up, middle fingers touching just below your navel. Take eight breaths.

MEDITATION AND PRACTICE

Ancient dervish sacred dancers raised their right palm to the heavens to receive god's blessings, which were transmitted through their bodies and into earth through the left hand pointing to the ground.

While they danced sacredly in their trance, they moved between the Universe of the Ethers and the concretized earth, becoming a conduit for divine blessings.

We must stop thinking me, me, me, and think we, we, we. For Westerners, this can feel like an impossible task since we're socialized to think only of self, winning, being first, competing, getting a lot, giving little, and so on. Many of us have been broken by this kind of socialization, as we constantly believe we don't measure up, or we feel like we are imposters in our own skins. We must change our focus to thankfulness, being in the present, and realizing we have a limited time on earth. We may not have been taught what we needed to learn, but we can learn now, go in the right direction, and come from a place of love and self-compassion in all our choices. Or if we have been going in a direction that we believed would lead us to a more fulfilled state, we can begin anew. We can always begin, change our course, and deepen our Practice when new information is provided. This breaks the cycle of going through motions without awareness and shows others they can do the same. We are never finished with refining our Practice.

November 19: Self-Perception Changes

———————————— SACRED DANCE ————————————

Lift the right leg, and place it well behind the left leg, while bending the left leg as if in a lunge. Swing the left arm across your body, and hold it there, while the right arm reaches behind you, palms are facing up. Hold the position for two breaths. Return to the center position, and hold that for two breaths. Repeat on the left. Hold for two breaths. Repeat four times on each side. Then bring the arms down, and allow the fingertips to touch, with palms facing upward, just below your navel. Breathe for a few beats. Then step to the right with your arm moving overhead, move clockwise to complete a full turn, and then step on the left to make a full counterclockwise turn. Bend your knees between each turn and bring the fingertips to touch just below your navel with each knee bend. Repeat this four times on the right and left. Conclude the sacred dance by bringing your fingertips together just below your navel.

MEDITATION AND PRACTICE

One of the ways that the ancient dervishes established themselves as followers of the Divine was by the evidence of the way they changed. As they danced, they removed aspects of their clothing to signal their progression from being self-oriented to being oriented toward love and egolessness, gracefully tossing aside that which no longer served their sacred dance.

Others can often see changes in yourself before you do. You can notice changes in your self-perception by realizing how much effort you put into focusing on your mantras, remaining calm in difficult or challenging conversations, or standing firmly but compassionately when you silence the inappropriate but habitual consumption voices inside your head. When you no longer give in to eating or drinking something that doesn't serve you or have any harsh voice telling you that you don't measure up, that marks a change in your self-perception. Generally, advances like this move you to a new plateau from which you won't regress.

November 20: Removal of Archetypes

SACRED DANCE

Practice and improvise the sacred dance given this week, bringing it fully into your body as yours. If you haven't done so already, memorize the choreography so that you're able to engage with the dance without referring to notes or the video.

MEDITATION AND PRACTICE

Led by a master sacred dancer, a group of dervishes entered communion with the Divine by first reciting prayers and then transitioning to Sacred Dance Meditation. Musicians played melodies that catalyzed the dancer's desire for mystic union. Each dance progressed through stating or dancing one's knowledge of the Higher Power, then imagining seeing the Creator. As the sacred dancer drew deeper into the trance, the union with the Higher Power became clear. Their self-image was transformed through the union, the power of the sacred dance, and the act of seeking full death of the self. Dervishes were trying to divest themselves of their archetypal patterns so they could commune with the Divine without filters. Psychologist Carl Gustav Jung and others believed that universal archetypes drive our perceptions and experiences.

While we have many pieces and parts moving around in us at one time, one archetype tends to lead. Sometimes archetypes get in the way of coming close to our Higher Self and remaining there. The idea is to stop acting automatically from archetypal patterns. We need to first acknowledge their existence and identify those aspects that keep us in patterns that don't serve our spiritual growth. What do you think your driving archetypes are? How are they hindering or helping you? Which would you like to change or move toward? Aim to remove your automatic and *unawakened* identification with archetypes that harm you or hold you back, or use the positive aspects of those archetypes to propel you.

November 21: Re-Creating from the Inside Out

SACRED DANCE

Trance the sacred dance today; improvise and move freely around your Sacred Dance Studio.

MEDITATION AND PRACTICE

Dervishes wanted to be closer to their Creator through sacred dance and sought reunion with their Higher Self through death of the lower self. To do this they re-created themselves slowly from the inside out.

Archetypes are everywhere, and they form who we are, individually and collectively. They are guiding, inspiring, possessing, ruling, and living through us each day. The statistics say that almost one hundred percent of our behavior is automatically driven by these archetypes. So, their influence is a given. It's a matter of what degree we will continue to allow them to have full rein. In this regard, we learn from the dervishes who sought to destroy them by their sacred dance.

To the extent you're aware of the archetypes operating within you gives you an idea of your level of spiritual awareness. Being awake and present in all situations allows you to change from reacting to responding from a place of connectedness. Like dervishes, you acknowledge the difficulty of this kind of personal re-creation. Yet, the change from the inside out is worth the effort. Make some notes in your journal about how you feel about this kind of spiritual work and which archetype is speaking to you the loudest.

※ ※ ※

NOVEMBER 22–30
Gratitude and Appreciation as Practice (Entry Point)

Character Development

Our essence precedes us, through Divine guidance.

For this week, you can wear your Sacred Dance Attire with a loose-fitting sheath on top of it and wear a head covering. If you're inclined, use some sacred flute music to ignite the soothing energy and connect with it. The usual east-facing beginning will be in place for each day, and each day will begin with the same movements. The sacred dance is meant to establish a deeper spiritual Practice that sits between you, your feelings and thoughts of gratitude, and your Higher Self.

November 22: Keeping the Practice of Watching Thinking

SACRED DANCE

Glide the palms up as you're pressing air away from you until the arms are up over the head, with the back of the wrists touching and elbows slightly bent. That is, in four slow pulses, press the palms away. Slowly bring the palms to your center with the wrists leading, right crossing in front of left, again with four waving pulses. Repeat this sequence, four times, alternating the right and left wrists crossing in front.

MEDITATION AND PRACTICE

A sacred caste of priests, the Magi, from the tribes of the Medes, led people to wholeness in ancient Persia. The Magi held sacred rites and ceremonies for the community, which included sacred Persian dance. In their position as priests, they mediated between the Supreme Being and the people. They were interpreters of omens and dreams and were the authorities for all religious matters. Beginning from the end of the 6th century BCE, the Magi functioned as official priests at all public and private services in Persia and its surrounding countries. They watched over the citizens and the leaders and foretold the future. Many people were very gracious in the presence of the Magi.

Though we are in the time of thanks around many areas of the world during this period of the year, the aim is to always be in touch with gratitude and appreciation. Good deeds embolden us to our higher purpose of creativity and uniting with the Higher Power. Every act of selflessness done with a thankful heart assists our Souls to move along the way, and it allows us to assist others.

November 23: Predicting the Future

SACRED DANCE

Glide the palms up in front of you as if you're pressing air away from you, and bring the back of the wrists together; elbows are bent, and knees are slightly bent. Lean the torso to the left and then to the right, and repeat that four times, alternating in each direction. Let your head and neck relax and move with your flow. Your lean is slow and deliberate, and you feel the air on your face, breathing deliberately with each shift of direction. Lean as far as you're comfortable. Bring the palms to your center with the wrists leading, right crossing in front of left.

MEDITATION AND PRACTICE

The ancient Persian Magi were known to have exceptional and extraordinary spiritual knowledge. As part of their Practice, the Magi developed and relied upon planetary and star movements and formations. Their abilities to predict the future were discussed throughout the known world, including the far reaches of Babylon. People sought the words of the Magi to help them make decisions, from determining where to live to whether to marry or when to embark on a journey.

Astronomy looks at what the stars and planets do, and astrology reviews the ways in which the planets and stars align to bring about actions. We can try our best to predict the future using a horoscope or other means. The most important thing we can do is to try to understand how we influence forces to bring about the future. In gratitude we can think about how the future might look for us and what we do each day to manifest it. However, no one can really know what the future holds, so it's best to be grateful for the day that we have.

November 24: Let Your Acts Be Yours

SACRED DANCE

Repeat the directions as given on November 23.

MEDITATION AND PRACTICE

The ancient Persian Magi accurately recorded the times of the motion of the stars. They documented the passage of the sun through twelve constellations, each constellation covering a thirty-degree section of the circular pathway that the sun forms. The Magi casted horoscopes based on the position of the planets and stars at the moment of one's birth. People came to the Magi to understand the nature of the child they were going to have.

The zodiac maps the heavens, and one's birth sign is derived from a specific location of the Earth during birth, based on where one was born. The positions of the planets are placed on a chart, with calculated factors such as the lunar nodes, the house cusps, other zodiac signs, and star positions. Angular relationships between the planets and other points, or aspects, are also located. The idea is that the placement of the stars at the time of birth reveals the person's strengths and weaknesses, driving motivations, and influencing aspects of elements.

Some have heard personal descriptions through zodiac study. If you'd like to get a reading and a zodiac birth chart, you can locate an astrologer through an internet search. After you've completed it, see which aspects of the report resonate with you!

We hear about our compatibility with other people based on their birth chart relative to ours. There is really something wonderful about this. Yet we must be careful that we aren't living to an expected way of being based on our birth sign.

November 25: Consider Being Viral on Social Media

SACRED DANCE

Repeat the dance as presented on November 23 up to and including leaning the torso. Turn counterclockwise, keeping your wrists together over your head. Bring the palms to your center with the wrists leading, right crossing in front of left.

MEDITATION AND PRACTICE

For the Magi, astrology included divination, determining celestial omens, and seeing the gods in the celestial formation of planets and stars. Relating celestial phenomena to human movements was based on the idea that what happened above the earth gave rise to outcomes. News of births and omens traveled by word of mouth throughout the community, and over time news reached the outlying countries, reported by travelers and messengers.

The old "newspaper test" is to ask yourself if you would be okay if any of your actions were reported in the newspaper. Nowadays the question is "How would you feel if your actions were posted and went viral on social media around the globe, instantly?" With hidden cameras and all sorts of tracking mechanisms, you can't be sure who's watching or listening. Awareness of how social media can make or break lives tends to mitigate negative acts. But negative motivations don't usually drive your behavior. Furthermore, some people might misinterpret even compassionate behavior or events that you celebrate, and they could post unsavory comments. Would you want a positive act to go viral on social media? How would you handle that? Make some notes in your journal about your feelings.

November 26: Parting Words Prose or Poem

SACRED DANCE

Repeat the dance as presented on November 23 up to and including leaning the torso. Turn clockwise. Bring the palms to your center with the wrists leading, left crossing in front of right.

MEDITATION AND PRACTICE

The Magi supposedly developed the zodiac, which is an area of the sky "extending 9 degrees on either side of the ecliptic, the plane of the earth's orbit and of the sun's apparent annual path. The orbits of the moon and of the principal planets also lie entirely within the zodiac."* The zodiac is divided into twelve signs corresponding to the constellations.

The Magi were called on not only for creating birth charts and developing astrological forecasts but also for divining the time and cause of death. From no birth chart or other reading from the stars can anyone know our time of death or that of others; thus, the basis for many religions is to prepare us for the unknown.

---

* *Encyclopaedia Britannica Online*, s.v. "Zodiac," accessed July 2, 2020, https://www.britannica.com/topic/zodiac.

We don't know why we are here. We can maybe guess or have someone surmise we will die within a certain period if illness has set in, or we can conjecture about why we have a human life or how many we may have. But we ultimately and eventually recall that we are immortal and determine to live fully. By not being afraid of death because we live in each moment, we can zero in on what we want our lives to create and how we express gratitude for it.

If you consider life as a gift or an opportunity to evolve and help others, what would you like for people to remember you by? What would you like people to say about you after you're moved on from earthly existence? How did you make the world a better place? Using these prompts, craft a couple paragraphs of prose, or a poem if you're a poet, and place it in a safe location you can easily refer to.

November 27: Teaching Others by Influence

SACRED DANCE

Glide the palms up as you're pressing air away from you, until the arms are up over the head, with the back of the wrists touching; elbows are slightly bent. In four slow pulses, press the palms away. Slowly bring the palms to your center with the wrists leading, right crossing in front of left. Repeat this sequence, four times, alternating the right and left wrists crossing in front. Glide the palms up in front of you again as if you're pressing air away from you and bring the back of the wrists together; elbows are bent, and knees are slightly bent. Lean the torso to the left and then to the right, and repeat four times, alternating in each direction. Let your head and neck relax and move with your flow. Your lean is slow and deliberate, and you feel the air on your face, breathing deliberately with each shift of direction. Lean as far as you're comfortable. Bring the palms to your center with the wrists leading, right crossing in front of left.

MEDITATION AND PRACTICE

The Greek word *magoi* was translated as "wise men," but this wasn't accurate. The word was closely translated as astrologer or priest. The Magi existed before the time of Zoroaster and the establishment of his Practices. Magi were known in the ancient world for not only interpreting celestial bodies and movements of the stars but as well for holding sacred dance ceremonies marking significant moments. They were said to be the men who visited Bethlehem to witness the arrival of a spiritual wonder, following the brightest star in the night sky. In any event, the Magi of ancient Persian Iran influenced the development of stories we hear in Judaism and Christianity.

What we do influences those who watch us, for better or for worse. Although no one is perfect, we nevertheless need to realize that we are role models to everyone. We can teach people how to be and how not to be. Practicing love and acting in alignment with how we'd want to be known can speak volumes to others. In our own way, we are the priests that others look to.

November 28: Anger Not Arising

SACRED DANCE

Perform the same motion with your palms, bringing the wrists together over your head. Lean the torso to the left and then to the right, keeping your arms over your head. Repeat four times, alternating the leaning in each direction. Let your head and neck relax and move with your flow. Your lean is slow and deliberate, and you feel the air on your face, breathing deliberately with each shift of direction. Lean as far as you're comfortable. Bring the palms to your center with the wrists leading, right crossing in front of left. Glide the palms up in front of you again as if you're pressing air away from you, and bring the back of the wrists together, with elbows bent and knees slightly bent. Lean the torso to the left and then to the right. Repeat four times, alternating the position of the crossing wrists. Turn counterclockwise, keeping your wrists together over your head. Bring the palms to your center with the wrists leading, right crossing in front of left.

MEDITATION AND PRACTICE

The Magi's divination played an important role in shaping sacred dance. The Magi helped people understand what would or might happen and showed them how their acts could influence it. With changes in empires and leaders, angry disputes broke out at court and within the community, as well as within families. The Magi played a significant role when mediating between the Divine and the people. Nevertheless, people had free will and exercised it, perhaps even ignoring the prophetic words of the Magi.

It's good not to be caught up in anger when it arises around you. Better is to be at a place where there is no anger but only compassion. Dealing with anger requires wisdom and selflessness, along with understanding that all is impermanent. Clearly stating your purpose and working within it helps to keep anger from taking hold. Anger, after all, is the final emotional position, stemming from attachment and ego. When you do feel anger, identify the source, and replace it with love. Anger only hurts you. When you notice any anger arising today, even just an inkling, please make a note of it in your journal.

November 29: Gratitude through the Mind-Body

SACRED DANCE

Review and repeat the sequence given this week, and memorize the movements. Let it live in your body, and find ways to improvise.

MEDITATION AND PRACTICE

The Magi were there to help people avoid negativity and to focus on the positive. They helped people to discern right courses of action.

What are your motives for speaking, acting, or doing? Do your best to answer before doing anything.

In many cases we must set aside the thinking mind and use the third eye and our Inner Mystic Dancer to help us. First, we must practice gratitude for the opportunity to act. Next, we need to think about the impact of our actions on all involved. Third, we must try to "divine" the impact on all concerned, looking at the outcomes from many perspectives. We must feel it in our bodies and work it through in Sacred Dance Meditation. Over time, this kind of contemplation becomes second nature. And we are thankful that we don't just consider what we want, but what is good for the whole.

November 30: Appreciation and Gratitude as Guidance

SACRED DANCE

Find your way into the trance state of the Sacred Dance Meditation today. Improvise, and feel it in your entire mind-body.

MEDITATION AND PRACTICE

During the ancient Persian Empire, the Magi were considered deeply profound, learned, and pious. There was only respect for them. The Magi were diligent in their thoughts, words, and deeds. They channeled Spirit within their mind-bodies.

We can hear the voice of the Creator in our mind-body if we will silence the other superfluous chatter we hear all day, every day, and if we let go of dogma that drives our thinking and acting. Yet, we are always well served to seek guidance from our trusted advisors. We should be aware that their guidance is a gift and show appreciation.

Write names of your trusted advisors in your journal. If you don't have any trusted advisors, you might want to begin to create a community of people you can turn to and share yourself with them. In this way you can also help them to advance on their spiritual path.

DECEMBER

We Are Light Beings

SACRED DANCE MEDITATION IN PERSONAL RETREAT

This month, the Season of Light is the theme, and you'll draw on some of the Sacred Dance Meditations studied over the time of your practicing. This month helps you prepare for the coming year and dance sacredly in reflection of your spiritual growth. The Sacred Dance Meditations will be incorporated into your returning to your ideas and plans, as this month provides four personal retreats that you engage with from your own home, or on a personal retreat site of your choosing.

Sacred dancers, you're encouraged to choreograph your own sacred dance movements, or you can select any of the ones covered throughout this year. Choreographing entails that you identify the moves you enjoy and bring them together in ways that allow you to feel free and embraced by Spirit, that allow you to live in divine communion with your entire mind-body. You may use music or not, as you wish, and if it resonates with the guidance you receive, you could retreat with another person whom you love and trust, and who will support you in your journey. It's also important that you support them in a very compassionate and equitable way.

The month is divided into three ten-day segments. If you have a spiritual affiliation, you may want to place the holiday dates on your calendar and, to the extent possible, incorporate the personal retreats so that they coincide with your Practices. During this month as in previous Sacred Dance Meditations, specific spiritual

Practices or traditions aren't identified or their rituals called out. But please do know that a tremendous amount of sameness is embodied in all these Practices, having descended from the root religion and being restatements or revisions of many shaman or other indigenous Sacred Dance Meditation Practices from eons ago.

Here are some of the themes and plans you may revisit to support the structure of the personal retreats, which you may recall from your Practice:

- Sacred Body Mandalas (June)
- Sacred Dance Mantras (September)
- Epiphanies (July)
- Being a Mystic (January)
- Harvesting Spirit (August)
- Creativity Plan (October)
- Provoking Spiritual Experiences (February)
- Sacred Giving Plan (April)
- Sacred Laughter Plan (May)
- Spiritual Journey Maps (March)
- Sacred Play Plan (May)
- Parting Words Prose or Poetry (November)

It may be a good idea to review your plans, ideas, and anything else related to creating directions in your spiritual growth. You may decide to choose different Sacred Dance Attire, or you may use any that you've already selected. Be aware that this Season of Light is being observed this month across the globe in some form, even by those who abstain from formal celebrations.

The month is divided into three ten-day personal retreats, with a separate day for the winter solstice, without specific entries for each day. Guidance is given for three, ten-day periods, and you can change the order to suit any of your commitments. Keep a couple ideas in mind: A great deal of food consumption may happen during this period. Consider what and how much you'll eat of foods that don't serve the body but will allow you to participate in ceremonies and rituals. Second, notice when you're affected by the perceived need to hurry. Take time to breathe through those moments, and slow down. And third, if you have difficulty with this time of the year, you can easily think of December as any other month, when the sun shines, the moon rises, the season changes, and we all dance sacredly through them.

DECEMBER 1–10
The Days of Silence

Over the next ten days, the Days of Silence, you will set aside time for Sacred Dance Meditation for a few periods throughout each day, preferably at the same time, such as upon awakening or just before you eat a meal. The idea is to find a time that isn't taxing for you.

You'll want to set aside as much time as you need for the Reflection Periods. If you've been following this work for a while, please have your journal nearby. You may want a fresh, blank journal that you can use for these personal retreats.

As you dance through the next ten days, the goal is to be silent as often as possible. If you need to participate in sacred days or feasts during this time, that's fine. But every time you must say something, speak from Spirit and use as few words as possible. Otherwise, eliminate conversation without being impolite and disengage with television, radio, or any mass communication. Stay away from news media of any kind and the internet, email, etc., unless you must. Even then, set limits on when you will get online. Lastly, keep your participation in the Days of Silence between you and your Higher Power.

Select the Sacred Dance Meditations from January, February, and March to aid your retreat. During the ten days, reflect on what you've learned from your Shadow, and embrace your inner mysticism. Here is the schedule:

- Reflection Period for Day 1, 2, and 3—Review the four cardinal directions and above and below in finding your location; also review the use of the sacred elements. Consider how these affect your body, and meditate on them.

- Reflection Period for Day 4, 5, and 6—For the next three days, feel and live the body mandala concept as you engage in your sacred dance, as you move throughout your day. Recall the body mandala when you lay down for bed at night.

- Reflection Period for Day 7 and 8—Review what you have learned from your Shadow.

- Reflection Period for Day 9—Have you fully grown into a mystic?

- Reflection Period for Day 10—How many spiritual experiences have you provoked? What can you say about the use of sacred and spiritual altars in your home? Have you engaged in sacred geometry?

DECEMBER 11–20
The Days of Presence and Contemplation

We continue with the personal retreat portion for the month of December. Follow the general directions for December 1–10.

For the next ten days, the goal is to continuously consider the presence of your Higher Power and contemplate your relationship to the Divine. That is, realize how the relationship has grown or deepened. Select the Sacred Dance Meditations from April, May, June, and August to aid your retreat. Here is the schedule:

- Reflection Period for Day 11 and 12—How have you harvested your Spirit?

- Reflection Period for Day 13 and 14—What are sacred portals? In what ways have you noticed and then walked through sacred portals?

- Reflection Period for Day 15 and 16—Note what has occurred in your life from your sacred giving plan. How have you manifested abundance from it? What has changed in you as a result? How does it inform your giving during the Season of Light? How have you changed by adhering to your sacred laughter plan?

- Reflection Period for Day 17 and 18—Review your spiritual journey map. What has transpired for you over the time you've been engaging with Sacred Dance Meditation? What can you add to your spiritual journey map?

- Reflection Period for Day 19 and 20—Is there anything you need to bring into the Light? From the notes you made earlier, or any new awareness you had lately, what aspects of you, your beliefs, and your relationship to others exist that you would like to release? Prepare this on a separate document that you can bring to the Winter Solstice Ceremony.

- December 21: Celebrate and Acknowledge the Winter Solstice.

Set up a fragrance bowl, large and visible in your home. Choose citrus, rose, eucalyptus, camphor, or whatever you have available, or what you can buy from your local market. Feel free to use essential oils and flowers too. Bless and charge the water. Ask the Universe to bless the scents and to remind you that you're dwelling amid powers greater than you who are here to aid your spiritual growth and make your journey fulfilling.

Today, select a Sacred Dance Meditation from the year that resonates with you. If you would prefer, you may choreograph a set of movements of your own. Determine what time of day the winter solstice will occur where you live. Invite people to celebrate with you, or go to a place where there will be celebrating.

Set aside time to acknowledge the moment when the day and night are the same length, and that next moment when we observe the Light. Wear Sacred Dance Attire if you have it, or claim as sacred whatever you will decide to wear; if possible, wear all white. If you're going in public, you can just wear something white that you have "charged" with Spirit.

Today, recall all the peoples of the ancient worlds who celebrate the winter solstice. Remember their efforts to build Medicine Wheels and pyramids to note the ways in which the planets moved and to be cognizant of the exact moment when the solstice occurred. Reflect on how amazing and wonderful it was that people in all and every cultural civilization celebrated and shared this remarkable moment.

Bring your notes from the reflection period of Day 19 and 20. Review them, and ask your Inner Mystic Dancer if all you need to be released is released. In a safe location where you will not cause a fire or trigger alarms, burn the paper containing your release.

Now, engage in your chosen Sacred Dance Meditation choreography, knowing that you have been moved onward into the Light with other beings who have gone before you and are surely coming behind you.

Using sacred vibrations of your gratitude, slowly pour the water out of your fragrance bowl. If you can, pour it outdoors into the soil.

❋ ❋ ❋

DECEMBER 22–31
Living in the Emergence of Light

The personal retreat for Living in the Emergence of Light helps you celebrate your divinity. You'll want to have as much light flowing into your space as possible for the next ten days, when you're awake. Continue to practice silence as you move forward over the next ten days. You can select Sacred Dance Meditations from July, September, and October to aid your retreat.

When you can, burn incense of your choice, but try to use natural resins. If you're able to do so, keep a fire burning in a fireplace, or you can even post a fireplace on your device if you would like. Light candles, and place them around your home or workspace, or use the LED kind. Light candles before your meals, and sit down to eat in peace and quiet. Continue sacred dancing at various points in your day.

Here are concepts covered in the last year that govern the next ten days of reflection as part of Living in the Emergence of Light:

- Reflection Period for Day 22 and 23—How has the use of spiritual altars and shrines aided you in recalling the acts of the Divine, as well as remembering you *are* the Divine with skin on? Also note what you have manifested because of acting upon your creativity plan.

- Reflection Period for Day 24 and 25—Have you had any epiphanies? What were they, and how did they help you or your community? What spiritual experiences were noteworthy for you?

- Reflection Period for Day 26 and 27—Who have you attracted to you by sowing seeds? By living good deeds? What kinds of disturbances have you experienced as a result? How have you reimagined yourself when gazing in a mirror?

- Reflection Period for Day 28 and 29—In your experience, how has truth or dharma helped you become more awakened?

- Reflection Period for Day 30 and 31—In what ways have you engaged in sacred play? Have you started taking yourself less seriously? How would this impact your draft of your parting words of prose or poetry? Before the end of the evening, quietly reflect.

As you move into the coming days, ease carefully into talking with people, and remember that you dance sacredly in the Light. Choose what to eat and give. Make certain that you remain connected to your Source, and vow to sacredly dance each day of your life. Also continue using the Practices of Being Awake in Your Mind-Body so that you can refine and realize all your intentions for the good of all for this life.

REFERENCES AND
FURTHER READING

Anwaruddin, Sardar M. "Emerson's Passion for Indian Thought." *International Journal of Literature and Arts* 1, no. 1 (2013): 1–6.

Arguelles, José, and Valum Votan. *Stopping Time 2.0: A Thirteen Moon Primer*. Edited by Stephanie South. Ashland, OR: Law of Time Press. https://lawoftime.org/wp-content/uploads/2016/10/StoppingTime2.0.pdf?dl=1.

Australian Institute of Parapsychological Research. "Psychic and Mystical Experiences of the Aborigines." AIPR. 2016. Accessed September 13, 2019. https://www.aiprinc.org/aboriginal/.

Aveni, Anthony F., Horst Härtung, and B. Buckingham. "The Pecked Cross Symbol in Ancient Mesoamerica." *Science* 202 (1978): 267–279.

Bresnan, Patrick. *Awakening: An Introduction to the History of Eastern Thought*. 4th ed. New York: Pearson Higher Education, 2009.

Bailey, Joseph A. "Yin/Yang Originated in Africa." Black Voice News. February 14, 2005. Accessed September 13, 2019. http://www.blackvoicenews.com/2005/02/14/yinyang-originated-in-africa/.

Caretta, M. Nicolás, and Achim Lelgemann. "Cross Circles: A Case of Northern Mexico." *Adoranten* (2011): 1–9. https://www.academia.edu/1778646/Cross_Circles_A_case_of_Northern_Mexico.

Cooper, Rabbi David A. *God Is a Verb: Kabbalah and the Practice of Mystical Judaism*. New York: Riverhead Books, an imprint of Penguin, 1997.

DeSilva, Freddy, dir. *Temple Making*. 2008; Awaken Productions. DVD Disc.

Díaz-Andreu, M. "Iberian Post-Palaeolithic Art and Gender: Discussing Human Representations in Levantine Art." *Journal of Iberian Archaeology* 1 (1998): 33–51.

Donnelly, Ignatius. *Atlantis: The Antediluvian World*. Mineola, NY: Dover Publications, 2011. First published 1882 by Harper.

Fillmore, Charles, and Cora Dedrick Fillmore. *The Twelve Powers*. Unity Village, MO: Unity Books, 2012. First published 1930 by Unity School of

Christianity. http://newthoughtlibrary.com/fillmoreCharles/TheTwelve-PowersOfMan/pages/twelve-powers-of-man-001.htm.

Gallagher, Shaun. *How the Body Shapes the Mind*. New York: Oxford University Press, 2006.

Garcia, Santiago Andres. "Early Representations of Mesoamerica's Feathered Serpent: Power, Identity, and the Spread of a Cult." Masters thesis, California State University, Fullerton, 2011.

Garcia, Ismael Arturo Montero. "Notes about Alta Vista in Chalchihuites Zacatecas." *Revista Mexicana de Astronomía y Astrofísica* 47 (2016): 37–50.

Georgios, Lykesas, Christina Papaioannou, Dania Aspasia, Maria Koutsuba, and Nikolaki Evgenia. "The Presence of Dance in Female Deities of the Greek Antiquity." *Mediterranean Journal of Social Sciences* 8, no. 2 (March 2017): 161–170.

Gillespie, Susan D. "Body and Soul among the Maya: Keeping the Spirits in Place." *Archaeological Papers of the American Anthropological Association* 11, no. 1 (January 2002): 67–78. https://doi.org/10.1525/ap3a.2002.11.1.67.

Harrison-Buck, Eleanor. "Maya Religion and Gods: Relevance and Relatedness in the Animic Cosmos." In *Tracing the Relational: The Archaeology of Worlds, Spirits, and Temporalities*, edited by M. E. Buchanan and B. J. Skousen, 113–127. Salt Lake City: University of Utah Press, 2015.

Haysom, Matthew. "The Double-Axe: A Contextual Approach to the Understanding of a Cretan Symbol in the Neopalatial Period." *Oxford Journal of Archeology* 29, no. 1 (January 2010): 35–55.

Hunt, Yvonne. "Traditional Dance in Greece." *The Anthropology of East Europe Review* 22, no. 1 (2004): 139–143.

Idang, Gabriel E. "African Culture and Values." *Phronimon* 16, no. 2 (2015): 97–111.

Kappelman, Julia Guernsey. "Sacred Geography at Izapa and the Performance of Rulership." In *Space, Power, and Poetics in Ancient Mesoamerica*, edited by Rex Koontz, Kathryn Reese-Taylor, and Annabeth Headrick, 83–102. Boulder, CO: Westview Press, 2001.

Kelbessa, Workineh. *Traditional Oromo Attitudes Towards the Environment: An Argument for Environmentally Sound Development*. Addis Ababa, Ethiopia: Organization for Social Science Research in Eastern and Southern Africa, 2001.

Koontz, Rex, Kathryn Reese-Taylor, and Annabeth Headrick, eds. *Space, Power, and Poetics in Ancient Mesoamerica*. Boulder, CO: Westview Press, 2001.

Lang, Curtis J., and Jane Sherry. "The Structure and Sacred Geometry of Quartz Crystals." Chap. 6 in *Spirits of Stone*. https://www.satyacenter.com/spirits-of-stone/chapter6-structure-and-sacred-geometry-of-quartz-crystals. Accessed September 13, 2019.

Levy, Fran J. *Dance and Other Expressive Art Therapies: When Words Are Not Enough*. New York: Routledge, 1995.

Looper, Matthew G. "Dance Performance at Quirigua." In *Space, Power, and Poetics in Ancient Mesoamerica*, edited by Rex Koontz, Kathryn Reese-Taylor, and Annabeth Headrick, 113–126. Boulder, CO: Westview Press, 2001.

Maron, Miriam. "The Healing Power of Sacred Dance." *Tikkun* 25, no. 2 (March/April 2010): 61.

Miller, Daniel. "Materiality: An Introduction." In *Materiality*, 1–50. Durham, NC: Duke University Press, 2005.

Morata Sáez, Javier, Juan Carlos, and Fernández Truan, "Physical Activities of the Iberos." *European Studies of Sports History* 2, no. 2 (Autumn 2009): 5–25.

Native Americans Online. "Sun Dance." https://www.native-americans-online.com/native-american-sun-dance.html. Accessed September 13, 2019.

Pearlman, Ellen. *Tibetan Sacred Dance: A Journey into the Religious and Folk Traditions*. Rochester, VT: Inner Traditions, 2002.

Pedersen, Traci. "Using Flowers to Enhance Chakra Energy Flow." *Spirituality & Health* (blog). https://spiritualityhealth.com/blogs/spirituality-health/2015/06/09/traci-pedersen-using-flowers-enhance-chakra-energy-flow#. Accessed June 12, 2020.

Penn Museum. "Revealing Masks." Accessed September 13, 2019. https://www.penn.museum/documents/education/penn-museum-africa.pdf.

Peterson, William. "Minangkabau Dance in West Sumatra: Tradition, Training and Tourism." *SPAFA Journal* 6, no. 1 (January-April, 1996): 5–12.

Queensland Government. "Aboriginal Ceremonies." Queensland Curriculum and Assessment Authority. Reviewed July 25, 2018. Accessed September 13, 2019. https://www.qcaa.qld.edu.au/about/k-12-policies/aboriginal-torres-strait-islander-perspectives/resources/aboriginal-ceremonies.

Regardie, Israel. *The Tree of Life: An Illustrated Study in Magic*, St. Paul, MN: Llewellyn Publications, 2001.

Rehak, Paul. "The 'Sphinx' Head from the Cult Center at Mycenae." In *Autochthon*. Papers Presented to O.T.P.K. Dickinson on the Occasion of His Retirement, edited by Anastasia Dakour-Hild and Susan Sherrat, 271–75. Oxford: British Archaeological Reports.

Sánchez, Edwin G. Mayoral, Francisco Laca Arocena, and Juan C. Mejía Ceballos. "Daily Spiritual Experience in Basques and Mexicans: A Quantitative Study." *Journal of Transpersonal Research* 2, no. 1 (2010): 10–25.

Shaw, Maria C. "The Lion Gate Relief at Mycenae Reconsidered." In *Archaeological Society of Athens, Greece*. Commemorative for Prof. G. Mylonas, 1986, 108–123. https://tspace.library.utoronto.ca/handle /1807/4306.

Simón, Francisco Marco. "Religion and Religious Practices of the Ancient Celts of the Iberian Peninsula." *e-Keltoi: Journal of Interdisciplinary Celtic Studies* 6, no. 6 (March 2005): 287–345. https://dc.uwm.edu/ ekeltoi/vol6/iss1/6/.

Stark, Alexander. "The Matrilineal System of the Minangkabau and Its Persistence Throughout History: A Structural Perspective." *Southeast Asia: A Multidisciplinary Journal* 13 (2013): 1–13.

Turaki, Yusufu. "Africa Traditional Religious System as Basis of Understanding Christian Spiritual Warfare." Lausanne Movement. Accessed September 13, 2019. https://www.lausanne.org/content/west-african-case -study?_sfm_wpcf-select-gathering=2000+Nairobi.

Wacks, David A. "Some Thoughts on Asturian Mythology." Lecture at the University of Oregon Osher Center for Lifelong Learning, Berkeley, CA, December 10, 2014. Accessed September 13, 2019. https://davidwacks .uoregon.edu/2014/12/12/asturian/.

Winton-Henry, Cynthia. *Dance—The Sacred Art: The Joy of Movement as a Spiritual Practice*. Nashville, TN: Skylight Paths Publishing, 2009.

INDEX

M

ABOUT THE AUTHOR

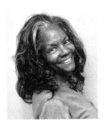 DR. CARLA STALLING WALTER writes about dance, spirituality, and well-being. Along with her doctorate, Dr. Walter holds certificates in Somatic Psychotherapy, Osteopathic Medicine, and Spiritual Counseling. She is the CEO and Founder of Dance in the Spirit, LLC. Her company provides personal and corporate retreats, classes, and workshops on Sacred Dance Meditation at locations around the globe. A practicing Zen Buddhist, she serves as a board member with the San Francisco Zen Center and is an active member of The Sacred Dance Guild. A native of Los Angeles, Walter lives in the San Francisco Bay Area.

About North Atlantic Books

North Atlantic Books (NAB) is an independent, nonprofit publisher committed to a bold exploration of the relationships between mind, body, spirit, and nature. Founded in 1974, NAB aims to nurture a holistic view of the arts, sciences, humanities, and healing. To make a donation or to learn more about our books, authors, events, and newsletter, please visit www.northatlanticbooks.com.

North Atlantic Books is the publishing arm of the Society for the Study of Native Arts and Sciences, a 501(c)(3) nonprofit educational organization that promotes cross-cultural perspectives linking scientific, social, and artistic fields. To learn how you can support us, please visit our website.